Non - Invasive Assessment of Airways Inflammation in Asthma & COPD

Stelios Loukides
Konstantinos Kostikas
Peter J. Barnes

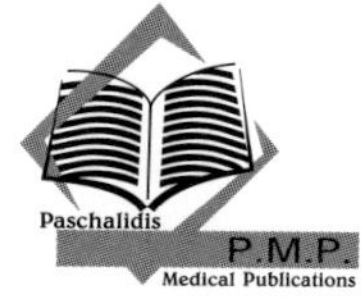

Paschalidis
P.M.P.
Medical Publications

PMP (Paschalidis Medical Publications)
14th, Tetrapoleos str., Athens, 115 27, Greece
Tel.: 003-210-7789125, 003-210-7793012, Fax: 003-210-7759421,
e-mail:
orders: Paschalidis@Medical-Books.gr
© information: GP@Medical-Books.gr, CP@Medical-Books.gr

ISBN: 978-960-489-104-7

Non-invasive assessment of airways inflammation

To our families, friends and co-workers,
for all the times of patience
during the creation of this book

Preface

Airway inflammation plays a central role in the pathogenesis of asthma and COPD and represents the underlying process of patients' symptoms and exacerbations. The long-standing Holy Grail for many researchers worldwide who are involved in the study of the mechanisms and clinical management of patients with inflammatory airway disorders is the development of methods for the effective monitoring of airway inflammation. Given the fact that the invasive assessment of lung inflammation, involving bronchoscopic and/or surgical techniques, is not always feasible, and definitely cannot be performed repeatedly, the Non-Invasive Assessment of Airways Inflammation in Asthma and COPD represents a timeless hot topic. This is especially important for patients with severe disease, who are not able to tolerate invasive procedures yet are the ones who may benefit the most from the monitoring of their airway inflammation. The decision for the making of this book emanated from the need to provide a collection of the rapid increase in recent knowledge by acknowledged international experts on this field, in order to define the grounds that we are currently standing and to attempt to shed some light on the evolution that we should be expecting in the near future. The topics covered include Exhaled Nitric Oxide, Induced Sputum, and Exhaled Breath Condensate, the three modalities that have been studied most extensively, in an attempt to provide information about Technical Considerations and "Normal" Values of candidate biomarkers, as well as insights on Application in Clinical Practice in Asthma and COPD. We could not neglect the special considerations of exhaled biomarkers in asthmatic children and the novel biomarkers that are emerging from ongoing research and the book is concluded by two perspectives evaluating whether "Non-Invasive Biomarkers Can Replace the Invasive Assessment of Airways Inflammation" and the "Future Directions for Non-Invasive Markers". What this book has definitely taught us is that the road towards the standardization and application of non-invasive monitoring of airway inflammation in clinical practice is still long and winding and there is still a lot of work to be done. Most important of all is the need for collaboration between working groups and this text represents a genuine step in that direction. With the hope that this book will be a useful reference for basic researchers and a guide for clinicians with special interest in clinical research, we now make it available to all of our colleagues in the field.

Stelios Loukides
Konstantinos Kostikas
Peter J. Barnes

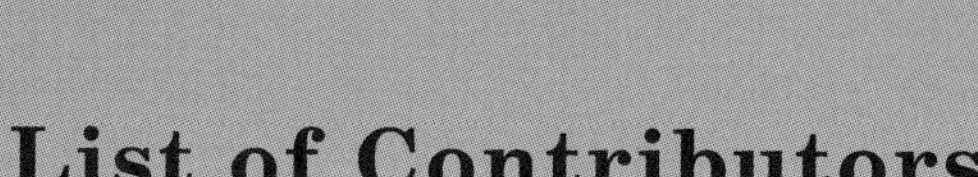

List of Contributors

Petros Bakakos
Lecturer in Respiratory Medicine
1st Respiratory Medicine
  Department
University of Athens Medical
  School
Sotiria Chest Hospital, Athens
Greece

Andrew Bush
Professor of Pediatric Respirology,
Imperial College, London and
Consultant Pediatric Chest
  Physician
Royal Brompton Hospital, London
United Kingdom

Peter J Barnes
Professor and Head of Respiratory
  Medicine
Imperial College London
Airway Disease Section
National Heart & Lung Institute,
  London
United Kingdom

Athanasios Chatzimichael
Professor of Pediatrics
Pediatric Department
University of Thrace, Alexandroupolis
Greece

Massimo Corradi MD
Department of Clinical Medicine,
  Nephrology and Health Sciences
University of Parma
Italy

Silvano Dragonieri
Fondazione Salvatore Maugeri
  IRCCS
Institute of Cassano Murge (BA)
Italy

Lieven J. Dupont
Associate Professor of Medicine
Department of Respiratory Medicine
Associate Professor of Medicine
University Hospital Gasthuisberg
Katholieke Universiteit Leuven
Belgium

Mina Gaga
Head of 7th Respiratory Medicine
  Department and Asthma Centre
Athens Chest Hospital, Athens
Greece

Petra Gergelova
Recearch Fellow
Department of Clinical Medicine,
  Nephrology and Health Sciences
University of Parma
Italy
Department of Public Health
Trnava University
Slovakia

Laurent Godinas
Research Fellow
Department of Pneumology, CHU
  Liege
GIGA Research Group Infection,
  Inflammation and Immunity
University of Liege
Belgium

Losonczy Gyorgy
Department Head
Semmelweis University, Department
  of Pulmonology, Budapest
Hungary

Georgios Hillas
SHO
Department of Respiratory and
  Critical Care Medicine
Sotiria Chest Hospital, Athens
Greece

Ildiko Horvath
Scientific advisor, Lecturer
  Pulmonologist

Semmelweis University,
  Department of Pulmonology,
  Budapest
Hungary

John Hunt
Associate Professor of Pediatrics
Pediatric Pulmonology, Allergy
  and Immunology
University of Virginia
Charlottesville, VA
United States of America

Konstantinos Kostikas
Respiratory Physician
2nd Respiratory Medicine
  Department
University of Athens Medical School
Attikon Hospital, Athens
Greece

Angela Koutsokera
Research Fellow
Respiratory Medicine Department
University of Thessaly Medical
  School, Larissa
Greece

Renaud Louis
Professor of Pneumology
Department of Pneumology, CHU
  Liege
GIGA Research Group Infection,
  Inflammation and Immunity
University of Liege
Belgium

Stelios Loukides
Lecturer in Respiratory Medicine
2nd Respiratory Medicine
  Department

University of Athens Medical
School
Attikon Hospital,
Athens
Greece

Neil Martin
Clinical Research Fellow
Institute for Lung Health
Department of Respiratory
medicine, Allergy and Thoracic
Surgery
Glenfield Hospital, University of
Leicester Hospitals NHS Trust,
Leicester
United Kingdom

Paolo Montuschi
Associate Professor
Department of Pharmacology
Faculty of Medicine
Catholic University of the Sacred
Heart, Rome
Italy

Antonio Mutti
Professor of Occupational
Medicine and Toxicology
Department of Clinical Medicine,
Nephrology and Health
Sciences
University of Parma
Italy

Anna-Carin Olin
Associate Professor
Occupational and Environmental
Medicine
Sahlgrenska University Hospital,
Gothenburg
Sweden

Emmanouil Paraskakis
Assistant Professor of Pediatrics
Respiratory Unit, Pediatric
Department
University of Thrace,
Alexandroupolis
Greece

Paolo Paredi
Airway Disease Section
National Heart and Lung Institute
Imperial College, London
United Kingdom

Koralia Paschalaki
Airway Disease Section
National Heart and Lung Institute
Imperial College, London
United Kingdom

Ian D. Pavord
Consultant Physician and
Honorary Professor of Medicine
Institute for Lung Health
Department of Respiratory
medicine, Allergy and Thoracic
Surgery
Glenfield Hospital, University of
Leicester Hospitals NHS Trust,
Leicester
United Kingdom

Nikoletta Rovina
Consultant in Respiratory
Medicine
1st Respiratory Medicine
Department
University of Athens Medical
School
Sotiria Chest Hospital, Athens
Greece

Florence Schleich
Research Fellow
Department of Pneumology, CHU
  Liege
GIGA Research Group
  Infection, Inflammation and
  Immunity
University of Liege
Belgium

Antonio Spanevello
Professor in Respiratory Medicine
Fondazione Salvatore Maugeri
  IRCCS
Institute of Tradate (VA) -
  University of Insubria, Varese
Italy

D. Robin Taylor
Professor of Respiratory Medicine
Dunedin School of Medicine,
University of Otago, Dunedin
New Zealand

Olga Toungoussova
Fondazione Salvatore Maugeri
  IRCCS
Institute of Cassano Murge (BA)
Italy

Andrea Zanini
Fondazione Salvatore Maugeri
  IRCCS
Institute of Tradate (VA)
Italy

Eleftherios Zervas
Consultant Physician
7th Respiratory Medicine
  Department
Athens Chest Hospital, Athens
Greece

Contents

PART III. EXHALED BREATH CONDENSATE

PART IV. OTHER CONSIDERATIONS IN EXHALED BIOMARKERS

Exhaled Biomarkers: Where do we Stand Today?

Stelios Loukides • *Konstantinos Kostikas* • *Peter J. Barnes*

Asthma is an inflammatory disorder of the airways associated with airflow obstruction and bronchial hyperresponsiveness that vary in severity across the spectrum of the disease. Although asthma is considered to be a chronic inflammatory disease, evaluation and therapy guidance are mainly based on clinical symptoms and lung function tests that remain the cornerstones of clinical practice (1). Chronic Obstructive Pulmonary Disease (COPD) is an inflammatory airways disorder mainly affected by smoking habit. It is considered as a preventable and treatable disease characterized by airflow limitation that is not fully reversible. COPD is a diverse disease entity with multiple dimensions that uniquely define the patient's performance, morbidity and mortality. FEV1 is both the traditional metric used to define the progression of COPD as well as the strongest spirometric predictor of mortality in COPD patients (2).

A large number of studies and reviews have addressed the in-

Correspondence

Dr. Stelios Loukides
Smolika 2, 16673 Athens, Greece
e-mail: ssat@hol.gr

flammatory profile of both COPD and asthma. Most of them conclude that invasive techniques such as bronchoscopy can clearly provide valuable information in relation to the underlying inflammation of these disorders (3, 4). Additional information has been provided by studies that have used tissue obtained during thoracic surgery for various reasons, with the latter providing a possible additional benefit mainly attributed to the size of obtaining samples and a clearer idea of the changes in both the airways and the lung parenchyma (5). Despite the above valuable information provided from invasive techniques, it s widely accepted that these techniques are not well tolerated by patients with more severe forms of both diseases. Moreover, they are not easily repeatable in such patients, mainly due to safety reasons.

The field of non-invasive techniques for the assessment of airways inflammation has developed rapidly since nitric oxide (NO) was recognized as an important mediator in exhaled air. The need for non-invasive assessment of airways inflammation is imperative, since inflammatory airway diseases, such as asthma and COPD, are characterized by variation in their clinical presentation throughout their course. Biomarkers in biological fluids and exhaled air have been the object of intense evaluation over the past few years, with some of them reaching their introduction in clinical practice, while others still remain research tools (6-9). The main question arising from all these non invasive procedures is whether the information obtained from measurements of mediators with these techniques fulfill the requirements of an appropriate biomarker (10). An ideal biomarker is required to be assessed with a standardized procedure, to present acceptable reproducibility, to demonstrate disease specificity and, last but not least, to have the ability to detect changes attributed either to therapeutic interventions or changes in health status (such as exacerbations). Summarizing the currently available techniques, which are mainly represented by sputum induction, and by measurements in exhaled air and exhaled breath condensate (EBC), it is difficult to identify the ideal biomarker which fulfills the above mentioned requirements.

Sputum induction is a semi-invasive technique that provided the opportunity to clinical researchers to elucidate the inflammatory process of many airway diseases including asthma and COPD. Its main advantage lies on the well-established methodology of collection, processing and analysis. The value of sputum induction is not restricted to sputum inflammatory cells, since inflammatory mediators can also be measured in the sputum supernatants. Its main clinical value today is related to the identification of eosinophilic inflammation and the use of eosinophils as a tool for guidance of treatment and the follow up of patients with both asthma and COPD (11, 12).

The major and most important representative of biomarkers measured in exhaled air is the fraction of exhaled nitric oxide (FeNO). FeNO is the most extensively studied exhaled biomarker today. The major limitation that it presents is the negative effect of smoking on its concentration. The main application of FeNO measurements has been established in asthma, since it provides rapid information regarding the presence of eosinophilic inflammation in the airways of asthmatic patients (13). Studies have shown that it can be used as a guide for the management of asthma, but with some conflict results(14, 15). However, it is the only technique today that is commercially available and applicable to everyday clinical practice. Finally, recently published data provide additional evidence that it may discriminate asthmatic and allergic rhinitis patients form those with non specific respiratory symptoms (16).

Exhaled breath condensate (EBC) is collected by cooling or freezing exhaled air. The large number of measurable molecules, the diversity of used methodologies regarding sample collection and processing, in addition to the lack of studies focusing on normal populations are some of the points that hamper its wide clinical use (17, 18). Despite the above limitations, it is a totally non-invasive technique that reflects biochemical changes of the airway lining fluid and as such it presents significant scientific interest.

What do we expect from biomarkers obtained by noninvasive methods in asthma and COPD? Both COPD and asthma are heterogeneous entities that encompass a variety of obstructive diseases differing significantly in terms of mechanisms and response to therapy. Therefore, the need for identification of different disease phenotypes within the range of these syndromes is crucial for the proper management of individual patients. The ideal approach is not to measure any single biomarker in order to detect elevated or decreased levels, but to try to identify the particular phenotype that is related to the specific biomarker and the underlying mechanism. Most likely a single biomarker is not sufficient and the combination of more than one biomarkers may approach more effectively the characterization of a specific phenotype. We believe that we are not close but we are definitely not that far from this achievement. We still have a lot to learn and improve in the field of biomarkers, but we always have to remember that the understanding of the pathophysiology of world epidemic diseases like asthma and COPD is essential to improve the management of these patients as well as to evaluate the plausible effects of new treatments, and non-invasive techniques may well contribute in that direction. Until now, and based on the available data, we believe that sputum induction is the most appropriate method for assessing in detail the cellular and biological profile of the underlying airway inflammation. The standardized methodology, the reproducibility of measurements, and the acceptable ranges of normal values establish it as the most valuable method. However, sometimes sputum induction is difficult to perform, involves some discomfort for the patient, requires dedicated personnel and special equipment, and may not be used repeatedly, in part because of its proinflammatory effect. In addition, sputum induction is associated with significant bronchoconstriction in a considerable portion of asthmatic patients, and all these factors render its introduction in everyday clinical practice difficult. The use of EBC is still promising because of its simplicity in sampling the airway-lining fluid to measure various biomarkers. However, its main limitation is the lack of a standard method of collection and procedure of measurements and the absence of established normal values for different mediators. We believe that data coming from the EBC studies regardless of the technical problems is essential because it provides evidence for the underlying pathophysiology of the two main inflammatory diseases. Additionally, FeNO seems to represent the most accurate biomarker for the non-smoking asthmatics, in terms of its properly validated technique and its ability to identify eosinophilic inflammation in such patients. However, it remains to be established in which patients it may be used as a guide for treatment.

Based on the available literature today, we believe that combining different noninvasive methods that sample different compartments of the airways may offer a more detailed evaluation of different mediators in relation to cellular components, and could provide valuable evidence for increasing sensitivity to certain interventions, such as the effectiveness of therapy. These differences may be exploited in the future as more markers are characterized, so that each disease phenotype may have a characteristic profile or fingerprint of different exhaled biomarkers. Treatments may additionally impose a characteristic effect on these biomarkers, and this may improve targeted treatment in the future, particularly as more potent and disease- or even phenotype-specific treatments become available.

The aim of this book is to attempt to evaluate thoroughly the evidence regarding all the available techniques of non-invasive assessment of airways inflammation that are currently available. For each of the aforementioned techniques, internationally acknowledged experts have provided detailed information regarding technical considerations, current "normal" values, application in clinical practice and future implications, both in asthma and COPD in general, and in specific phenotypes of the two diseases.

References

1. Bateman ED, Hurd SS, Barnes PJ, Bousquet J, Drazen JM, FitzGerald M, et al. Global strategy for asthma management and prevention: GINA executive summary. Eur Respir J. 2008 Jan;31(1):143-78.

2. Rabe KF, Hurd S, Anzueto A, Barnes PJ, Buist SA, Calverley P, et al. Global strategy for the diagnosis, management, and prevention of chronic obstructive pulmonary disease: GOLD executive summary. Am J Respir Crit Care Med. 2007 Sep 15;176(6):532-55.

3. Fabbri LM, Romagnoli M, Corbetta L, Casoni G, Busljetic K, Turato G, et al. Differences in airway inflammation in patients with fixed airflow obstruction due to asthma or chronic obstructive pulmonary disease. Am J Respir Crit Care Med. 2003 Feb 1;167(3):418-24.

4. Gamble E, Grootendorst DC, Hattotuwa K, O'Shaughnessy T, Ram FS, Qiu Y, et al. Airway mucosal inflammation in COPD is similar in smokers and ex-smokers: a pooled analysis. Eur Respir J. 2007 Sep; 30(3):467-71.

5. Tomaki M, Sugiura H, Koarai A, Komaki Y, Akita T, Matsumoto T, et al. Decreased expression of antioxidant enzymes and increased expression of chemokines in COPD lung. Pulm Pharmacol Ther. 2007;20(5):596-605.

6. Hillas G, Loukides S, Kostikas K, Bakakos P. Biomarkers obtained by non-invasive methods in patients with COPD: where do we stand, what do we expect? Curr Med Chem. 2009; 16(22):2824-38.

7. Kharitonov SA, Barnes PJ. Exhaled biomarkers. Chest. 2006 Nov;130(5): 1541-6.

8. Barnes PJ, Chowdhury B, Kharitonov SA, Magnussen H, Page CP, Postma D, et al. Pulmonary biomarkers in chronic obstructive pulmonary disease. Am J Respir Crit Care Med. 2006 Jul 1;174(1):6-14.

9. Brightling CE. Clinical applications of induced sputum. Chest. 2006 May;129(5):1344-8.

10. Biomarkers and surrogate endpoints: preferred definitions and conceptual framework. Clin Pharmacol Ther. 2001 Mar;69(3):89-95.

11. Green RH, Brightling CE, McKenna S, Hargadon B, Parker D, Bradding P, et

al. Asthma exacerbations and sputum eosinophil counts: a randomised controlled trial. Lancet. 2002 Nov 30; 360(9347):1715-21.

12. Siva R, Green RH, Brightling CE, Shelley M, Hargadon B, McKenna S, et al. Eosinophilic airway inflammation and exacerbations of COPD: a randomised controlled trial. Eur Respir J. 2007 May;29(5):906-13.

13. Taylor DR, Pavord ID. Biomarkers in the assessment and management of airways diseases. Postgrad Med J. 2008 Dec;84(998):628-34; quiz 33.

14. Smith AD, Cowan JO, Brassett KP, Herbison GP, Taylor DR. Use of exhaled nitric oxide measurements to guide treatment in chronic asthma. N Engl J Med. 2005 May 26;352(21):2163-73.

15. Shaw DE, Berry MA, Thomas M, Green RH, Brightling CE, Wardlaw AJ, et al. The use of exhaled nitric oxide to guide asthma management: a randomized controlled trial. Am J Respir Crit Care Med. 2007 Aug 1;176(3): 231-7.

16. Kostikas K, Papaioannou AI, Tanou K, Koutsokera A, Papala M, Gourgoulianis KI. Portable exhaled nitric oxide as a screening tool for asthma in young adults during pollen season. Chest. 2008 Apr;133(4):906-13.

17. Horvath I, Hunt J, Barnes PJ, Alving K, Antczak A, Baraldi E, et al. Exhaled breath condensate: methodological recommendations and unresolved questions. Eur Respir J. 2005 Sep; 26(3):523-48.

18. Koutsokera A, Loukides S, Gourgoulianis KI, Kostikas K. Biomarkers in the exhaled breath condensate of healthy adults: mapping the path towards reference values. Curr Med Chem. 2008;15(6):620-30.

Exhaled Nitric Oxide - Technical Considerations

Paolo Paredi

Koralia Paschalaki

Airway inflammation plays a central role in the pathogenesis of lung disease. However, because lung function tests may not reflect the activity of inflammation in the airways, there is a need for surrogate markers. The measurement of nitric oxide (NO) in the exhaled breath has received a lot of interest because it is completely non-invasive, quick and reproducible.

Crucially, contrary to other non-invasive methods such as induced sputum and exhaled breath condensate, the single exhalation measurement of exhaled NO has been carefully standardised in a joint recommendation by the European and American respiratory societies(1). This has made the measurements more reliable and has reduced the variability of fractional exhaled NO levels that was initially observed in health and disease and was most probably related to the different techniques of measurement used in different laboratories across the world.

The potential usefulness of exhaled NO in a clinical setting was

Correspondence

Dr. Paolo Paredi

Airway Disease Section, National Heart and Lung Institute, Imperial College School of Science, Technology and Medicine, Dovehouse Street, London SW3 6LY, UK
e-mail: p.paredi@imperial.ac.uk

further acknowledged by the Food and Drug Administration in the United States which approved the use of this gas for the monitoring of anti-inflammatory therapy in asthma.

The single expiratory technique measures predominantly larger airway-derived NO and may only partially reflect peripheral inflammation. A novel method for the measurement of NO allows the partitioning of alveolar and bronchial NO by analysing mathematically the levels of this gas in the exhaled breath obtained at different exhalation flow rates (2). This technique confirmed the notion that the majority of NO measured at the mouth derives from the central airways with only a small contribution deriving from the periphery of the lung (3). Contrary to the single breath measurement of NO, the use of the multiple breath test has not been thoroughly standardised.

We will discuss the factors that affect the single breath measurement of NO and the methods used to control them. We will also describe the multiple breath method for the measurement of NO and its limitations

Source of NO in Exhaled Air

Nitric oxide synthases. Endogenous NO is derived from L-arginine by the enzyme NO synthase (NOS), of which at least three distinct isoforms exist (4). Two of these enzymes are constitutively expressed and are activated by small rises in intracellular calcium concentration, secondary to cell activation. Neuronal NOS (NOS1, nNOS) is predominantly expressed in neurones and endothelial NOS (NOS3, eNOS) mainly in endothelial cells, although other cell types also express both of these isoforms including epithelial cells. A third enzyme is inducible (NOS2, iNOS), has a much greater level of activity, and is independent of calcium concentration. NOS2 may be induced by inflammatory cytokines, endotoxin, and viral infections and may show increased expression in inflammatory diseases (5). Genetic polymorphisms of all three isoforms of NOS have been detected.

Cellular sources in the airways. The cellular source of NO gas in the lower respiratory tract is not yet certain. Studies with perfused porcine lungs suggest that exhaled NO originates at the alveolar surface, rather than from the pulmonary circulation (6), and it may be derived from NOS3 expressed in the alveolar walls of normal lungs. Studies in ventilated perfused lungs of guinea pigs have shown that exhaled NO is reduced during perfusion with calcium-free solutions, suggesting that NO is derived from a constitutive NOS, which is calcium-dependent. Airway epithelial cells may express both NOS3 and NOS1 and therefore may contribute to NO in the lower respiratory tract. There is some expression of NOS2 even in airway epithelial cells from normal subjects, and NOS2 appears to be an important isoform contributing to exhaled NO in healthy mice. In inflammatory diseases such as asthma it is likely that the increase in exhaled NO reflects further induction of NOS2 in response to inflammatory signals such as proinflammatory cytokines. Indeed, increased NOS activity has been demonstrated in lung tissue of patients with asthma, cystic fibrosis, and obliterative bronchiolitis(5). In asthmatic patients there is evidence for increased expression of NOS2 in airway epithelial cells, and this is likely to be due to increased transcription mediated via the transcription factors STAT-1 and nuclear factor-κB (NF-κB), and increased availability of L-arginine (7). Proinflammatory cytokines induce the expression of NOS2 in cultured human airway epithelial cells, and it is likely that these same cytokines are released in asthmatic inflammation. NOS2 may be expressed in other cell types, such as alveolar macrophages, eosinophils, and other inflammatory cells. Further evidence that the increase in exhaled NO is derived from increased NOS2 expression is the observation that corticosteroids inhibit inflammatory induction of NOS2 in epithelial cells (8), decrease expression in bronchial biopsies (9) and reduce exhaled NO concentrations in asthmatic patients (10).

Anatomic origin. NO is produced along the entire length of human airways. The conducting airways secrete NO into the lumen, which mixes with alveoli NO during exhalation, resulting in the observed expiratory concentration. The levels of NO derived from the upper respiratory tract (20 to 1000ppb) and sinuses (100 to 3000ppb) are a hundred-fold higher than exhaled NO measured in the lower respiratory tract (1 to 7 ppb) (11).

The source of NO in the lower respiratory tract is also of mixed origin and may be derived from airway and alveolar epithelial cells, which express both NOS3 and NOS1. The contribution of endothelial-derived NO is minimal, as inhaled NOS inhibitors are able to reduce exhaled NO by 4 to 70% without any effect on the systemic circulation. By contrast, L-NMMA infusion modulates blood pressure and heart rate but has only a minimal effect on exhaled NO (12).

Simultaneous measurement of expired CO_2 and NO demonstrate that exhaled NO precedes the peak value of CO_2 (end-tidal), suggesting that NO is derived from airways rather than from alveoli. Direct sampling via fiberoptic bronchoscopy in normal subjects shows similar levels of NO in trachea and main bronchi to that recorded at the mouth, thus indicating that there is NO derived from the lower airways (11). Exhaled NO is therefore most likely to be of epithelial rather than of endothelial origin, and most NO is derived from airways rather than from alveoli.

A novel method for the measurement of NO allows the partitioning of alveolar and bronchial NO by analysing mathematically the levels of this gas in the exhaled breath obtained at different exhalation flow rates (2). This technique confirmed the notion that the majority of NO measured at the mouth derives from the central airways with only a small contribution deriving from the more distal airways (3).

NO Measurement

Factors affecting exhaled NO levels

Exhalation flow rate
Exhaled NO concentrations are remarkably expiratory flow dependent (13) (Figure 1). This is due to the continuous production of NO in the

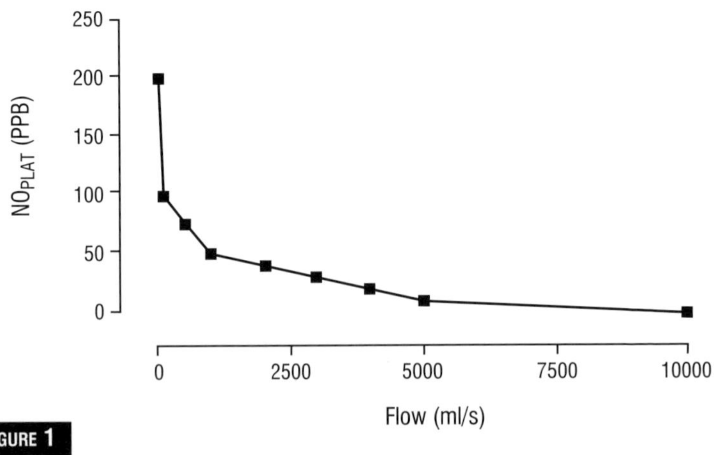

FIGURE 1

Flow dependency of exhaled NO. Modified from reference 13.

airways which enriches the low NO air coming from the periphery of the lung. Faster exhalation flows will minimise the NO transfer time in the airways reducing the final NO concentrations in the breath.

Exhaled NO levels are particularly exhalation flow dependent at lower exhalation flow rates, making the measurements more variable in this range of flows. In view of this strong relationship, exhalation flow rates should always be standardised as indicated by the ATS/ERS guidelines (1) (45-55 ml/s).

Nasal NO contamination

The concentration of NO in the nasal cavities is about one hundred times higher compared to the lung periphery. Therefore, it is important to prevent the contamination of exhaled breath with nasal air(14). This can be achieved by exhaling against a resistance of at least 5 cm H_2O which generates sufficient back pressure to push the soft palate upwards sealing the nasal cavities form the pharynx (Figure 2).

Breath hold

Breath hold produces NO accumulation in the lung and in the airways resulting in higher concentrations of the gas in the exhaled breath(1). Because the degree of gas accumulation may vary in different subjects depending on the volume of the anatomical dead space and lung volumes, this manoeuvre should be discouraged.

Ambient contamination

High environmental NO concentrations (>40ppb) may affect exhaled NO levels. This is because high concentrations of NO in the inhaled air may produce an early NO peak which is related to environmental NO

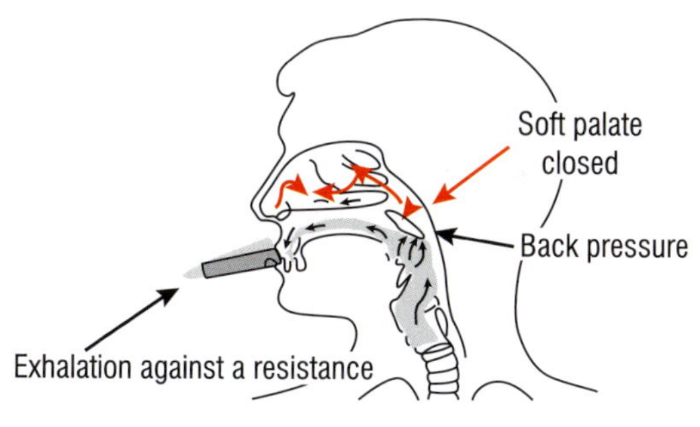

FIGURE 2

Flow dependency of exhaled NO. Modified from reference 14

in the instrument and in the subjects' dead space. This initial peak NO may take some time to "wash out" and may affect the final NO plateau readings normally interpreted as representative of the central airways.

Smoking

Cigarette smoke chronically reduces the levels of exhaled NO(15, 16). This may be due to reduced iNOS expression and NO production from lung epithelial cells due to cigarette smoke(17). For this reason, exhaled NO may be a less informative marker in current smokers. Subjects should not smoke for at least an hour before NO measurement.

Spirometry

Repeated forced vital capacity (FVC) manoeuvres such as those performed during spirometry reduce exhaled NO by 36%(18). The lower levels of NO may result from a reduction in neurally derived nitric oxide (NO) originating from the lower airway. For this reason, it is advisable to measure exhaled NO before spirometry.

Other factors

Diet and medications may also alter the levels of exhaled NO. For this reason, patients should be instructed to fast for at least an hour before the measurement and the use of medications, particularly corticosteroids and anti leukotrienes should be recorded.

Single breath NO measurement

Online measurement

The nitric oxide concentration in exhaled air is usually measured by the ozone-chemiluminescence method. This method is based on the reaction between NO and ozone (O_3) to form nitrogen dioxide (NO_2), some of which is in excited state (NO_2^*). Red and infrared light (~640 - 3000 nm) is emitted as the excited form of nitrogen dioxide regains its stable ground state ($NO_2^* \rightarrow NO_2 + h\nu$). The amount of light can be quantified by a photomultiplier and is proportional to the amount of NO in the specimen gas (Figure 3).

Even though most NO analysers are based on the chemiluminescence principle, other technologies such as laser absorption spectrometry and laser magnetic resonance are under investigation. It is

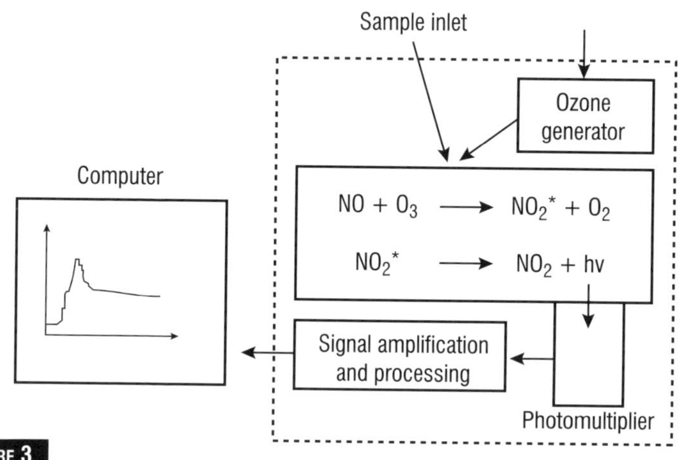

FIGURE 3

Schematic illustration of an ozone-chemiluminescence NO analyser. Red and infrared light is emitted as NO reacts with ozone. The NO concentration in the sample gas can be calculated by quantifying the amount of light emitted

hoped that the development of new technologies will increase the portability and reliability of the devices.

During online measurements the concentration of NO in the exhaled breath is displayed continuously as the patient blows into the analyser. Most NO analysers, besides NO, also provide mouth pressure, exhaled volume, exhalation flow rate and CO_2 tracings (Figure 4). This allows the quality control of the exhalation ma-

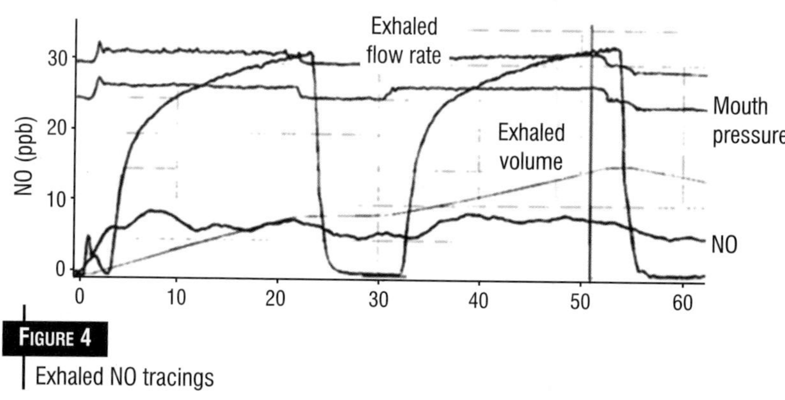

FIGURE 4

Exhaled NO tracings

noeuvre by enabling the operator to verify that the mouth pressure was sufficient to close the soft palate and that the exhalation flow rate was stable during the exhalation.

Exhalation manoeuvre
Subjects inhale slowly over the course of 2 to 3 seconds through the mouth to total lung capacity (TLC) without wearing nose clips. However, nose clips should be worn if the subject is unable to avoid nasal inhalation or exhalation. The exhalation manoeuvre should be performed without breath hold, at a constant exhalation flow rate (45-55ml/s) and against a mild resistance (>5 cm H_2O). This is necessary to avoid nasal contamination and for standardization purposes as discussed above.

The online NO tracings consist of a "wash out phase" representing air coming from the upper airways, followed by a plateau phase reflecting alveolar air. NO measurements are calculated on the plateau phase subject to it being longer than 6 seconds. Repeated, reproducible exhalations should be performed to obtain at least two NO plateau values that are within 10% agreement, exhaled NO is then calculated as the mean between these two values. At least 30 seconds of relaxed tidal breathing off the NO measurement circuit should elapse between exhalations to allow subjects to rest.

Offline measurement
Chemiluminescence NO analysers are bulky and not transportable. However, exhaled breath can be collected remotely offline into a reservoir during a single exhalation (Figure 5). The breath samples can be later analysed where the NO device is available.

The same factors affecting the online measurement of NO may equally affect NO measured offline, therefore, only when the single exhalation into the reservoir is pressure and flow-controlled and the dead space is discarded, the two techniques are in agreement and can be used interchangeably (19).

Like for the online measurement, the exhalation manoeuvre is performed without nose clips and breath hold. The addition of silica gel in the reservoir reduces the humidity and allows to store the breath samples for up to 48h without significant changes in NO concentrations.

Because the offline method allows remote NO collection and delayed NO analysis, it may be the method of choice for home monitoring of inflammatory lung diseases and epidemiological studies (1).

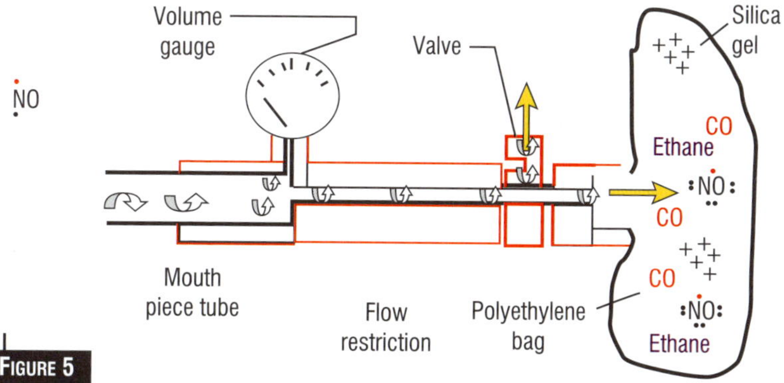

Schematic diagram of the portable equipment for collection of exhaled NO. The arrows indicate the direction of air flow. The three way valve is in the closed position for reservoir collection of exhaled breath.

Multiple breath NO measurement

In order to explain the dynamics of NO production and recovery in the exhaled breath, a number of mathematical models have been developed. In 1997, Hyde and colleagues introduced a model based on one compartment which described NO dynamics in the alveolar region only (20) but did not take into account NO exchange in the airways. They proposed that NO in the alveolar spaces reaches a certain concentration (C_{Alv}) as a result of its continuous production in the alveolar tissues and its diffusion into the alveolar air at a certain rate ($J_{NO,Alv}$). Once in the alveolar air, NO can be either exhaled or back diffuse into the pulmonary blood circulation because of its high affinity for haemoglobin. The diffusion rate of alveolar NO to the pulmonary capillaries is a product of the alveolar diffusing capacity of NO ($D_{NO,Alv}$) and alveolar NO concentration. After inhalation of air with a low NO concentration, NO from the alveolar tissue diffuses into the alveolar air and a steady-state dynamic equilibrium between tissue and gas phase is soon achieved. During the steady state, the diffusion of NO into the capillaries equals the diffusion of NO from the tissue to luminal air (20) (Figure 6), giving:

$$C_{Alv} \times D_{NO,Alv} = J_{NO,Alv} \qquad (1)$$

One compartment model (1997). NO produced in the alveoli diffuses to alveolar air ($J_{NO,Alv}$), causing a certain concentration of NO in the alveolar air (C_{Alv}). The diffusion of NO from alveolar air to the pulmonary circulation equals the product of Calv and the alveolar diffusing capacity of NO ($D_{NO,Alv}$).

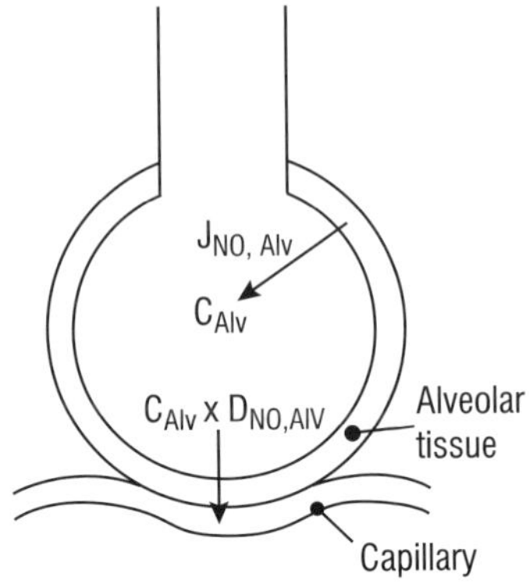

C_{Alv} can be assessed by measuring the end-exhalation NO plateau at a high exhalation flow rate (minimal airway contribution to exhaled NO concentration), and $D_{NO,Alv}$ can be measured using NO as the tracer gas in determining pulmonary diffusing capacity. With equation (1), $J_{NO,Alv}$ can be calculated based on these measurements, allowing approximation of alveolar NO production.

The one compartment model described above does not explain the flow dependency of exhaled NO levels, this is because it does not take into account the airway contribution to exhaled NO which is the cause of exhalation flow dependency (13). To better explain NO dynamics and clinical findings, the two compartment model was introduced. This model (2) describes both a flexible alveolar compartment which includes the respiratory bronchioles to generation 18 and beyond according to Weibel et al (21) and the bronchial compartments. Gas exchange occurs in the alveolar compartment while the bronchial compartment is seen as a single rigid cylindrical tube representing conducting airways larger than respiratory bronchioles [from trachea to generation 17 according to Weibel et al (21)]. Both compartments are capable of producing NO and washing NO away in the pulmonary or bronchial circulation (Figure 7).

In both compartments NO diffusion between tissue and gas phases depends on the relative concentrations of NO and C_{Alv} depends on alveolar NO dynamics as described in the one compartment model.

The final NO concentration in the exhaled air is dependent on NO concentration in alveolar air and its conditioning as it travels through

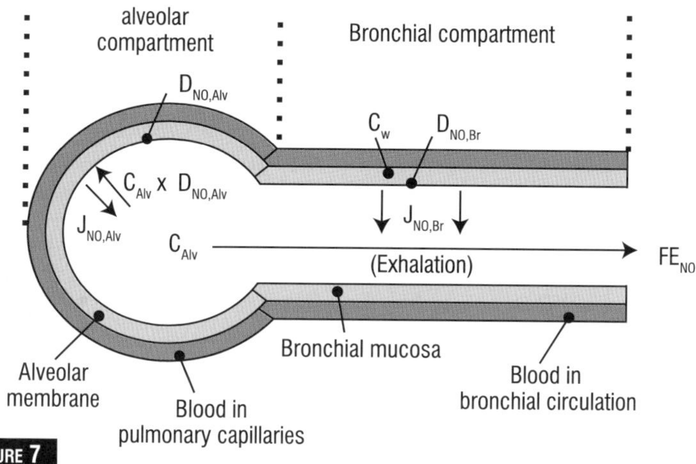

FIGURE 7

Schematic illustration of the two-compartment model of pulmonary NO dynamics (Reproduced after permission from reference 2). See text for details.

the bronchial compartment. The conductive airways can be modelled as composed of infinitely small units, each of these adjacent units produce NO and contribute to the final NO concentrations measured at the mouth. As it approaches the bronchial compartment, the luminal air NO concentration equals the alveolar NO concentration, however, as it travels in the airways more proximally and reaches the first unit, NO diffuses from the bronchial wall to the luminal air, and at the entry to the second unit the luminal NO concentration equals the alveolar NO concentration plus NO diffused in the first unit, and so on. The exhaled air becomes more and more enriched in NO as it reaches the mouth and more units have contributed their share of NO to the total final NO concentration measured in the breath. The diffusion rate is determined by the bronchial diffusing capacity of NO ($D_{NO,Br}$). Conditioning of alveolar air in the bronchial compartment depends on the transit time of the alveolar air through conducting airways during exhalation (inverse to exhalation flow rate), the airway wall NO concentration (CW), and the bronchial diffusing capacity of NO ($D_{NO,Br}$). The final NO concentration in exhaled air (FENO) can be expressed as a function of alveolar NO concentration (C_{Alv}), bronchial wall NO concentration (CW), bronchial diffusing capacity of NO ($D_{NO,Br}$) and exhalation flow rate ($\dot{V}$), as follows (2, 22).

$$FE_{NO} = Cw \left[1 - e^{-\frac{D_{NO,Br}}{\dot{V}}} \right] + C_{Alv} \times e^{-\frac{D_{NO,Br}}{\dot{V}}} \qquad (2)$$

As the total NO output from the lower respiratory tract is a product of exhaled NO concentration and exhalation flow rate ($\dot{V}_{NO} = FE_{NO} \times \dot{V}$), the total NO output can be written based on equation (2) as follows:

$$\dot{V}_{NO} = \left[Cw \left[1 - e^{-\frac{D_{NO,Br}}{\dot{V}}} \right] + C_{Alv} \times e^{-\frac{D_{NO,Br}}{\dot{V}}} \right] \times \dot{V} \qquad (3)$$

These fundamental equations of the two compartment model are able to simulate the experimentally demonstrated inverse relationship between FENO and $\dot{V}$ which was not explained by the one compartment model. After measuring the exhaled NO concentration (FE$_{NO}$) at several different known flow rates ($\dot{V}$), the unknown parameters (C_{Alv}, CW and $D_{NO,Br}$) can be solved using the basic equations. This allows separate assessment of alveolar and bronchial NO dynamics. At sufficiently high exhalation flow rates, when $\dot{V} >> D_{NO,Br}$, the exponential function can be substituted with its approximate

$$e^{-\frac{D_{NO,Br}}{\dot{V}}} = 1 - \frac{D_{NO,Br}}{\dot{V}}$$

Equation (3) is then rearranged to give:

$$\dot{V}_{NO} = C_{Alv} \times \dot{V} + (Cw - C_{Alv})D_{NO,Br} \qquad (4)$$

Equation (4) presents NO output as a sum of NO produced in the alveoli ($C_{Alv} \times \dot{V}$) and NO diffused from the bronchial wall to the luminal air (($CW - C_{Alv})D_{NO,Br}$). The latter term describes the theoretical maximum bronchial NO flux ($J_{NO,Br}$) reached at an infinitely high exhalation flow rate when the bronchial luminal NO concentration does not rise above the alveolar NO concentration. By introducing JNO,Br into equation (4), it can be rearranged to give:

$$\dot{V}_{NO} = C_{Alv} \times \dot{V} + J_{NO,Br} \qquad (5)$$

Equation (5) is a linear regression where $\dot{V}_{NO}$ as a function of $\dot{V}$, C_{Alv} is the slope of the line and JNO,Br is the intercept with the y axis. $\dot{V}_{NO}$

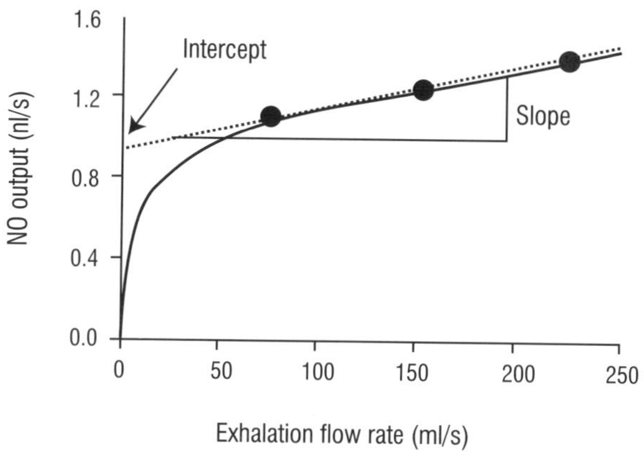

FIGURE 8

Plot of three NO output measurements (•) against flow rate. At higher flow rates (>50 ml/s), where NO output (solid curve) is almost linear, the bronchial NO flux approaches its theoretical maximum and can be considered constant. The slope and intercept of a regression line (dotted line) between NO output and flow rate are approximates of bronchial NO flux and alveolar NO concentration, respectively (Reproduced after permission from reference 2).

and $\dot{V}$ are known ($\dot{V}_{NO}$ =FE_{NO} x $\dot{V}$) therefore C_{Alv} and $J_{NO,Br}$ can thus be solved by means of a regression line. After measuring the exhaled NO concentration at several different exhalation flow rates, VNO is calculated for each $\dot{V}$ used. $\dot{V}_{NO}$ is then plotted against V and a regression line is set. The slope of the regression line is an approximate of C_{Alv} and the intercept is an approximate of $J_{NO,Br}$ (2, 22) (Figure 8).

If the exhaled NO is measured only at a single exhalation flow rate, as recommended by current guidelines(1), the presence of pulmonary inflammation can be detected based on an increased NO concentration in exhaled air. However, this method cannot be used to differentiate between alveolar and bronchial sources of NO, nor to differentiate between alveolar and bronchial inflammation. The mathematical models suggest that we could partition alveolar and bronchial inflammation by measuring the exhaled NO concentration at multiple exhalation flow rates.

Limitations of the multiple breath NO measurement

The major limitation of the multiple breath mathematical model described above is that it does not take into account the axial back diffusion of NO from the conductive airways to the alveoli. Because NO has a high affinity for haemoglobin, the pulmonary circulation acts as a "sink" for this gas washing it away and producing a concentration gradient favouring NO diffusion to the alveoli from the conductive airways. Condorelli et al. (3) have studied the axial diffusion of NO and have generated simple equations that account for this effect:

$$C_{alv} = S\text{-}Ix\{(0.00078\ s/ml)/0.57\}=S\text{-}I/740ml/s$$
$$J_{NO} = 1.7xI$$

(where S is the slope and I the y-intercept in the linear regression described above)

The C_{alv} equation is of special interest because it illustrates that the concentration of NO in the alveoli is very low. It also sensitises the clinical researcher to the fact that any changes in C_{alv} due to local inflammatory processes may not be detected because the pulmonary circulation may remove the NO produced in excess. This may limit the use of exhaled NO as a marker of airway inflammation in diseases such as COPD where most of the changes occur in the periphery of the lung.

Another important limitation in the use of the multiple breath NO method is that, contrary to the single breath method, it has not been standardised. More specifically, the choice of different sets of exhalation flow rates causes major variations of the slope and intercept of the regression line resulting in different C_{alv} and Jno measuremnts. Furthermore, including low exhalation flow rates (<50 ml/s) increases the variability of the measurements due to the steep shape of the flow/NO concentration curve at slow exhalation flow rates. These points need to be investigated further and standardization is required.

A number of other variables are not taken into consideration by the mathematical model described above. For example it is assumed that the airways are rigid and do not change diameter throughout the respiratory cycle, and that the inhaled and exhaled air flows do not vary from linear to turbulent and that the diffusion of NO remains the constant.

All these limitations are difficult to address with a mathematical model which, as such, may not have the flexibility required to interpret the complex dynamics of NO exchange in the lung. However, the multiple breath NO measurement has the advantage of providing and "estimate" of the concentrations of NO in the airways and its production in the alveoli, and therefore may have some use in research. Its use in clinical practice will have to be explored once the technique has been appropriately standardised.

Conclusions

Measuring exhaled NO is simple, non-invasive and repeatable and may be applied to children and to patients with severe disease. A large number of studies have used exhaled NO to monitor airway inflammation providing an insight into the relationship between inflammation and lung disease. The measurement of exhaled NO using the single exhalation manoeuvre has been standardised by the European and American Respiratory Societies and produces reproducible and reliable results. The Food and Drug Administration in the United States approved the use of this gas for the monitoring of anti-inflammatory therapy in asthma.

The measurement of exhaled NO at multiple exhalation flow rates allows to partition NO produced in the central airways and peripheral lung. Unfortunately the measurements have not been standardised and a number of limitations related to the mathematical model on which this technique is based on, have not been addressed. For these reasons, the use of the multiple exhalations flows technique remains to this date a research tool.

Longitudinal studies are required to investigate the usefulness of these measurements in a clinical setting, furthermore, less sophisticated and cheaper devices are required to allow the day to day use of these techniques in the clinical management of inflammatory lung diseases.

References

1. ATS/ERS recommendations for standardized procedures for the online and offline measurement of exhaled lower respiratory nitric oxide and nasal nitric oxide, 2005. Am J Respir Crit Care Med2005 Apr 15;171(8): 912-30.
2. Tsoukias NM, George SC. A two-compartment model of pulmonary nitric oxide exchange dynamics. J Appl Physiol1998 Aug;85(2):653-66.
3. Condorelli P, Shin HW, Aledia AS, Silkoff PE, George SC. A simple technique to characterize proximal and peripheral nitric oxide exchange using constant flow exhalations and an axial

diffusion model. J Appl Physiol2007 Jan;102(1):417-25.

4. Nathan C, Xie QW. Regulation of biosynthesis of nitric oxide. J Biol Chem1994 May 13;269(19):13725-8.

5. Belvisi M, Barnes PJ, Larkin S, Yacoub M, Tadjkarimi S, Williams TJ, et al. Nitric oxide synthase activity is elevated in inflammatory lung disease in humans. Eur J Pharmacol1995 Sep 5;283(1-3):255-8.

6. Cremona G, Higenbottam T, Takao M, Hall L, Bower EA. Exhaled nitric oxide in isolated pig lungs. J Appl Physiol1995 Jan;78(1):59-63.

7. Guo FH, Comhair SA, Zheng S, Dweik RA, Eissa NT, Thomassen MJ, et al. Molecular mechanisms of increased nitric oxide (NO) in asthma: evidence for transcriptional and post-translational regulation of NO synthesis. J Immunol2000 Jun 1;164(11):5970-80.

8. Nightingale JA, Rogers DF, Barnes PJ. Effect of repeated sputum induction on cell counts in normal volunteers. Thorax1998 Feb;53(2):87-90.

9. Saleh D, Ernst P, Lim S, Barnes PJ, Giaid A. Increased formation of the potent oxidant peroxynitrite in the airways of asthmatic patients is associated with induction of nitric oxide synthase: effect of inhaled glucocorticoid. FASEB J1998 Aug;12(11):929-37.

10. Kharitonov SA, Yates D, Robbins RA, Logan-Sinclair R, Shinebourne EA, Barnes PJ. Increased nitric oxide in exhaled air of asthmatic patients. Lancet1994 Jan 15;343(8890):133-5.

11. Kharitonov SA, Chung KF, Evans D, O'Connor BJ, Barnes PJ. Increased exhaled nitric oxide in asthma is mainly derived from the lower respiratory tract. Am J Respir Crit Care Med1996 Jun;153(6 Pt 1):1773-80.

12. Sartori C, Lepori M, Busch T, Duplain H, Hildebrandt W, Bartsch P, et al. Exhaled nitric oxide does not provide a marker of vascular endothelial function in healthy humans. Am J Respir Crit Care Med1999 Sep;160(3):879-82.

13. Silkoff PE, McClean PA, Slutsky AS, Furlott HG, Hoffstein E, Wakita S, et al. Marked flow-dependence of exhaled nitric oxide using a new technique to exclude nasal nitric oxide. Am J Respir Crit Care Med1997 Jan; 155(1):260-7.

14. Kharitonov SA, Barnes PJ. Nasal contribution to exhaled nitric oxide during exhalation against resistance or during breath holding. Thorax1997 Jun;52(6):540-4.

15. Kharitonov SA, Robbins RA, Yates D, Keatings V, Barnes PJ. Acute and chronic effects of cigarette smoking on exhaled nitric oxide. Am J Respir Crit Care Med1995 Aug;152(2):609-12.

16. Schilling J, Holzer P, Guggenbach M, Gyurech D, Marathia K, Geroulanos S. Reduced endogenous nitric oxide in the exhaled air of smokers and hypertensives. Eur Respir J1994 Mar; 7(3):467-71.

17. Hoyt JC, Robbins RA, Habib M, Springall DR, Buttery LD, Polak JM, et al. Cigarette smoke decreases inducible nitric oxide synthase in lung epithelial cells. Exp Lung Res2003 Jan-Feb;29(1):17-28.

18. Deykin A, Halpern O, Massaro AF, Drazen JM, Israel E. Expired nitric oxide after bronchoprovocation and repeated spirometry in patients with

asthma. Am J Respir Crit Care Med 1998 Mar;157(3 Pt 1):769-75.

19. Paredi P, Loukides S, Ward S, Cramer D, Spicer M, Kharitonov SA, et al. Exhalation flow and pressure-controlled reservoir collection of exhaled nitric oxide for remote and delayed analysis. Thorax1998 Sep;53(9):775-9.

20. Hyde RW, Geigel EJ, Olszowka AJ, Krasney JA, Forster RE, 2nd, Utell MJ, et al. Determination of production of nitric oxide by lower airways of humans--theory. J Appl Physiol1997 Apr;82(4):1290-6.

21. Weibel ER, Gomez DM. Architecture of the human lung. Use of quantitative methods establishes fundamental relations between size and number of lung structures. Science1962 Aug 24;137:577-85.

22. Hogman M, Drca N, Ehrstedt C, Merilainen P. Exhaled nitric oxide partitioned into alveolar, lower airways and nasal contributions. Respir Med2000 Oct;94(10):985-91.

Exhaled Nitric Oxide - Towards Normal Values

Anna-Carin Olin
D. Robin Taylor

The GINA definition of asthma emphasizes the chronic inflammatory processes which are pivotal to the pathophysiology of asthma (1). Controlling airway inflammation is a key element in reducing airway hyper-responsiveness and its associated symptoms. Assessing airway inflammation in the long term management of asthma is an important way to improve overall clinical outcomes including reducing exacerbations (2).

Asthma is heterogeneous, with a range of pathological phenotypes. A recent review proposed four important cytological subtypes: eosinophilic, neutrophilic, pauci-granulocytic and mixed-cell types (3). Identifying the inflammatory subtype in asthma is potentially helpful. In particular, eosinophilic airway inflammation, as assessed by sputum induction, has been shown to be related to exacerbations of asthma and corticosteroid responsiveness (2).

Correspondence ——
Dr. Anna-Carin Olin
Occupational and Environmental Medicine Department, Sahlgrenska University Hospital, Box 414, 405 30 Gothenburg, Sweden
e-mail: anna-carin.olin@amm.gu.se

However, sputum induction is cumbersome to perform. Hence there is a need for an easy, non-invasive measurement of airway inflammation, both to explore the aetiology of respiratory symptoms, to monitor the effects of treatment, and to identify the contribution of airway inflammation to apparently poor asthma control.

In airways disease, the fraction of nitric oxide in exhaled air (FeNO) has been developed as a biomarker of airway inflammation. In most asthmatics, FeNO levels increase when control is poor, and decrease with the administration of steroid treatment and control is established (4). More particularly, FeNO may be used as surrogate marker for eosinophilic inflammation, although it is important to stress that the association between eosinophilia in induced sputum and FeNO is modest (Figure 1) (5). This may in part be because eosinophils and nitric oxide reflect different aspects of a complex in-

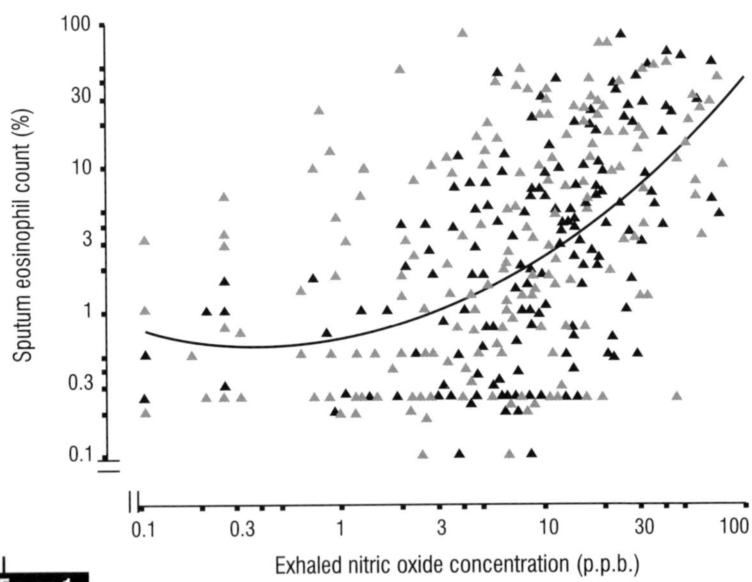

Scatter plot of sputum eosinophil count vs. exhaled nitric oxide concentration in 405 non-smokers with quadratic regression line; males are shown in black triangles and females in grey triangles. Flow-rate measuring FeNO was 250 mL/s achieving lower FeNO levels as compared to present method recommending 50 mL/s. (Reproduced after permission from reference 5).

flammatory process. Also, a number of factors, mediated via the nitric oxide synthase enzymes, influence nitric oxide dynamics in addition to airway inflammation. Exogenous factors are important: FeNO is increased in viral infections in which neutrophils are the predominant inflammatory cell type, even though in stable asthma there seems to be no association between FeNO and the presence of neutrophils in induced sputum.

The Utility of "Normal" Values

"Normal values" for a biomarker like FeNO serve two important purposes. Firstly, predicted values derived from reference equations may be used to describe the range of values in the general population. They are based on the statistical distribution of measurements obtained in large numbers of randomly selected healthy individuals. For spirometry normal values obtained in healthy populations are used to provide the 5th-95th percentiles or 5th-95th confidence intervals for that population, and these are modified by factors which have been shown to significantly affect lung function, notably age, sex, and height. The calculation of percent predicted values is based on these factors being incorporated into prediction equations. Using this same approach, several sets of "normal values" for FeNO, in which major modifying biological factors are taken into account, have been published (see Table 1 and 2). Only those published by Travers et al. and Olin et al. have been derived from population-based samples.

Secondly, a biological test may be used to distinguish individuals affected by a disease state from those who are not. This requires that values for the biomarker obtained in disease differ significantly from those obtained in health. The greater the difference, the more likely it is that the biomarker will be both sensitive and specific for one or more patho-physiological features of the disease in question. Historically, distinguishing asthma from COPD has largely evolved as a result of spirometric test methodology. The presence of an obstructive pattern with or without reversibility over time or with treatment has been used to define the clinical entity. Unfortunately the sensitivity and specificity of spirometric changes is poor, especially for asthma, and thus the diagnostic utility of spirometry is limited. For FeNO, the diagnostic use of population-based reference values is also problematic. Variation of FeNO in a healthy population is large, and bio-

STUDIES OF NORMAL VALUES IN HEALTHY NON-SMOKING SUBJECTS

Author and reference	Groups for which reference values are given	"Normal values" (ppb)
Olivieri et al. 2005 (17)	Male, non-smoker, non-asthmatic Female, non-smoker, non-asthmatic (note: atopy not considered)	4.5 to 20.6 3.6 to 18.2 (note: values quoted are 5th and 95th centiles)
Travers et al. (15)	Male, non-smoker, non-atopic Male, non-smoker, atopic Female, non-smoker, non-atopic Female, non-smoker, atopic	9.5 to 47.4 11.2 to 56.5 7.5 to 37.4 8.8 to 44.6 (note: values quoted are 90% confidence interval)
Olin et al.(13)	Random population 1 131 never-smoking subjects not reporting any asthma symptom, dry cough or the use of inhaled glucocrticoids	See Table 2.
Dressel et al (16)	Male, non-smoker, non-atopic, 165cm. Male, non-smoker, atopic, 165 cm. Female, non-smoker, non-atopic, 160cm. Female, non-smoker, atopic, 160cm.	8.2 to 47.6 12.2 to 71.0 6.6 to 38.3 9.9 to 57.3 (note: values quoted are 5th and 95th centiles)

logical factors like age and height only explain a minor part of this variation. Against this background, it has proved better to develop optimal cut-points based on the distribution of FeNO in patients *with current respiratory symptoms* rather than healthy controls. In symptomatic individuals, the distribution of FeNO is likely to be different (Figure 2) (6-9). However, studies providing informative data have been small with a limited number of subjects. As such while they may be helpful in distinguishing disease from non-disease, they will be underpowered to identify biological factors which explain a large

TABLE 2

UPPER CUT-OFF LIMITS FOR FENO (PPB) IN HEALTHY SUBJECTS, CALCULATED FROM THE ADONIX STUDY(13)

A. Subjects without atopy (n= 845)

Height	Age 25-49 years		Age 50-75 years	
(cm)	Women	Men	Women	Men
150-59	25	27	34	32
160-69	26	30	36	35
170-79	28	33	39	39
180-89	30	37	41	44
190-99	–	42	–	49

B. Subjects with atopy (n=286)

Height	Age 25-49 years		Age 50-75 years	
(cm)	Women	Men	Women	Men
150-59	30	58	37	65
160-69	36	63	45	63
170-79	43	54	53	62
180-89	51	50	64	57
190-99	–	50	–	56

part of the variation. Thus in clinical studies, factors affecting FeNO which have been identified in large populations, may still need to be controlled for when assessing the diagnostic utility of a single FeNO measurement in the disease state.

Defining the clinical relevance of cut-points for FeNO in relation to population-based "normal values" is still in its infancy. While we have sought to provide up-to-date data on this topic, significant work still needs to be done to clarify these issues.

Biological Factors Influencing FeNO

In large healthy populations, FeNO levels range from 2 to 200ppb, but with marked skewing to the right (Figure 2) (10). Factors that affect FeNO levels even in asymptomatic individuals have been identi-

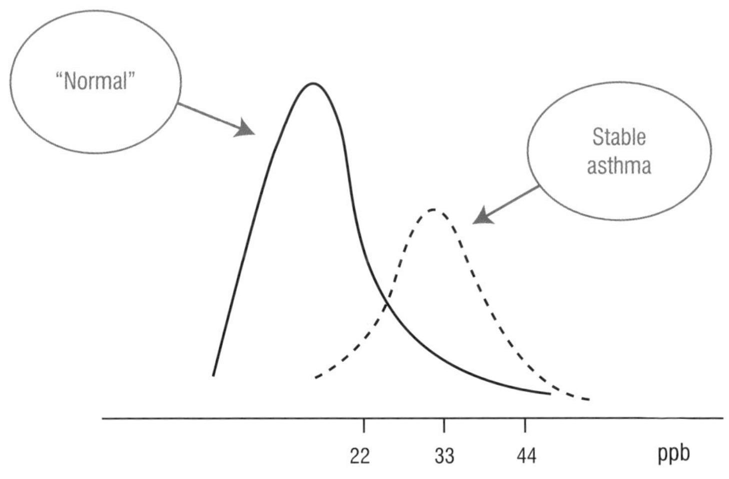

The distribution of FeNO in healthy subjects, depicted as a dotted line, and a stable asthmatic population (dotted line), all examined in a random population study by Olin et al (10). The figures on the x-axis show the mean and 95% confidence intervals for the asthmatic group.

fied, and include genetic factors, sex, age, height and atopy. Other possible factors have been identified including ethnicity and body mass index (BMI), but the data are inconsistent

Genetic factors

Genetic factors were shown to account for about 57% of the variation in FeNO (11) in a study of 377 adult twins in Norway. Among the included subjects, 35% were atopic and 21% had airway hyperresponsiveness. Furthermore a common heritable origin for atopy and FeNO was indicated.

Ethnicity

Consistent with the Norwegian twin study, FeNO levels appear to differ with ethnicity, even though the studies so far are small and have used different nitric oxide analyzers, making direct comparisons difficult.

Levasque et al. (12) examined 429 healthy, non-smoking adult university students and teachers, and among those who were African-American, the geometric mean FeNO was 19.9 parts per billion ppb. This compared with 17.0ppb in the ADONIX-study (13) in which the majority were Caucasian subjects from a random Swedish population.

Stuber et al. have examined Aymara children (n=200), living at high altitude, and found that FeNO tended to be lower than in European children living at the same altitude (12.4 $\pm$ 8.8 (SD) ppb vs 16.1 $\pm$ 11.1 ppb, p = 0.06). This may be an adaptive rather than a purely ethnic effect.

In Chinese children, Wong et al reported that FeNO levels were higher than in Caucasian controls, with the differences appearing to be greater in males (median 17.0ppb versus 11.6ppb, p=0.01) than females (median 19.8 versus 9.1ppb, p=0.04). The sex-related differences were just as significant as the ethnic ones (14).

Ethnicity is not reported in any of the studies by Olin et al. (13), Travers et al (15), Dressel et al. (16) or Olivieri et al (17), presumably because their populations were ethnically uniform.

Sex

Sex is likely to influence FeNO although the reasons are not entirely clear. Various explanations have been suggested including the effects of body size on the airway surface area and female hormonal effects on nitric oxide flux. The majority of studies examining this relationship have reported that FeNO levels are higher in males than in females. In a recent study by Taylor et al. (18), FeNO was measured in 895 members of the Dunedin Multidisciplinary Health and Development Study all aged 32. The FeNO levels were approximately 25% less in females (males 15.3ppb versus females 11.6ppb, p <0.0001). After controlling for height, weight, lung function indices, smoking, atopy, asthma and rhinitis, the between-sex differences remained significant. Travers et al. (12), found a similar difference between the sexes; male subjects (100 of a total of 193 subjects) had 24% higher FeNO levels than females. Levesque et al. have reported that in a population of 895 healthy African American adults, males exhibited higher FeNO levels than females (19). Dressel et al. also reported an independent effect of sex from a pre-employment examination of 897 subjects (383 males) free of respiratory symptoms: men had 17% higher

FeNO values (20.5 versus 17.5ppb) (16). There are a number of other studies describing lower levels of FeNO in females but they all include a relative small number of subjects and may be prone to bias; Olivieri et al: n= 204, 9.9 vs 11.7ppb (17); Tsang et al.: n=121, 23.1ppb vs. 35.4ppb (20); and Jilma et al.: n=43; 20ppb vs 43ppb (21). In contrast to these results, Olin et al. have reported in population-based study including 1131 healthy never-smoking subjects (13) that there were no significant sex-related d-ifferences in FeNO after controlling for height and weight. In a further analysis which included a much larger sample, there was an effect of sex that seemed age dependent (manuscript in preparation). For present purposes, data from the study (13) have been re-analyzed, stratified for sex and atopy. Separate upper-limit FeNO levels for men and women, based on upper cut-off limits for that population, are presented in Table 2.

Age

FeNO levels increase throughout childhood to age 12 (22) at a rate of approximately 5% per annum. The mean FeNO levels obtained in children aged 12 years or less are approximately 5ppb less than for adults. FeNO has also been reported to increase with age in adults (10) although data are conflicting (15-17, 20). The study by Olin et al. (10) includes a larger number of subjects (n=2200), making it less prone to bias, although the studies by Dressel et al. (16) and Travers et al. also include substantial number of subjects (n=987 and n=193 respectively).

Height

There seems to be an increase in FeNO with height that is inde-pendent of lung function (10). The magnitude of the increase is substantial; in healthy non-atopic male of 155cm the upper 95% confidence interval for FeNO is 27ppb and for a taller male of 195cm the corresponding value is 42ppb (Table 2). However, based on re-analyzed data from the study by Olin et al., this trend seems to be absent in atopic men (see Table 2). This may reflect that other factors, such as allergen exposure, are more important for predicting the FeNO values, and height only explains a minor part of the total variation. In atopic women the trend was still pre-sent (see Table 2).

Atopy

Data from a large number of studies consistently show that increased FeNO levels occur with atopy. There also seems to be a correlation between the extent of atopy, as measured by the number and size of skin prick test reactions, and the magnitude of the increase in FeNO (23-26). Even in asymptomatic atopic subjects FeNO levels are higher than in non-atopics (10). It has been suggested that this may be explained by subclinical airway inflammation, although this is speculative (27).

Whether or not separate reference values should be used for atopics or non-atopics is a matter of debate. A very reasonable and practical approach is suggested by Dressel et al. (16), in which different reference values are used for those who report hay-fever. A similar approach is suggested by Travers et al. (15). This allows a direct comparison of measured FeNO levels against reference values which are specific for atopic subjects, avoiding the need to define atopic status by either a blood test for total IgE or a skin-prick test, which may not be easily available.

Body Mass Index

In healthy subjects, BMI has not been associated with FeNO. This was examined in the population-based study by Olin et al. (10, 13). However it may be that in subjects with morbid obesity (BMI greater than $40kg/m^2$) FeNO levels are lower. In subjects with co-existing obesity and asthma the situation may be different. In a study by Komakula et al (28), BMI was negatively associated with FeNO in 67 subjects with asthma, but not in controls.

At present we do not recommend any adjustment for weight or BMI when measuring FeNO in subjects with ongoing respiratory symptoms. However, there may be a subpopulation of asthmatic subjects with very high BMI in whom FeNO is falsely low.

Exogenous Factors Affecting FeNO

Smoking

Smoking is associated with lower FeNO levels (10, 29, 30) and there are several possible explanations for this such as down-regulation of nitric oxide synthases (31) or enhanced local nitric oxide clearance from the airways (32). The magnitude of the smoking effect has been reported to be approximately 35% (18). Only one study has suggested that the effect is directly related to the number of cigarettes smoked (33). McSharry et al. provide a correction factor for measuring FeNO in current smokers, but the application of this correction factor may only be appropriate in patients with current asthma (33). In the studies by Travers et al. (15) and Dressel et al. (16), appropriate adjustments for the calculation of "normal values" in asymptomatic smokers are provided but are untried. In general, clinical decisions based on a FeNO result obtained from a current symptomatic smoker should be cautious, as the result may be falsely low.

Diet

Nitrate rich foods have been shown to influence FeNO (34); (35). Vints et al found a maximal increase in FeNO of 60% two hours after a nitrate rich meal (equivalent to 230 mg nitrate) which still remained significant (+22%) 15 hours after the food-intake. The values were only back to normal after 20 hours.

Whether intake of caffeine leads altered FeNO is still unclear. Two different randomized placebo-controlled studies have provided contradictory results. Taylor et al. found no effect of caffeine (36) whereas Bruce et al. found a significant decrease of FeNO 1 hour after intake of caffeinated coffee (mean -19%) or a caffeine capsule (mean -13%) (37).

The magnitude of effect for each of the above factors may be statistically significant, but is unlikely to be of clinical importance. However, in research studies which focus on FeNO as a primary endpoint, taking account of nitrate-rich food intake may be appropriate. Examples of nitrate rich foodstuffs are green vegetables like salad and spinach, and ham and sausages.

Cut-Off Points for FeNO

It remains unclear as to what constitute clinically relevant cut-off points for FeNO. In healthy asymptomatic populations, and given that high rather than low values are more clinically relevant (except in the rare situation of primary ciliary dyskinesia) arguably the chosen value should be the upper limit of the 95% confidence interval. In individuals with a confirmed diagnosis of asthma, the situation is more complex, and reference ranges for patients with stable asthma as well as those for healthy populations may have to be considered simultaneously.

The overall aim must be to construct reference values that are clinically relevant and easy to use. So far no study has examined the value of adjusting cut-points for FeNO for the diagnosis of asthma in relation to biological factors like age, height and sex. In the absence of this information particular recommendations cannot be made. The exception is in children where there is substantial evidence that it is important to control for age, atopy and possibly height.

For the time being we recommend the use of cut-points which are of clinical importance for diagnosis and monitoring of airway inflammation rather than a specific disease entity. These are pragmatic and based on reference ranges reported from mixed population studies as well as clinically important values obtained from groups of patients with asthma or non-specific respiratory symptoms.

Assessing Patients with Asthma-Like Symptoms

Diagnosis always begins with evaluating the clinical history. The diagnosis of asthma cannot be based solely on FeNO measurements. Indeed FeNO is not a diagnostic test for asthma! If symptoms are typical for asthma, FeNO measurements may help in ruling in or out eosinophilic airway inflammation as a cause of the patient's symptoms. High or low values are particularly helpful.

With that proviso, early studies have examined optimal cut-points for FeNO in relation to asthma diagnosis (38-40). Deykin et al used an off-line method to measure FeNO and the results are not generalisable. Smith et al, used the presently recommended measurement technique (39), examined 47 subjects of whom only 17 subjects were diagnosed with asthma using conventional criteria, and concluded that a FeNO of 20ppb was the optimum cut-point for asthma diagnosis. Dupont et al, examined 240 subjects of whom 160 were diagnosed with asthma using an exhalation flow (200 mL/s). Receiver operator curve analyses revealed that 16ppb was optimal for diagnosing asthma, achieving both positive and negative predictive values for asthma diagnosis of >90%. However, these authors reported that the accuracy of the test was low at intermediate FeNO levels, and they suggested a dual diagnostic interpretation i.e. low values rule out asthma and high values support a diagnosis. Subjects with intermediate values need further evaluation. Our recommended strategy for interpreting FeNO is based on this approach.

If FeNO is <25ppb (in adults) symptoms are unlikely to be due to eosinophilic airway inflammation, and atopic asthma is unlikely (5). In a *symptomatic patient,* a low FeNO level points to reasons other than active eosinophilic airway inflammation as the cause of the patient's symptoms e.g. gastro-esophageal reflux, anxiety, vocal cord dysfunction, obesity. It is important to note that many of these entities may complicate asthma or even supervene as the principal cause of the patient's symptoms. However, given that none is amenable to inhaled steroid therapy, a low FeNO result is clinically helpful in guiding the clinician away from inappropriate use of ICS to treat the patient's symptoms. In steroid naive patients with asthma (typical symptoms with airway hyper-responsiveness and/or variable airflow obstruction) but a low FeNO, their asthma may be due to non-eosinophilic inflammation, and similarly, they are less likely to respond to steroid therapy.

FeNO values between 25 and 50ppb require cautious interpretation, and may often indicate that further diagnostic testing is necessary. One may consider sex, age, and height to further interpret the results. Where serial measurements have been obtained over time, the trends into and out of this range may be helpful in the overall interpretation of the current result.

FeNO values >50ppb are indicative of active eosinophilic airway inflammation, and in the context of typical symptoms and variable airflow limitation, would justify a diagnosis of asthma. Further testing is not needed. Once again one may consider age, sex, height and smoking history to further interpret the results; e.g. in an elderly or tall, non-smoking male a high FeNO may be normal value. The magnitude of the FeNO level is not usually related to the clinical severity.

The evidence to support the use of 50ppb as a clinically relevant cut-off point comes from a number of sources. In the ADONIX study (10) the upper limit of the 95% confidence interval for FeNO in the subgroup of patients with stable asthma was 43.6ppb. In patients with chronic non-specific airway symptoms, an optimal cut-off point of 47ppb was related to the likelihood of steroid responsiveness (41). In patients with established asthma, Pijnenburg et al., showed that if inhaled steroid therapy was withdrawn from patients whose asthma is well controlled, subsequent relapse occurred in those whose FeNO was greater than 49ppb two weeks after the withdrawal of therapy (42). More recently Michils et al. have shown that in ICS-naive patients, a FeNO of greater than 35ppb predicted improved asthma control in response to steroid treatment with a positive predictive value of 68% (43).

Monitoring Asthma

In patients with stable, well-controlled asthma, the upper limit of "normal" is approximately 35 to 50ppb in adults. This has been established in both cross-sectional (7, 10, 15) as well as longitudinal studies (44). However, persistently high FeNO (>50ppb) may occur despite apparently adequate anti-inflammatory treatment (45). The most common cause is poor compliance with ICS therapy. Occasionally it represents poor drug delivery to the airways. In some cases the high FeNO is alveolar in origin, and oral steroid treatment may be indicated (46). Only rarely does it signal truly steroid resistant asthma. If the patient is asymptomatic, then no change in treatment is required, because, as stated previously, reducing or withdrawing ICS therapy is likely to be followed by relapse (47).

Smith et al. have recently highlighted that achieving a normal FeNO value, based on reference values from a healthy population, is not necessary for adequate asthma control (48). In that study of 73 patients with asthma, the patients were given 14 days of treatment with oral prednisone 30 mg/day, and FeNO decreased to 17.7ppb (95% C.I. 15.5-20.2). The post-prednisone values approximated to the predicted values derived from the equation of Olin et al. (13). However, when the patients' inhaled fluticasone dose was adjusted to achieve optimal asthma control, the subjects/ geometric mean FeNO was higher, at 20.2ppb (95% C.I. 17.1-22.2ppb). This indicated that achieving predicted normal values for FeNO is not clinically necessary. Indeed, there are no data to support lowering FeNO by increased doses of inhaled or oral steroids once acceptable asthma control has been achieved. The situation may be somewhat different in the subgroup of patients with difficult asthma. Van Veen et al. (49) have shown in a longitudinal study of 98 subjects with difficult-to-treat asthma that increased FeNO (above 20ppb at an exhalation rate of 100 mL/s) was associated with an excess decline in FEV_1 of 43 mL/year. The risk was highest among those with a baseline FEV_1 $\geq$80 percent predicted. Whether it is beneficial to try to reduce airway inflammation and normalize FeNO in this subgroup is an open question.

Low FeNO values (<25ppb in adults, 20ppb in children), against a background of an established diagnosis of asthma and increased FeNO prior to commencing inhaled steroid therapy, signal adequate control of airway inflammation. This may be as a result of or in spite of anti-inflammatory therapy (i.e. the asthma is in remission). Treatment may be reduced or, depending on the history, withdrawn altogether at least on a trial basis. Relapse is less likely with a low FeNO which remains low 4 weeks after withdrawing ICS treatment (50).

In individual patients, serial measurements may indicate that these cut-off points are inappropriate. For example, in a patient whose FeNO at the time of asthma diagnosis is 120ppb, good control may be achieved when FeNO is reduced to and maintained at 70ppb. On the other hand, some patients may experience an increase in symptoms with FeNO at 40ppb, with good control at 25ppb. The inter-patient variability emphasizes that cut-points based on group mean data are a guide and not absolute as to their clinical relevance.

What is a Clinically Revelant Change in FeNO?

It is difficult to judge what constitutes a clinically important change in individual patients except by obtaining serial FeNO measurements. The within-subject coefficient of variation for FeNO in healthy subjects is approximately 15% or up to 4ppb (7). This increases to approximately 25% in patients with asthma (7, 51). In one study, FeNO levels during acute asthma were 50% higher when asthma was unstable compared to when stability was restored (52).

Data obtained from steroid withdrawal studies show that the mean increase in FeNO associated with the advent of loss of control ranges from 16ppb (53) to 25ppb (44), the latter representing a 60% increase from baseline. However, the range of the increase in FeNO between stability and loss of control is high, from -10 to +141ppb. An acute rise (over 12-24 hours) in FeNO may occur following intense exposure to an allergen to which the patient is sensitized. The magnitude of the rise may be as high as 150 ppb (54).

The predictive values of a single measurement of FeNO for loss of asthma control are insufficiently sensitive or specific to justify their use for this purpose (44, 55). As a prognostic indicator for imminent loss of control, FeNO is no better than more conventional lung function testing (44).

Conclusions

The interpretation of FeNO measurements requires to be undertaken with reference to the patient's current symptoms. Reference ranges provide a guide as to which factors may be relevant when using FeNO for diagnostic purposes. The most important are age (children), sex, smoking status and atopy. However, at present it is unclear how reference ranges should be used in relation to assessing currently active airway inflammation. The use of cut-points (less than 25ppb or greater than 50ppb in adults) is pragmatic but also has limitations. Further work is needed to refine our current levels of knowledge in this area so that the results of serial FeNO measurements may be interpreted more appropriately. Using FeNO measurements, the management of airways disease is improved, particularly in patients with complex asthma whose symptoms are of multifactorial etiology.

References

1. Bousquet J, Clark TJ, Hurd S, Khaltaev N, Lenfant C, O'Byrne P, et al. GINA guidelines on asthma and beyond. Allergy. 2007 Feb;62(2):102-12.
2. Green RH, Brightling CE, McKenna S, Hargadon B, Parker D, Bradding P, et al. Asthma exacerbations and sputum eosinophil counts: a randomised controlled trial. Lancet. 2002 Nov 30;360 (9347):1715-21.
3. Wenzel SE. Asthma: defining of the persistent adult phenotypes. Lancet. 2006 Aug 26;368(9537):804-13.
4. Taylor DR, Pijnenburg MW, Smith AD, De Jongste JC. Exhaled nitric oxide measurements: clinical application and interpretation. Thorax. 2006 Sep; 61(9): 817-27.
5. Berry MA, Shaw DE, Green RH, Brightling CE, Wardlaw AJ, Pavord ID. The use of exhaled nitric oxide concentration to identify eosinophilic airway inflammation: an observational study in adults with asthma. Clin Exp Allergy. 2005 Sep;35(9):1175-9.
6. van der Lee I, van den Bosch JM, Zanen P. Reduction of variability of exhaled nitric oxide in healthy volunteers. Respir Med. 2002 Dec;96(12): 1014-20.
7. Kharitonov SA, Gonio F, Kelly C, Meah S, Barnes PJ. Reproducibility of exhaled nitric oxide measurements in healthy and asthmatic adults and children. Eur Respir J. 2003 Mar;21(3): 433-8.
8. Olin AC, Alving K, Toren K. Exhaled nitric oxide: relation to sensitization and respiratory symptoms. Clin Exp Allergy. 2004 Feb;34(2):221-6.
9. Buchvald F, Baraldi E, Carraro S, Gaston B, De Jongste J, Pijnenburg MW, et al. Measurements of exhaled nitric oxide in healthy subjects age 4

to 17 years. J Allergy Clin Immunol. 2005 Jun;115(6):1130-6.

10. Olin AC, Rosengren A, Thelle DS, Lissner L, Bake B, Toren K. Height, age, and atopy are associated with fraction of exhaled nitric oxide in a large adult general population sample. Chest. 2006 Nov;130(5):1319-25.

11. Lund MB, Kongerud J, Nystad W, Boe J, Harris JR. Genetic and environmental effects on exhaled nitric oxide and airway responsiveness in a population-based sample of twins. Eur Respir J. 2007 Feb;29(2):292-8.

12. Kippelen P, Caillaud C, Robert E, Masmoudi K, Prefaut C. Exhaled nitric oxide level during and after heavy exercise in athletes with exercise-induced hypoxaemia. Pflugers Arch. 2002 Jun;444(3):397-404.

13. Olin AC, Bake B, Toren K. Fraction of exhaled nitric oxide at 50 mL/s: reference values for adult lifelong never-smokers. Chest. 2007 Jun;131(6): 1852-6.

14. Wong GW, Liu EK, Leung TF, Yung E, Ko FW, Hui DS, et al. High levels and gender difference of exhaled nitric oxide in Chinese schoolchildren. Clin Exp Allergy. 2005 Jul;35(7):889-93.

15. Travers J, Marsh S, Aldington S, Williams M, Shirtcliffe P, Pritchard A, et al. Reference ranges for exhaled nitric oxide derived from a random community survey of adults. Am J Respir Crit Care Med. 2007 Aug 1;176(3):238-42.

16. Dressel H, de la Motte D, Reichert J, Ochmann U, Petru R, Angerer P, et al. Exhaled nitric oxide: independent effects of atopy, smoking, respiratory tract infection, gender and height. Respir Med. 2008 Jul;102(7):962-9.

17. Olivieri M, Corradi M, Malerba M. Gender and exhaled nitric oxide. Chest. 2007 Oct;132(4):1410; author reply

18. Taylor DR, Mandhane P, Greene JM, Hancox RJ, Filsell S, McLachlan CR, et al. Factors affecting exhaled nitric oxide measurements: the effect of sex. Respir Res. 2007;8:82.

19. Levesque MC, Hauswirth DW, Mervin-Blake S, Fernandez CA, Patch KB, Alexander KM, et al. Determinants of exhaled nitric oxide levels in healthy, nonsmoking African American adults. J Allergy Clin Immunol. 2008 Feb;121(2):396-402 e3.

20. Tsang KW, Ip SK, Leung R, Tipoe GL, Chan SL, Shum IH, et al. Exhaled nitric oxide: the effects of age, gender and body size. Lung. 2001;179(2):83-91.

21. Jilma B, Kastner J, Mensik C, Vondrovec B, Hildebrandt J, Krejcy K, et al. Sex differences in concentrations of exhaled nitric oxide and plasma nitrate. Life Sci. 1996;58(6):469-76.

22. Buchvald F, Hermansen MN, Nielsen KG, Bisgaard H. Exhaled nitric oxide predicts exercise-induced bronchoconstriction in asthmatic school children. Chest. 2005 Oct;128(4):1964-7.

23. Gratziou C, Lignos M, Dassiou M, Roussos C. Influence of atopy on exhaled nitric oxide in patients with stable asthma and rhinitis. Eur Respir J. 1999 Oct;14(4):897-901.

24. Ho LP, Wood FT, Robson A, Innes JA, Greening AP. Atopy influences exhaled nitric oxide levels in adult asthmatics. Chest. 2000 Nov;118(5):1327-31.

25. Jouaville LF, Annesi-Maesano I, Nguyen LT, Bocage AS, Bedu M, Caillaud D. Interrelationships among asthma, atopy, rhinitis and exhaled nitric oxide in a population-based sample of children. Clin Exp Allergy. 2003 Nov;33(11):1506-11.

26. van Amsterdam JG, Janssen NA, de Meer G, Fischer PH, Nierkens S, van Loveren H, et al. The relationship between exhaled nitric oxide and allergic sensitization in a random sample of school children. Clin Exp Allergy. 2003 Feb;33(2):187-91.

27. van den Toorn LM, Overbeek SE, de Jongste JC, Leman K, Hoogsteden HC, Prins JB. Airway inflammation is present during clinical remission of atopic asthma. Am J Respir Crit Care Med. 2001 Dec 1;164(11):2107-13.

28. Komakula S, Khatri S, Mermis J, Savill S, Haque S, Rojas M, et al. Body mass index is associated with reduced exhaled nitric oxide and higher exhaled 8-isoprostanes in asthmatics. Respir Res. 2007;8:32.

29. Persson MG, Zetterstrom O, Agrenius V, Ihre E, Gustafsson LE. Single-breath nitric oxide measurements in asthmatic patients and smokers. Lancet. 1994 Jan 15;343(8890):146-7.

30. Kharitonov SA, Robbins RA, Yates D, Keatings V, Barnes PJ. Acute and chronic effects of cigarette smoking on exhaled nitric oxide. Am J Respir Crit Care Med. 1995 Aug;152(2):609-12.

31. Hoyt JC, Robbins RA, Habib M, Springall DR, Buttery LD, Polak JM, et al. Cigarette smoke decreases inducible nitric oxide synthase in lung epithelial cells. Exp Lung Res. 2003 Jan-Feb;29(1):17-28.

32. Balint B, Donnelly LE, Hanazawa T, Kharitonov SA, Barnes PJ. Increased nitric oxide metabolites in exhaled breath condensate after exposure to tobacco smoke. Thorax. 2001 Jun;56(6):456-61.

33. McSharry CP, McKay IC, Chaudhuri R, Livingston E, Fraser I, Thomson NC. Short and long-term effects of cigarette smoking independently influence exhaled nitric oxide concentration in asthma. J Allergy Clin Immunol. 2005 Jul;116(1):88-93.

34. Olin AC, Aldenbratt A, Ekman A, Ljungkvist G, Jungersten L, Alving K, et al. Increased nitric oxide in exhaled air after intake of a nitrate-rich meal. Respir Med. 2001 Feb;95(2):153-8.

35. Vints AM, Oostveen E, Eeckhaut G, Smolders M, De Backer WA. Time-dependent effect of nitrate-rich meals on exhaled nitric oxide in healthy subjects. Chest. 2005 Oct;128(4):2465-70.

36. Taylor ES, Smith AD, Cowan JO, Herbison GP, Taylor DR. Effect of caffeine ingestion on exhaled nitric oxide measurements in patients with asthma. Am J Respir Crit Care Med. 2004 May 1;169(9):1019-21.

37. Bruce C, Yates DH, Thomas PS. Caffeine decreases exhaled nitric oxide. Thorax. 2002 Apr;57(4):361-3.

38. Deykin A, Massaro AF, Drazen JM, Israel E. Exhaled nitric oxide as a diagnostic test for asthma: online versus offline techniques and effect of flow rate. Am J Respir Crit Care Med. 2002 Jun 15;165(12):1597-601.

39. Smith AD, Cowan JO, Filsell S, McLachlan C, Monti-Sheehan G, Jackson P, et al. Diagnosing asthma: comparisons between exhaled nitric oxide measurements and conventional tests. Am J Respir Crit Care Med. 2004 Feb 15;169(4):473-8.

40. Dupont LJ, Demedts MG, Verleden GM. Prospective evaluation of the validity of exhaled nitric oxide for the diagnosis of asthma. Chest. 2003 Mar;123(3):751-6.

41. Smith AD, Cowan JO, Brassett KP, Filsell S, McLachlan C, Monti-Sheehan G, et al. Exhaled nitric oxide: a predic-

tor of steroid response. Am J Respir Crit Care Med. 2005 Aug 15;172(4): 453-9.

42. Pijnenburg MW, Bakker EM, Hop WC, De Jongste JC. Titrating steroids on exhaled nitric oxide in children with asthma: a randomized controlled trial. Am J Respir Crit Care Med. 2005 Oct 1;172(7):831-6.

43. Michils A, Baldassarre S, Van Muylem A. Exhaled nitric oxide and asthma control: a longitudinal study in unselected patients. Eur Respir J. 2008 Mar;31(3):539-46.

44. Jones SL, Kittelson J, Cowan JO, Flannery EM, Hancox RJ, McLachlan CR, et al. The predictive value of exhaled nitric oxide measurements in assessing changes in asthma control. Am J Respir Crit Care Med. 2001 Sep 1;164(5):738-43.

45. Pijnenburg MW, Bakker EM, Lever S, Hop WC, De Jongste JC. High fractional concentration of nitric oxide in exhaled air despite steroid treatment in asthmatic children. Clin Exp Allergy. 2005 Jul;35(7):920-5.

46. Berry M, Hargadon B, Morgan A, Shelley M, Richter J, Shaw D, et al. Alveolar nitric oxide in adults with asthma: evidence of distal lung inflammation in refractory asthma. Eur Respir J. 2005 Jun;25(6):986-91.

47. Pijnenburg MW, Hofhuis W, Hop WC, De Jongste JC. Exhaled nitric oxide predicts asthma relapse in children with clinical asthma remission. Thorax. 2005 Mar;60(3):215-8.

48. Smith A, Cowan, JO, Taylor, DR. Exhaled nitric oxide levels in asthma:"personal best" versus reference values. JACI. 2009;In press.

49. van Veen IH, Ten Brinke A, Sterk PJ, Sont JK, Gauw SA, Rabe KF, et al. Exhaled nitric oxide predicts lung function decline in difficult-to-treat asthma. Eur Respir J. 2008 Aug;32(2):344-9.

50. Zacharasiewicz A, Wilson N, Lex C, Erin EM, Li AM, Hansel T, et al. Clinical use of noninvasive measurements of airway inflammation in steroid reduction in children. Am J Respir Crit Care Med. 2005 May 15;171(10):1077-82.

51. Ekroos H, Karjalainen J, Sarna S, Laitinen LA, Sovijarvi AR. Short-term variability of exhaled nitric oxide in young male patients with mild asthma and in healthy subjects. Respir Med. 2002 Nov;96(11):895-900.

52. Massaro AF, Gaston B, Kita D, Fanta C, Stamler JS, Drazen JM. Expired nitric oxide levels during treatment of acute asthma. Am J Respir Crit Care Med. 1995 Aug;152(2):800-3.

53. Beck-Ripp J, Griese M, Arenz S, Koring C, Pasqualoni B, Bufler P. Changes of exhaled nitric oxide during steroid treatment of childhood asthma. Eur Respir J. 2002 Jun;19(6):1015-9.

54. Hewitt RS, Smith AD, Cowan JO, Schofield JC, Herbison GP, Taylor DR. Serial exhaled nitric oxide measurements in the assessment of laboratory animal allergy. J Asthma. 2008 Mar;45(2):101-7.

55. Gelb AF, Flynn Taylor C, Shinar CM, Gutierrez C, Zamel N. Role of spirometry and exhaled nitric oxide to predict exacerbations in treated asthmatics. Chest. 2006 Jun;129(6):1492-9.

Exhaled Nitric Oxide - Application in Clinical Practice in Asthma

Lieven J. Dupont

Asthma is a chronic inflammatory disorder characterized by the presence of inflammatory cells and the release of several inflammatory mediators in the airways (1). Airway inflammation is thought to result in airway obstruction, bronchial hyperresponsiveness and remodelling of the airways (2). The diagnosis and monitoring of asthma is based on conventional measurements consisting of a combination of frequency and severity of symptoms, use of reliever medication as reported by the patient and measurements of airway obstruction (PEF or FEV_1), assessment of bronchodilator response and bronchial challenge tests to assess bronchial hyperresponsiveness(3).

However, self-reporting of symptoms is dependent on perception of symptoms with the potential for both under- and over-perception (4) which may lead to under- and over- treatment using the current

Correspondence

Prof. Lieven J. Dupont

Division of Respiratory Medicine, University Hospital Gasthuisberg, 49 Herestraat, B-3000 Leuven, Belgium

e-mail lieven.dupont@uz.kuleuven.ac.be

symptom-based approach to determine doses of anti-inflammatory medication. Selfmonitoring of PEFR requires cooperation in producing maximal expiration and performing the measurements daily for several weeks. Although airway inflammation may be reflected by the degree of airway obstruction, the relationship of the pulmonary function tests with objective indices of inflammation is not a simple one (5) and patients with mild asthma frequently have normal baseline values of FEV_1. Challenge testing to metacholine or histamine is a reliable diagnostic test for airway hyperresponsiveness, with positive results in nearly all individuals, but the relationship to the degree of inflammation is not unique (6).

Failing to obtain adequate information with regard to airway inflammation may put the patients at risk of frequent exacerbations or progressive airway remodelling which may lead to non-reversible airflow obstruction (7). As inflammation is a central feature of bronchial asthma, directly measuring airway inflammation may be more appropriate for the diagnosis and monitoring of asthma, especially in patients with severe asthma where the disease is often more complicated and difficult to control. Before the advent of exhaled markers, only invasive techniques such as bronchoscopy could directly sample bronchial tissue and fluids for the presence of inflammatory cells and mediators. Examination of induced sputum produces valuable information on airway inflammation and may be beneficial in guiding therapy in patients with asthma. Green et al. have shown that therapy guided by eosinophil count in induced sputum leads to a four- to five-fold reduction in exacerbation rate compared with a guideline-defined approach (8) and findings in keeping with this observation have subsequently been reported by Jayaram et al. (9). However, in spite of this convincing evidence, induced sputum analysis is impractical (requiring skilled technicians), time-consuming, and expensive which prevents it from being implemented in routine clinical practice. In addition, sputum induction may produce temporary decrements in lung function. The measurement of nitric oxide in exhaled air (FeNO) features as a non-invasive, simple way to assess airway inflammation.

Gaseous NO was detected in exhaled breath in 1991 (10) and in 1993 the first report was published linking elevated NO to asthma (11). The association between increased fraction of nitric oxide in exhaled air (FeNO) and asthma was soon replicated in numerous reports (12-14). The discovery of this potential biomarker for asthma stimulated a concerted research effort evaluating the application of

FeNO levels in clinical practice. This chapter outlines the data supporting the added clinical value of measuring FeNO in asthma.

Basis for Measuring FeNo in Asthma

Analysis of FeNO has been found to be highly reproducible, relatively quick and simple to perform and equipment is becoming more affordable (15, 16). Analysis of FeNO only requires a steady exhalation from the patient into the mouthpiece of the NO analyser to allow measurement (15). As FeNO values are dependent on the expiratory flow rate, standardization of measurement technique is extremely important to allow comparisons across different studies (15). The technique is simple to use and provides repeatable and reproducible results in adults and in children as young as 4 years old (17). Although the measurement of NO in the exhaled air is non-invasive and simple, the equipment used to measure FeNO is expensive. Widespread clinical use of FeNO as a diagnostic test will certainly be more practicable if technological advances result in the development of smaller and cheaper analysers, which can then be used in an out-hospital setting. Currently, such technologies are being increasingly used in secondary and tertiary care settings.

Normative values for FeNO have been reported in a number of different populations, listed in Table 1, using the standard methodology (18-32). The upper limit of normal is between 30 to 50 parts per billion (ppb) depending on the definition of upper limit. Predictive equations for FeNO have been derived and include adjustments for previously described confounders including smoking in adults (24) and height in children (31).

The following evidence can summarize the rationale behind the concept of using FeNO as a guide in the diagnosis and management of asthma. 1. Increased FeNO in asthmatics is highly correlated with eosinophilic airway inflammation. 2. The use of inhaled corticosteroids (ICS) in asthma results in a fall in FeNO and there is a dose response relationship between ICS and FeNO. 3. Raised FeNO predicts steroid responsiveness in patients with non-specific respiratory symptoms.

Association with airway inflammation in asthma

The origin for the 'excess' NO in asthma has been related to the pro-

TABLE 1

STUDIES THAT HAVE REPORTED NORMAL VALUES FOR FeNO IN NON-ASTHMATIC POPULATIONS WHERE THE STANDARD METHODOLOGY AT A FLOW RATE OF 50 ML/S WAS USED

Study	Number of study subjects	FeNO mean ± SD (ppb)
Adults		
El Halawani 2003 (18)	42	**19.9 ± 18.4**
de Winter-de Groot 2005 (19)	24	**18.1 ± 7.4**
Haight 2006 (20)	23 (<30 years)	median **18.7**
	25 (>60 years)	median **36.9**
Olivieri 2006 (21)	204	**10.8 ± 4.7**
Olin 2006 (22)	2295	**16.0** (25-75: 11-22)
Travers 2007 (23)	193	**17.9**
	(24% atopy 10% smokers)	(90% CI 8-41)
Olin 2007 (24)	1131	**16.6** (95% CI 6-47)
	845 non-atopic	**16.0**
	286 atopic	**18.8**
Taylor 2007 (25)	236	M **20.2** (18.6, 21.9)
	264	F **13.7** (12.8, 14.7)
Maestrelli 2007 (26)	122	M **21.6** [1.06]
		F **16.3** [1.07]
Children		
Scollo 2000 (27)	23	**10.1 ± 4.1**
Jöbsis 2001 (28)	73	**10.5 ± 1.1**
Kharitonov 2003 (17)	20	**15.6 ± 9.2**
Malmberg 2003 (29)	62	**5.3 ± 0.4**
Santamaria 2005 (30)	40	**10.0 ± 4.2**
Buchvald 2005 (31)	405	**9.7**
		(95%UL=25 ppb)
Malmberg 2006 (32)	114	**10.3**
		(age dependent)

duction of NO from the substrate L-arginine by the activity of a family of enzymes collectively termed nitric oxide synthases (NOSs) (33). The inducible isotype of NOS (iNOS) is usually present in the airways of asthmatic individuals (34) and is upregulated in direct proportion with FeNO concentrations (34, 35). The relevance of iNOS in proximal airways to FeNO values in asthma is highlighted by a study where a relatively selective iNOS inhibitor was inhaled, which reduced NO release in the proximal airways by an average of 80% whereas NO production in the distal airways was not affected (36). There is also increased diffusivity of NO in the asthmatic airway, possibly due to increased constitutive NO synthase expression, which is not suppressed by steroids (37). One non-enzymatic source of FeNO is the pH-dependent conversion of NO_2 to NO where acidic conditions favour NO release. The airway fluid of asthmatics is acidic and normalization of airway fluid pH with inhalation of phosphate-buffered saline reduces FeNO and in particular the NO production in the proximal airways (38).

FeNO is increased in asthma, and correlates well with measures of eosinophilic airway inflammation (39-52). In most studies, FeNO is found to be elevated two- to three-fold in asthma compared with normal controls (11-14). FeNO is raised in most cases of corticosteroid-naive, and in 40-60% of ICS-treated, patients with asthma (53).

FeNO correlates with the number of eosinophils in induced sputum (39-45), bronchoalveolar lavage fluid (46) and bronchial biopsies (42). In another study a significant relationship between FeNO and the number of circulating IL-4 producing CD4+ T-cells was reported (47). A positive correlation between FeNO and activated eosinophils, as assessed by major basic protein density on endobronchial biopsy specimens, was noted in asthmatic subjects using only short-acting beta 2-agonists and in asymptomatic subjects with asthma (48). Payne et al. showed similar results using endobronchial biopsies from children with difficult-to-control asthma who had recently used oral steroids (49). FeNO is also related to other indices of airway inflammation in asthma, including blood eosinophils (50, 51), sputum eosinophilic cationic protein (52), the degree of airway hyperresponsiveness (13, 40) and bronchial wall thickness, assessed by computed tomography scanning (50, 54, 55).

FeNO may also be influenced by factors other than eosinophilic airway inflammation. These include age, atopy, gender, smoking, body size, and genetic variation (19, 20, 22, 24, 25). This results in false-positive and false-negative FeNO results when compared against a gold standard. In Shaw et al., the relationship between FeNO and sputum eosinophils was imperfect, resulting in many false-positive results (56). Persistently high NO levels have been reported in spite of high doses of ICS (57), "Atopic asthmatic" subjects who are in remission for many years but who nevertheless have eosinophilic airway inflammation in bronchial biopsies (48), FeNO levels remain increased. High allergen load or peripheral airways inflammation resulting in an increased FeNO, necessitate proper phenotyping to achieve optimal utility of exhaled NO measurements in the management of asthma patients.

Response to anti-inflammatory treatment for asthma

Treatment with inhaled glucocorticosteroids efficiently reduces the high FeNO levels in asthmatics (58-64). A linear dose-response relationship is seen for sputum eosinophils, and changes in FeNO correlated significantly with these changes in sputum eosinophils (53). Silkoff et al. found that FeNO was able to detect a dose-dependent effect between 100 and 800 mg beclomethasone, whereas FEV_1 did not, and that this response effect was reproducible (62-64). In a study by Jatakanon et al, the suppression of FeNO by corticosteroid therapy appears to reach a plateau at a dose equivalent to budesonide 400µg daily (61).

Currie et al. evaluated the addition of montelukast to ICS in asthmatics (65). Although montelukast did not improve lung function, a significant reduction in FeNO was seen when montelukast was added to ICS (65). Similar results were seen in a pediatric population in which the addition of montelukast to ICS did not alter FEV_1, but significantly decreased FeNO levels when compared with placebo (66). FeNO levels increased to baseline levels 2 weeks after withdrawal of montelukast. A second pediatric study with montelukast failed to show a significant reduction in FeNO (67). As a result, FeNO may also serve as a marker of treatment response and compliance with controller medication, particularly inhaled corticosteroids.

FeNO levels predict steroid responsiveness

The clinical benefit of increased steroid treatment in patients with asthma is greatest in patients with raised FeNO levels (68, 69). Smith et al evaluated the predictive accuracy of FeNO measurements in adult patients with undiagnosed respiratory symptoms (68). The positive and negative predictive values for a range of outcomes following a trial of inhaled fluticasone were superior for FeNO as a predictor than spirometry, bronchodilator response, and measurements of airway hyperresponsiveness. This study also identified an optimum cut point for steroid response at an FeNO of 47 ppb (68). This outcome was largely independent of the final diagnosis. A similar result has been reported by Szefler et al. who showed that children with high FeNO values are more likely to respond to ICS than children with lower FeNO values (70).

Taken together, these data provide sufficient evidence that FeNO measurements may have a potentially important role in evaluating and treating patients with asthma. FeNO may be used as a surrogate marker for airway eosinophilia and FeNO levels have a role in predicting the response to ICS treatment. These associations between FeNO with both airway inflammation & steroid responsiveness suggest that FeNO might be used as an online inflammometer in clinical practice.

FeNO in the Diagnosis of Asthma

Several studies have used FeNO to discriminate between asthmatics and non-asthmatics (Table 2) (29, 71-78) and confirm that FeNO value has better test accuracy than commonly used diagnostic strategies for asthma (73).

In adults, FeNO is helpful in discriminating asthma from non-asthma (71, 73-78). Evidence from prospective trials confirms high sensitivity and specificity for FeNO as a diagnostic test for asthma in patients presenting with chronic non-specific respiratory symptoms (71, 73). In a study by Dupont et al. among 240 non-smoking steroid naive individuals of whom 160 (67%) fulfilled the criteria for the diagnosis of asthma, FeNO levels were highly predictive of asthma with a sensitivity and specificity of 85% and 90%, respectively (71). Smith et al. obtained similar sensitivity and specificity in 47 patients of whom 17 had asthma (73). Predictive values were almost identical to those obtained using induced sputum cell counts. In addition, FeNO is superior to conventional tests including spirometry and peak flow in the diagnosis of asthma, probably reflecting the fact that the majority of unselected patients presenting with non-specific respiratory symptoms will have mild disease with normal lung function (73). In this setting FeNO measurements may be more relevant than traditional lung function tests (29, 73, 74, 77). The combination of a raised FeNO (>33 ppb) and abnormal spirometry (FEV_1<80% predicted) provides even greater sensitivity (94%) and specificity (93%) for the diagnosis of asthma (73, 79). However, it is advisable to limit FeNO evaluation to patients with chronic respiratory symptoms (>6 weeks), to minimize potential

TABLE 2

STUDIES EVALUATING DIAGNOSTIC VALUE OF FeNO MEASUREMENTS IN ASTHMA

Author	Design	Pretest probability	Cut-off FeNO	Sensitivity	Specificity	PPV	NPV
Dupont 2003 (71)	240 adults $FeNO_{200}$	67%	> 13 pb	85%	90%	80%	90%
Narang 2002 (72)	88 children (5-19y) $FeNO_?$	39%	> 25 pb	NR	NR	100%	80%
Malmberg 2003 (73)	96 children $FeNO_{50}$	25%	> 10ppb	86%	92%	78%	95%
Smith 2004 (74)	47 adults $FeNO_{50}$	36%	> 20 ppb	88%	79%	70%	92%
Berkman 2005 (75)	85 adults $FeNO_{250}$	47%	> 7 ppb	83%	88%	89%	86%
Arora 2006 (76)	172 adults $FeNO_{50}$	80%	>17 ppb	63%	59%	86%	28%
Fortuna 2007 (77)	50 adults $FeNO_{50}$	44%	> 20 ppb	77%	64%	62%	78%
Meidinger 2007 (78)	62 adults	56%	47 ppb	72%	76%		
Menzies 2007 (79)	151 aduls (63% on ICS) $FeNO_{50}$	67%	>13 ppb	83%	27%	NR	NR

false positive results in patients presenting with viral respiratory tract infection (73).

Measuring FeNO in preschool children using modifications of the standard online technique to offline tidal breathing methods without flow control are less sensitive in discriminating between asthmatic and nonasthmatic subjects (15, 80). As a result, the overall diagnostic usefulness of FeNO measurements in young children is less well defined (29, 72). In an unselected population of preschool children too young to perform spirometric tests, FeNO performed poorly in distinguishing between asthma and non-asthma (81). In the differential diagnosis of non-specific respiratory symptoms in children, the same issues are encountered (82, 83). During an acute episode of wheezing, FeNO was significantly higher in those with recurrent wheeze than in controls, while in children with their first episode of wheezing FeNO levels did not differ from normal children (82). Treating infants and young children with recurrent wheeze and increased FeNO levels with corticosteroids improved symptoms and reduced FeNO to normal or near normal values (82, 84).

An important drawback to the implementation of exhaled NO as a diagnostic test for asthma is the large number of confounding factors which might influence the FeNO level (15). Active smoking results in a significant reduction of the FeNO levels, both in normal subjects as well as in patients with asthma (15). Administration of inhaled steroids also results in a significant reduction of the FeNO levels in patients with asthma (58-64). It is also important to take into account that patients may fulfill conventional clinical criteria for the diagnosis of asthma and yet FeNO levels will be normal, especially in non-atopic subjects. Normal values do not exclude the diagnosis of asthma and in these patients, measuring AHR may reveal a positive clinically relevant result. FeNO measurements thus complement AHR both in population surveys (85) as in patients presenting with symptoms suggestive of asthma (71, 73, 74). On the other hand, eosinophilic bronchitis and cough variant asthma, which are also characterized by eosinophilic airway inflammation, similarly present with increased FeNO levels, and a positive response to a trial of steroid treatment is likely (41, 86). For other diagnoses such as vocal cord dysfunction presenting as "asthma", which clinicians often treat empirically with steroids with little meaningful benefit (87), it is just as helpful to have a low normal FeNO level indicating a condition which is not characterised by eosinophilic airway inflammation and, in turn, is less likely to respond to steroids.

Although more work is required to confirm optimum cut points, it is possible to offer general guidelines for interpreting FeNO levels.

Low FeNO levels (<20ppb if 12 years or younger; <25ppb for adults) are unlikely to be associated with eosinophilic airway inflammation, and in symptomatic patients clinicians should consider non-eosinophilic pathologies such as neutrophilic asthma, vocal cord dysfunction, rhinosinusitis, anxiety/hyperventilation, gastro-oesophageal reflux, etc.

High FeNO (>50 ppb) in an individual with an appropriate symptom history is compatible with a diagnosis of atopic asthma. Intermediate FeNO levels (25-50 ppb) may reflect mild eosinophilic airway inflammation but interpretation should be based on clinical presentation.

FeNO in the Management of Asthma

There are two areas in which FeNO may provide helpful information in the management of asthma. 1. The prognostic significance of FeNO as predictor of asthma exacerbations or when considering reduction or withdrawal of ICS therapy. 2. The role of FENO in optimizing corticosteroid therapy in asthma.

Prognostic significance of FeNO by predicting exacerbations

Although FeNO and eosinophilic inflammation do not relate closely to markers of asthma control (i.e. symptoms and disordered airway function), they do relate somewhat to asthma exacerbations (88, 89) implying that assessment of inflammation in the detection of exacerbations provides information about asthma not available through other means.

Using a steroid reduction protocol to induce an exacerbation, Jatakanon et al., (88) demonstrated changes in sputum eosinophils to be superior to FeNO measurements in predicting loss of asthma control. In the study by Jones et al. (89), FeNO ranked similar to sputum eosinophils and measurements of airway hyperreponsiveness to hypertonic saline in predicting loss of asthma control after withdrawal of ICS therapy. An increase in FeNO of >60% after ICS withdrawal provided a sensitivity of only 50% but a positive predictive value of 83% for loss of control. These 2 studies (88, 89) used a steroid withdrawal protocol to mimic a clinical exacerbation and are not necessarily ideal. In a much smaller study, Harkin et al. reported that, in routine practice, increased levels of FeNO predicted an exacerbation within the following 2 weeks (90). In adults with mild stable asthma, Gelb et al. could demonstrate that a baseline FeNO of >29 ppb predicted relapse (sensitivity 59% and specificity 82%) over a follow-up period of 18 months. Combining FeNO results with FEV_1 results improved the sensitivity: none of the patents with FeNO <28 ppb and FEV_1 >76% experienced a relapse (91). Overall, the prognostic value of FeNO measurements to predict deteriorating asthma appears thus limited.

Prognostic significance of FeNO by predicting successful reduction of steroids

A number of studies evaluated whether markers of airway inflammation can be used to predict the successful reduction or withdrawal of ICS treatment.

In a paediatric dose-reduction study, a normal FeNO reading was able to predict successful ICS dose reduction, and raised FeNO predicted loss of control even in children who were initially clinically stable (92). FeNO at a cut-point of 22 ppb or less provided a negative predictive value of 92% for asthma relapse after ICS withdrawal. In another study by Pijnenburg et al. (93), FeNO levels measured at 2 and 4 weeks following steroid withdrawal were highly predictive of relapse in asthma, with an optimum cut-point of 49 ppb above which asthma relapse was likely with a sensitivity of 71% and specificity of 93%. In another randomized study, ICS were discontinued in eight stable asthmatics and continued in 10 (94). The findings in this small study were that FeNO and peripheral blood eosinophils increased in the ICS withdrawal group where three children relapsed, in contrast with none in the control arm.

In contrast to these data and while sputum eosinophils >0.8% prior to steroid withdrawal were shown to predict asthma relapse, no significant prognostic value could be derived from FeNO measurements in studies by Leuppi et al. (95) and Deykin et al. (96). However, in the former study, baseline rather than sequential FeNO values were used in the calculations and in the latter study, the number of patients in whom FeNO values were obtained was limited, which makes it difficult to draw valid conclusions from these studies.

Taken together, sputum eosinophil counts probably offer superior prognostic accuracy when evaluating whether or not patients require ongoing ICS treatment. In circumstances where induced sputum cannot be obtained, a high FeNO level (>50 ppb) is likely to predict asthma relapse and a low FeNO level (<20 ppb in children, <25 ppb in adults) is likely to predict asthma stability if measured at least 4 weeks after ICS treatment is reduced/withdrawn in a currently asymptomatic patient. The outcome in those with an intermediate result (FeNO 20-50 ppb) is less certain.

FeNO measurements are made in clinic at regular intervals on an outpatient basis, but it might be that with portable home FeNO monitoring, daily measurements of FeNO may prove to be beneficial in anticipating deteriorating asthma (97).

FeNO as a guide to adjustment of corticosteroid therapy

Traditionally, adjustment of asthma therapy with ICS has been based on current asthma control and physiological testing such as spirometry and peak flows. However, there is a poor association between these markers and the degree of underlying airway inflammation, which is the prime target for ICS therapy (5, 9, 10). Titrating ICS against the level of airway inflammation, as determined by sputum eosinophils, has been shown to significantly reduce asthma exacerbations and hospital admissions compared with the conventional approach (9, 10).

This has prompted a number of studies (56, 60, 97-99) to assess whether FeNO, as a surrogate marker of eosinophilic airway inflammation, can improve outcomes using ICS therapy in asthma (Table 3). The first report by Smith et al. (97), revealed that ICS doses could be reduced by over 40% when using only FeNO as a guide, compared to the conventional clinical approach, without compromising asthma control and with a non-significant difference in exacerbation rate between the two groups. Pijnenburg et al. (60) reported that, in a group of asthmatic children, titrating ICS dose to both FeNO levels and symptoms as compared with a clinical approach, resulted in reduced levels of airway inflammation and a significant reduction in the severity of airway hyperresponsiveness. The FeNO group showed a concomitant (but non-significant) reduction in exacerbations requiring oral prednisone. Cumulative ICS use did not differ between the FeNO and symptoms based treated groups and FeNO increased in the symptom group. A third study allocated 25 children to a control group, where

TABLE 3

STUDIES EVALUATING FeNO TO GUIDE ASTHMA THERAPY

Study design	Dose adjustment ICS based on	Main results
Smith 2005 (98) n=94 12-75 y 13% on LABA	$FeNO_{250}$ (>15 ppb) vs. asthma control	Non-singinficant reduction in exacerbations in FeNO group Significant reduction in cumulative steroid dose in FeNO group
Pijnenburg 2005 (99) n=85 6-18 y no LABA	$FeNO_{50}$ (≥30 ppb) and symptoms vs. symptoms only	AHR improved in FeNO group NS reduction in exacerbations Increased dose of ICS in both groups
Fritsch 2005 (100) n=49 children no LABA	$FeNO_{50}$ (> 20 ppb) and symptoms/FEV_1 vs. symptoms/FEV_1 only	No significant outcome differences with FeNO based strategy Improved MMEF in FeNO group
Shaw 2007 (101) n=119 >18 y 52 wks 14% on LABA	$FeNO_{50}$ (> 26 ppb) and ACQ (>1.57) vs. ACQ (> 1.57) only	No significant outcome differences achieved with FeNO based strategy. Reduced ICS dose and reduced FeNO in FeNO group.
Szefler 2008 (102) n=546 12-20 y 46wks LABA acc. to AC	$FeNO_{50}$ (4 levels) and AC (4 levels) vs. AC (4 levels)	No significant change in asthma control or exacerbations ICS dose higher in FeNO group

treatment was based on symptoms, beta-agonist use and lung function, and 25 children to a FeNO group where, in addition, FeNO influenced treatment decisions (98). After 5 visits in 6 months children in the FeNO group had better MEF50%, although at the cost of higher ICS doses. A cut-off point of 22.9 ppb had the best predictive value for exacerbations in the next 6 weeks. Shaw et al. (56) reported that using FeNO measurements to titrate ICS dose did not improve outcomes when compared to a clinical algorithm, which was confirmed in a large randomized trial at ten centers in the USA in patients, aged 12-20 years, who had persistent asthma (99). During the 46-week treatment period, the mean number of days with asthma symptoms did not differ between standard treatment, based on asthma guidelines or standard treatment modified on the basis of measurements of FeNO. Other symptoms, pulmonary function, and asthma exacerbations did not differ either and patients in the NO monitoring group received higher doses of inhaled corticosteroids (99).

These studies do not show that the addition of FeNO as an indicator of airway inflammation to conventional asthma management resulted in clinically important improvements in symptomatic asthma control.

What are the pitfalls in these studies? First, all used a single cut-off level for FeNO to prompt either an increase or a decrease in ICS dose. Clearly this is an area that requires further investigation. Although single cut-points are appropriate in 'back-titration' studies with high ICS starting doses, two cut-points defining three management choices (increase, no change or decrease in dose) may be more effective as algorithm for the management of asthma.

Second, the "one size fits all" approach used may not be appropriate in regular clinical practice. An alternative method of dealing with FeNO in individual patients might be using "personal best values" as baseline or individual target FeNO levels.

Third, substantially different criteria to guide ICS dose adjustment were applied. The cut-point for FeNO being different between the different dose-adjustment strategy studies in addition to variations in the dose titration algorithms in these studies might explain the apparently different outcomes. Overall the results of these intervention studies are negative, but further work is required.

An important issue that has emerged is whether FeNO should be used for both upwards as well as downward titration of inhaled steroids. These studies (56, 60, 97-99) have highlighted that unnecessarily high doses of ICS may be safely reduced in those patients in whom FeNO levels are consistently low (<25 ppb). This was not necessarily achievable in the conventional strategy groups, where ongoing asthma symptoms (which are not necessarily due to airway inflammation) would prevent a reduction in ICS dose. By providing objective evidence of airway inflammation, FeNO can provide reassurance that successful dose reduction is likely in these patients (100). On the other hand, it is not clear if a high FeNO (>50 ppb), especially in an asymptomatic patient, should prompt an increase in ICS dose. In some cases, it is not possible to normalize FeNO levels in patients with persistently high FeNO levels despite maximum doses of ICS therapy (57). Therefore, until further studies are carried out, the current role for FeNO would seem to be to facilitate reduction of ICS doses in patients with low FeNO levels (<25ppb). Only if asthma is poorly controlled and issues of patient compliance and inhaler technique have been addressed should a high FeNO prompt an increase in ICS dose. An alternative approach could consist of measuring FeNO levels when asthma is stable and to use this value as the baseline reference point for individual patients against which subsequent measurements are weighed (53).

FeNO in patients with severe asthma

The value of measuring FeNO in patients with severe asthma and the way these values should be incorporated in the clinical work-up and guidance of these patients is not yet clear. Subgroups of patients with severe asthma who are on high doses of inhaled or oral corticosteroid treatment still have high FeNO levels (101, 102). This might be due to relative steroid resistance, persistent systemic eosinophilic inflammation or persistence of inflammation in regions of the airways which are insufficiently reached by inhaled steroids such as the sinonasal region or the peripheral airways (101, 103).

In a longitudinal study by Van Veen et al. in 136 patients with severe asthma the predictive value of inflammatory markers (exhaled nitric oxide, blood and sputum eosinophils and bronchial hyperresponsiveness) on the decline in FEV_1 over 5 years was investigated (104). The results of this study showed that patients with high FeNO levels ($\geq$20ppb) and a normal lung function at baseline ($FEV_1 \geq 80\%$ predicted) had a 90% risk of having an accelerated decline in lung function ($\geq$25 ml/year) as compared to 30% in those with FeNO levels <20 ppb at baseline. The study demonstrates that FeNO measurements can help to identify patients with severe asthma who are at risk of developing persistent airflow limitation and who might benefit from novel asthma treatment or individualized treatment strategies (53, 105).

Conclusion

Asthma remains a prevalent disease with significant morbidity and mortality. Traditional measures of asthma control do not necessarily reflect ongoing airways inflammation and may not provide optimal assessment for guiding therapy. FeNO is a potential surrogate for airways inflammation that is easy to obtain and comfortable for the patient. The clinical utility of routinely measuring FeNO remains unclear, although current studies are encouraging that it parallels ongoing eosinophilic inflammation in a wide range of patients. Additional prospective randomized studies utilizing clinical outcomes as primary endpoints are necessary to evaluate the utility of FeNO. Widespread clinical use of exhaled NO as a diagnostic test will certainly be more practicable since technological advances resulted in the development of smaller and cheaper analysers, which can be used in an out-hospital setting.

References

1. Djukanovic R, Roche WR, Wilson JW, Beasley CR, Twentyman OP, Howarth RH, et al. Mucosal inflammation in asthma. Am Rev Respir Dis1990 Aug; 142(2):434-57.
2. Barnes PJ. Pathophysiology of asthma. Br J Clin Pharmacol 1996 Jul; 42(1):3-10.
3. National Asthma Education and Prevention Program. Expert Panel Report 2: Guidelines for the diagnosis and management of asthma. Publication No. 97-4051. 1997.
4. Teeter JG, Bleecker ER. Relationship between airway obstruction and respiratory symptoms in adult asthmatics. Chest 1998 Feb;113(2):272-7.
5. Sont JK, Han J, van Krieken JM, Evertse CE, Hooijer R, Willems LN, et al. Relationship between the inflammatory infiltrate in bronchial biopsy specimens and clinical severity of asthma in patients treated with inhaled steroids. Thorax 1996 May; 51(5): 496-502.
6. Goldstein MF, Veza BA, Dunsky EH, Dvorin DJ, Belecanech GA, Haralabatos IC. Comparisons of peak diurnal expiratory flow variation, post-bronchodilator FEV(1) responses, and methacholine inhalation challenges in the evaluation of suspected asthma. Chest 2001 Apr;119(4):1001-10.
7. Ulrik CS, Backer V. Nonreversible airflow obstruction in life-long non-smokers with moderate to severe asthma. Eur Respir J1999 Oct;14(4): 892-6.
8. Green RH, Brightling CE, McKenna S, Hargadon B, Parker D, Bradding P, et al. Asthma exacerbations and sputum eosinophil counts: a randomised controlled trial. Lancet 2002 Nov 30; 360(9347):1715-21.
9. Jayaram L, Pizzichini MM, Cook RJ, Boulet LP, Lemiere C, Pizzichini E, et al. Determining asthma treatment by monitoring sputum cell counts: effect on exacerbations. Eur Respir J2006 Mar;27(3):483-94.
10. Gustafsson LE, Leone AM, Persson MG, Wiklund NP, Moncada S. Endogenous nitric oxide is present in the exhaled air of rabbits, guinea pigs and humans. Biochem Biophys Res Commun1991 Dec 16;181(2):852-7.
11. Alving K, Weitzberg E, Lundberg JM. Increased amount of nitric oxide in

exhaled air of asthmatics. Eur Respir J1993 Oct;6(9):1368-70.

12. Kharitonov SA, Yates D, Robbins RA, Logan-Sinclair R, Shinebourne EA, Barnes PJ. Increased nitric oxide in exhaled air of asthmatic patients. Lancet1994 Jan 15;343(8890):133-5.

13. Dupont LJ, Rochette F, Demedts MG, Verleden GM. Exhaled nitric oxide correlates with airway hyperresponsiveness in steroid-naive patients with mild asthma. Am J Respir Crit Care Med1998 Mar;157(3 Pt 1):894-8.

14. Kharitonov SA, Barnes PJ. Exhaled markers of pulmonary disease. Am J Respir Crit Care Med 2001 Jun;163 (7): 1693-722.

15. ATS/ERS recommendations for standardized procedures for the online and offline measurement of exhaled lower respiratory nitric oxide and nasal nitric oxide, 2005. Am J Respir Crit Care Med2005 Apr 15;171(8):912-30.

16. Hemmingsson T, Linnarsson D, Gambert R. Novel hand-held device for exhaled nitric oxide-analysis in research and clinical applications. J Clin Monit Comput2004 Dec;18(5-6):379-87.

17. Kharitonov SA, Gonio F, Kelly C, Meah S, Barnes PJ. Reproducibility of exhaled nitric oxide measurements in healthy and asthmatic adults and children. Eur Respir J2003 Mar;21(3):433-8.

18. ElHalawani SM, Ly NT, Mahon RT, Amundson DE. Exhaled nitric oxide as a predictor of exercise-induced bronchoconstriction. Chest 2003 Aug;124 (2):639-43.

19. De Winter-de Groot KM, Van der Ent CK, Prins I, Tersmette JM, Uiterwaal CS. Exhaled nitric oxide: the missing link between asthma and obesity? J Allergy Clin Immunol 2005 Feb; 115 (2): 419-20.

20. Haight RR, Gordon RL, Brooks SM. The effects of age on exhaled breath nitric oxide levels. Lung 2006 Mar-Apr;184(2):113-9.

21. Olivieri M, Talamini G, Corradi M, Perbellini L, Mutti A, Tantucci C, et al. Reference values for exhaled nitric oxide (reveno) study. Respir Res 2006;7:94.

22. Olin AC, Rosengren A, Thelle DS, Lissner L, Bake B, Toren K. Height, age, and atopy are associated with fraction of exhaled nitric oxide in a large adult general population sample. Chest 2006 Nov;130(5):1319-25.

23. Travers J, Marsh S, Aldington S, Williams M, Shirtcliffe P, Pritchard A, et al. Reference ranges for exhaled nitric oxide derived from a random community survey of adults. Am J Respir Crit Care Med2007 Aug 1;176(3):238-42.

24. Olin AC, Bake B, Toren K. Fraction of exhaled nitric oxide at 50 mL/s: reference values for adult lifelong never-smokers. Chest 2007 Jun;131(6): 1852-6.

25. Taylor DR, Mandhane P, Greene JM, Hancox RJ, Filsell S, McLachlan CR, et al. Factors affecting exhaled nitric oxide measurements: the effect of sex. Respir Res 2007;8:82.

26. Maestrelli P, Ferrazzoni S, Visentin A, Marian E, Dal Borgo D, Accordino R, et al. Measurement of exhaled nitric oxide in healthy adults. Sarcoidosis Vasc Diffuse Lung Dis 2007 Mar; 24(1):65-9.

27. Scollo M, Zanconato S, Ongaro R, Zaramella C, Zacchello F, Baraldi E. Exhaled nitric oxide and exercise-in-

duced bronchoconstriction in asthmatic children. Am J Respir Crit Care Med 2000 Mar;161(3 Pt 1):1047-50.

28. Jobsis Q, Schellekens SL, Kroesbergen A, Hop WC, de Jongste JC. Offline sampling of exhaled air for nitric oxide measurement in children: methodological aspects. Eur Respir J 2001 May;17(5):898-903.

29. Malmberg LP, Pelkonen AS, Haahtela T, Turpeinen M. Exhaled nitric oxide rather than lung function distinguishes preschool children with probable asthma. Thorax 2003 Jun;58(6):494-9.

30. Santamaria F, Montella S, De Stefano S, Sperli F, Barbarano F, Valerio G. Relationship between exhaled nitric oxide and body mass index in children and adolescents. J Allergy Clin Immunol2005 Nov;116(5):1163-4; author reply 4-5.

31. Buchvald F, Baraldi E, Carraro S, Gaston B, De Jongste J, Pijnenburg MW, et al. Measurements of exhaled nitric oxide in healthy subjects age 4 to 17 years. J Allergy Clin Immunol 2005 Jun;115(6):1130-6.

32. Malmberg LP, Petays T, Haahtela T, Laatikainen T, Jousilahti P, Vartiainen E, et al. Exhaled nitric oxide in healthy nonatopic school-age children: determinants and height-adjusted reference values. Pediatr Pulmonol 2006 Jul; 41(7): 635-42.

33. Ricciardolo FL, Sterk PJ, Gaston B, Folkerts G. Nitric oxide in health and disease of the respiratory system. Physiol Rev2004 Jul;84(3):731-65.

34. Hamid Q, Springall DR, Riveros-Moreno V, Chanez P, Howarth P, Redington A, et al. Induction of nitric oxide synthase in asthma. Lancet 1993 Dec 18-25;342(8886-8887):1510-3.

35. Lane C, Knight D, Burgess S, Franklin P, Horak F, Legg J, et al. Epithelial inducible nitric oxide synthase activity is the major determinant of nitric oxide concentration in exhaled breath. Thorax 2004 Sep;59(9):757-60.

36. Brindicci C, Ito K, Barnes PJ, Kharitonov SA. Effect of an inducible nitric oxide synthase inhibitor on differential flow-exhaled nitric oxide in asthmatic patients and healthy volunteers. Chest 2007 Aug;132(2):581-8.

37. Silkoff PE, Sylvester JT, Zamel N, Permutt S. Airway nitric oxide diffusion in asthma: Role in pulmonary function and bronchial responsiveness. Am J Respir Crit Care Med 2000 Apr;161 (4 Pt 1): 1218-28.

38. Shin HW, Shelley DA, Henderson EM, Fitzpatrick A, Gaston B, George SC. Airway nitric oxide release is reduced after PBS inhalation in asthma. J Appl Physiol 2007 Mar;102(3):1028-33.

39. Jatakanon A, Lim S, Kharitonov SA, Chung KF, Barnes PJ. Correlation between exhaled nitric oxide, sputum eosinophils, and methacholine responsiveness in patients with mild asthma. Thorax 1998 Feb;53(2):91-5.

40. Berlyne GS, Parameswaran K, Kamada D, Efthimiadis A, Hargreave FE. A comparison of exhaled nitric oxide and induced sputum as markers of airway inflammation. J Allergy Clin Immunol 2000 Oct;106(4):638-44.

41. Brightling CE, Symon FA, Birring SS, Bradding P, Wardlaw AJ, Pavord ID. Comparison of airway immunopathology of eosinophilic bronchitis and asthma. Thorax 2003 Jun;58(6):528-32.

42. Tsujino I, Nishimura M, Kamachi A, Makita H, Munakata M, Miyamoto K,

et al. Exhaled nitric oxide--is it really a good marker of airway inflammation in bronchial asthma? Respiration 2000; 67(6): 645-51.

43. Piacentini GL, Bodini A, Costella S, Vicentini L, Mazzi P, Sperandio S, et al. Exhaled nitric oxide and sputum eosinophil markers of inflammation in asthmatic children. Eur Respir J 1999 Jun;13(6):1386-90.

44. Berry MA, Shaw DE, Green RH, Brightling CE, Wardlaw AJ, Pavord ID. The use of exhaled nitric oxide concentration to identify eosinophilic airway inflammation: an observational study in adults with asthma. Clin Exp Allergy 2005 Sep;35(9):1175-9.

45. Pontin J, Blaylock MG, Walsh GM, Turner SW. Sputum eosinophil apoptotic rate is positively correlated to exhaled nitric oxide in children. Pediatr Pulmonol 2008 Nov;43(11):1130-4.

46. Warke TJ, Fitch PS, Brown V, Taylor R, Lyons JD, Ennis M, et al. Exhaled nitric oxide correlates with airway eosinophils in childhood asthma. Thorax 2002 May;57(5):383-7.

47. Shirai T, Inui N, Suda T, Chida K. Correlation between peripheral blood T-cell profiles and airway inflammation in atopic asthma. J Allergy Clin Immunol 2006 Sep;118(3):622-6.

48. van den Toorn LM, Overbeek SE, de Jongste JC, Leman K, Hoogsteden HC, Prins JB. Airway inflammation is present during clinical remission of atopic asthma. Am J Respir Crit Care Med 2001 Dec 1;164(11):2107-13.

49. Payne DN, Adcock IM, Wilson NM, Oates T, Scallan M, Bush A. Relationship between exhaled nitric oxide and mucosal eosinophilic inflammation in children with difficult asthma, after treatment with oral prednisolone. Am J Respir Crit Care Med 2001 Oct 15; 164(8 Pt 1):1376-81.

50. Strunk RC, Szefler SJ, Phillips BR, Zeiger RS, Chinchilli VM, Larsen G, et al. Relationship of exhaled nitric oxide to clinical and inflammatory markers of persistent asthma in children. J Allergy Clin Immunol 2003 Nov;112(5): 883-92.

51. Silvestri M, Sabatini F, Sale R, Defilippi AC, Fregonese L, Battistini E, et al. Correlations between exhaled nitric oxide levels, blood eosinophilia, and airway obstruction reversibility in childhood asthma are detectable only in atopic individuals. Pediatr Pulmonol 2003 May;35(5):358-63.

52. Mattes J, Storm van's Gravesande K, Reining U, Alving K, Ihorst G, Henschen M, et al. NO in exhaled air is correlated with markers of eosinophilic airway inflammation in corticosteroid-dependent childhood asthma. Eur Respir J 1999 Jun;13(6): 1391-5.

53. Taylor DR, Pijnenburg MW, Smith AD, De Jongste JC. Exhaled nitric oxide measurements: clinical application and interpretation. Thorax 2006 Sep;61(9): 817-27.

54. Ketai L, Harkins M, Fiato KL, Iwamoto GK. Exhaled nitric oxide and bronchial wall thickening in asthmatics during and after acute exacerbation: evidence of bronchial wall remodeling. J Asthma 2005 Oct;42(8):667-71.

55. Nishio K, Odajima H, Motomura C, Nakao F, Nishima S. Effect of inhaled steroid therapy on exhaled nitric oxide and bronchial responsiveness in children with asthma. J Asthma 2006 Dec;43(10):739-43.

56. Shaw DE, Berry MA, Thomas M, Green RH, Brightling CE, Wardlaw AJ, et al. The use of exhaled nitric oxide to guide asthma management: a randomized controlled trial. Am J Respir Crit Care Med2007 Aug 1;176(3):231-7.

57. Pijnenburg MW, Bakker EM, Lever S, Hop WC, De Jongste JC. High fractional concentration of nitric oxide in exhaled air despite steroid treatment in asthmatic children. Clin Exp Allergy 2005 Jul;35(7):920-5.

58. Kharitonov SA, Yates DH, Barnes PJ. Inhaled glucocorticoids decrease nitric oxide in exhaled air of asthmatic patients. Am J Respir Crit Care Med 1996 Jan;153(1):454-7.

59. Beck-Ripp J, Griese M, Arenz S, Koring C, Pasqualoni B, Bufler P. Changes of exhaled nitric oxide during steroid treatment of childhood asthma. Eur Respir J2002 Jun;19(6): 1015-9.

60. Pijnenburg MW, Bakker EM, Hop WC, De Jongste JC. Titrating steroids on exhaled nitric oxide in children with asthma: a randomized controlled trial. Am J Respir Crit Care Med 2005 Oct 1;172(7):831-6.

61. Jatakanon A, Kharitonov S, Lim S, Barnes PJ. Effect of differing doses of inhaled budesonide on markers of airway inflammation in patients with mild asthma. Thorax 1999 Feb;54(2):108-14.

62. Silkoff PE, McClean P, Spino M, Erlich L, Slutsky AS, Zamel N. Dose-response relationship and reproducibility of the fall in exhaled nitric oxide after inhaled beclomethasone dipropionate therapy in asthma patients. Chest 2001 May;119(5):1322-8.

63. Kharitonov SA, Donnelly LE, Montuschi P, Corradi M, Collins JV, Barnes PJ. Dose-dependent onset and cessation of action of inhaled budesonide on exhaled nitric oxide and symptoms in mild asthma. Thorax 2002 Oct;57(10):889-96.

64. Jones SL, Herbison P, Cowan JO, Flannery EM, Hancox RJ, McLachlan CR, et al. Exhaled NO and assessment of anti-inflammatory effects of inhaled steroid: dose-response relationship. Eur Respir J 2002 Sep;20(3):601-8.

65. Currie GP, Lee DK, Haggart K, Bates CE, Lipworth BJ. Effects of montelukast on surrogate inflammatory markers in corticosteroid-treated patients with asthma. Am J Respir Crit Care Med 2003 May 1;167(9):1232-8.

66. Ghiro L, Zanconato S, Rampon O, Piovan V, Pasquale MF, Baraldi E. Effect of montelukast added to inhaled corticosteroids on fractional exhaled nitric oxide in asthmatic children. Eur Respir J 2002 Sep;20(3):630-4.

67. Strauch E, Moske O, Thoma S, Storm Van's Gravesande K, Ihorst G, Brandis M, et al. A randomized controlled trial on the effect of montelukast on sputum eosinophil cationic protein in children with corticosteroid-dependent asthma. Pediatr Res 2003 Aug;54(2): 198-203.

68. Smith AD, Cowan JO, Brassett KP, Filsell S, McLachlan C, Monti-Sheehan G, et al. Exhaled nitric oxide: a predictor of steroid response. Am J Respir Crit Care Med 2005 Aug 15;172(4): 453-9.

69. Little SA, Chalmers GW, MacLeod KJ, McSharry C, Thomson NC. Non-invasive markers of airway inflammation as predictors of oral steroid respon-

siveness in asthma. Thorax 2000 Mar; 55(3):232-4.

70. Szefler SJ, Phillips BR, Martinez FD, Chinchilli VM, Lemanske RF, Strunk RC, et al. Characterization of within-subject responses to fluticasone and montelukast in childhood asthma. J Allergy Clin Immunol 2005 Feb;115 (2): 233-42.

71. Dupont LJ, Demedts MG, Verleden GM. Prospective evaluation of the validity of exhaled nitric oxide for the diagnosis of asthma. Chest 2003 Mar;123(3):751-6.

72. Narang I, Ersu R, Wilson NM, Bush A. Nitric oxide in chronic airway inflammation in children: diagnostic use and pathophysiological significance. Thorax 2002 Jul;57(7):586-9.

73. Smith AD, Cowan JO, Filsell S, McLachlan C, Monti-Sheehan G, Jackson P, et al. Diagnosing asthma: comparisons between exhaled nitric oxide measurements and conventional tests. Am J Respir Crit Care Med 2004 Feb 15;169(4):473-8.

74. Berkman N, Avital A, Breuer R, Bardach E, Springer C, Godfrey S. Exhaled nitric oxide in the diagnosis of asthma: comparison with bronchial provocation tests. Thorax 2005 May; 60(5):383-8.

75. Arora R, Thornblade CE, Dauby PA, Flanagan JW, Bush AC, Hagan LL. Exhaled nitric oxide levels in military recruits with new onset asthma. Allergy Asthma Proc 2006 Nov-Dec;27(6): 493-8.

76. Fortuna AM, Feixas T, Gonzalez M, Casan P. Diagnostic utility of inflammatory biomarkers in asthma: exhaled nitric oxide and induced sputum eosinophil count. Respir Med 2007 Nov;101(11):2416-21.

77. Miedinger D, Chhajed PN, Tamm M, Stolz D, Surber C, Leuppi JD. Diagnostic tests for asthma in firefighters. Chest 2007 Jun;131(6):1760-7.

78. Menzies D, Jackson C, Mistry C, Houston R, Lipworth BJ. Symptoms, spirometry, exhaled nitric oxide, and asthma exacerbations in clinical practice. Ann Allergy Asthma Immunol 2008 Sep;101(3):248-55.

79. Smith AD, Taylor DR. Is exhaled nitric oxide measurement a useful clinical test in asthma? Curr Opin Allergy Clin Immunol 2005 Feb;5(1):49-56.

80. Baraldi E, de Jongste JC. Measurement of exhaled nitric oxide in children, 2001. Eur Respir J 2002 Jul;20 (1):223-37.

81. Brussee JE, Smit HA, Kerkhof M, Koopman LP, Wijga AH, Postma DS, et al. Exhaled nitric oxide in 4-year-old children: relationship with asthma and atopy. Eur Respir J2005 Mar;25(3): 455-61.

82. Baraldi E, Dario C, Ongaro R, Scollo M, Azzolin NM, Panza N, et al. Exhaled nitric oxide concentrations during treatment of wheezing exacerbation in infants and young children. Am J Respir Crit Care Med 1999 Apr;159(4 Pt 1):1284-8.

83. Ratjen F, Kavuk I, Gartig S, Wiesemann HG, Grasemann H. Airway nitric oxide in infants with acute wheezy bronchitis. Pediatr Allergy Immunol 2000 Nov;11(4):230-5.

84. Moeller A, Franklin P, Hall GL, Turner S, Straub D, Wildhaber JH, et al. Inhaled fluticasone dipropionate decreases levels of nitric oxide in recurrenty wheezy infants. Pediatr Pulmonol 2004 Sep;38(3):250-5.

85. Henriksen AH, Lingaas-Holmen T,

Sue-Chu M, Bjermer L. Combined use of exhaled nitric oxide and airway hyperresponsiveness in characterizing asthma in a large population survey. Eur Respir J 2000 May;15(5):849-55.

86. Chatkin JM, Ansarin K, Silkoff PE, McClean P, Gutierrez C, Zamel N, et al. Exhaled nitric oxide as a noninvasive assessment of chronic cough. Am J Respir Crit Care Med 1999 Jun; 159(6):1810-3.

87. Mikita JA, Mikita CP. Vocal cord dysfunction. Allergy Asthma Proc2006 Jul-Aug; 27(4):411-4.

88. Jatakanon A, Lim S, Barnes PJ. Changes in sputum eosinophils predict loss of asthma control. Am J Respir Crit Care Med 2000 Jan;161(1):64-72.

89. Jones SL, Kittelson J, Cowan JO, Flannery EM, Hancox RJ, McLachlan CR, et al. The predictive value of exhaled nitric oxide measurements in assessing changes in asthma control. Am J Respir Crit Care Med 2001 Sep 1;164(5):738-43.

90. Harkins MS, Fiato KL, Iwamoto GK. Exhaled nitric oxide predicts asthma exacerbation. J Asthma 2004 Jun;41 (4):471-6.

91. Gelb AF, Flynn Taylor C, Shinar CM, Gutierrez C, Zamel N. Role of spirometry and exhaled nitric oxide to predict exacerbations in treated asthmatics. Chest 2006 Jun;129(6):1492-9.

92. Zacharasiewicz A, Wilson N, Lex C, Erin EM, Li AM, Hansel T, et al. Clinical use of noninvasive measurements of airway inflammation in steroid reduction in children. Am J Respir Crit Care Med 2005 May 15;171(10):1077-82.

93. Pijnenburg MW, Hofhuis W, Hop WC, De Jongste JC. Exhaled nitric oxide predicts asthma relapse in children with clinical asthma remission. Thorax 2005 Mar;60(3):215-8.

94. Lonnkvist K, Anderson M, Hedlin G, Svartengren M. Exhaled NO and eosinophil markers in blood, nasal lavage and sputum in children with asthma after withdrawal of budesonide. Pediatr Allergy Immunol 2004 Aug;15(4):351-8.

95. Leuppi JD, Salome CM, Jenkins CR, Anderson SD, Xuan W, Marks GB, et al. Predictive markers of asthma exacerbation during stepwise dose reduction of inhaled corticosteroids. Am J Respir Crit Care Med 2001 Feb;163 (2):406-12.

96. Deykin A, Lazarus SC, Fahy JV, Wechsler ME, Boushey HA, Chinchilli VM, et al. Sputum eosinophil counts predict asthma control after discontinuation of inhaled corticosteroids. J Allergy Clin Immunol 2005 Apr;115(4): 720-7.

97. Smith AD, Cowan JO, Brassett KP, Herbison GP, Taylor DR. Use of exhaled nitric oxide measurements to guide treatment in chronic asthma. N Engl J Med 2005 May 26;352(21): 2163-73.

98. Fritsch M, Uxa S, Horak F, Jr., Putschoegl B, Dehlink E, Szepfalusi Z, et al. Exhaled nitric oxide in the management of childhood asthma: a prospective 6-months study. Pediatr Pulmonol 2006 Sep;41(9):855-62.

99. Szefler SJ, Mitchell H, Sorkness CA, Gergen PJ, O'Connor GT, Morgan WJ, et al. Management of asthma based on exhaled nitric oxide in addition to guideline-based treatment for inner-city adolescents and young adults: a randomised controlled trial. Lancet 2008 Sep 20;372(9643):1065-72.

100. Prieto L, Bruno L, Gutierrez V, Uixera S, Perez-Frances C, Lanuza A, et al. Airway responsiveness to adenosine 5'-monophosphate and exhaled nitric oxide measurements: predictive value as markers for reducing the dose of inhaled corticosteroids in asthmatic subjects. Chest 2003 Oct; 124(4):1325-33.

101. Silkoff PE, Lent AM, Busacker AA, Katial RK, Balzar S, Strand M, et al. Exhaled nitric oxide identifies the persistent eosinophilic phenotype in severe refractory asthma. J Allergy Clin Immunol 2005 Dec;116(6): 1249-55.

102. Stirling RG, Kharitonov SA, Campbell D, Robinson DS, Durham SR, Chung KF, et al. Increase in exhaled nitric oxide levels in patients with difficult asthma and correlation with symptoms and disease severity despite treatment with oral and inhaled corticosteroids. Asthma and Allergy Group. Thorax 1998 Dec;53(12): 1030-4.

103. Van Veen I, Ten Brinke A, Gauw SA, et al. Patients with severe asthma and high levels of exhaled nitric oxide despite treatment: a seperate phenotype. Am J Respir Crit Care Med 2006;A577.

104. van Veen IH, Ten Brinke A, Sterk PJ, Sont JK, Gauw SA, Rabe KF, et al. Exhaled nitric oxide predicts lung function decline in difficult-to-treat asthma. Eur Respir J 2008 Aug; 32 (2):344-9.

105. Heaney LG, Robinson DS. Severe asthma treatment: need for characterising patients. Lancet 2005 Mar 12-18;365(9463):974-6.

Exhaled Nitric Oxide in COPD: Application in Clinical Practice

Massimo Corradi • *Petra Gergelova* • *Antonio Mutti*

everal studies have demonstrated that the analysis of the fraction of exhaled nitric oxide (FeNO) is a potentially valuable non-invasive method for the measurement and monitoring of inflammation in the respiratory tract. Like a variety of other lung diseases, chronic obstructive pulmonary disease (COPD) is associated with pulmonary inflammatory response; in particular, there is accumulation of inflammatory mucous exudates in the lumen and infiltration of the small airway wall and lung parenchyma by inflammatory cells. In these patients, there is also a high level of expression of inducible NO synthase (iNOS) in sputum macrophages, alveolar walls, small airway epithelium and vascular smooth muscle. Since COPD is characterised by airway inflammation with enhanced iNOS cellular expression, assessing FeNO in patients with COPD may be

Correspondence

Dr. Massimo Corradi

Department of Clinical Medicine, Nephrology and Health Sciences, University of Parma, Italy

e-mail: massimo.corradi@unipr.it

useful in the evaluation, management and prediction of outcome, similarly to what is done in asthma patients.

Unfortunately, the relatively normal levels of FeNO found in exhaled breath of COPD patients, together with inconsistencies as to whether FeNO is raised in patients with COPD and/or in patients with worsening COPD, have cast doubt on the usefulness of this marker in the assessment of COPD airway inflammation, in marked contrast to asthma, where there is general consensus that FeNO is high, increases during exacerbation, and falls after anti-inflammatory therapy. Therefore, FeNO test in COPD patients is still mainly a research tool.

In this chapter we will revise factors affecting FeNO levels in COPD patients, and some possible, though still uncertain, clinical applications of FeNO in COPD patients.

Factors Affecting FeNO Levels in COPD Patients

Here described are those factors, relatively common in COPD patients, which may affect FeNO values, thus explaining, at least in part, normal FeNO levels observed in clinically stable COPD population.

Cigarette Smoke

Possible explanations for contradictory results in FeNO data obtained in COPD patients could be due to different smoking histories of patients in various studies. Cigarette smoking is a relevant confounding factor for FeNO values, a significant negative correlation between smoking history (pack years) and levels of FeNO having been repeatedly reported (1-3). Smoking COPD patients have FeNO values lower that those observed in ex smokers with COPD (1, 3). Therefore, FeNO usefulness in current smokers with COPD is limited, owing to the opposite effects of tobacco smoke and inflammation. In smoking COPD patients, it is possible that potential increases in NO due to airway inflammation is counteracted by the inhibitory effect of smoking habits on endogenous NO production. Decreased NO levels in smokers are considered to be a result of several factors, including self-regulation of NOS expression by the high NO concentrations in cigarette smoke, inactivation of NO by oxidants in cigarette smoke like superoxide anions, and finally tobacco smoke-induced toxic damage to NO-producing cells (4).

Whatever the mechanism affecting NO levels in smokers is, it does appear to be reversible. The study of Hogman et al. showed that FeNO levels increased after just 1 week of not smoking and had increased again by 8 weeks (5). Despite that, ex smokers with COPD have FeNO values still within normal range or only slightly increased in comparison with controls. In addition, whereas smoking significantly influences FeNO and negatively affects its concentration also in asthma, FeNO levels still distinguish steroid-naive asthmatic smokers from nonasthmatic smokers, and cigarette smoking does not obviate the clinical value of measuring FeNO in asthma among smokers (6). Therefore, it is possible that other factors, not strictly related to tobacco smoke, may explain why FeNO levels are not elevated in ex smoking COPD patients.

Type of Inflammation

It is well known that in asthma chronic airway inflammation is predominantly eosinophilic, whereas in COPD it is mainly characterised by the presence of increased numbers of macrophages and neutrophils (7). NO production has been shown to increase mainly in those clinical conditions (asthma, rhinitis, atopy) associated with eosinophilic airway inflammation, with such a strong correlation that FeNO is now considered a surrogate biomarker of eosinophilic inflammation in the airways (8).

The presence of a mild eosinophilic inflammation in COPD could explain why FeNO values are not increased in COPD, similarly to what observed in cystic fibrosis – another clinical condition implying a predominant non eosinophilic inflammation – in which FeNO levels either normal or even lower than reference values have been reported (9). Consistent with this hypothesis is the typically high increase in FeNO values seen in atopic asthmatic patients, whereas some studies have shown that normal levels of FeNO can be detected in non-atopic asthmatic subjects (10). This observation may be explained by the fact that, in non-atopic asthma, neutrophilic inflammation is sometimes seen instead of the characteristic eosinophilic inflammation observed in atopic asthma, and elevation in FeNO is closely associated with the eosinophilic count but not with neutrophils.

Although the airway inflammation and the accompanying cytokine production are different in COPD from those found in asthma, expression of both constitutive and inducible NOS synthase isoforms have been reported to be elevated in macrophages and other cell lines in

COPD (11). In addition, it has been shown that the percent neutrophils in induced sputum and FeNO are mildly correlated (12), thus suggesting that FeNO is also a marker of neutrophilic inflammation, or may arise from neutrophils, in keeping with reports of iNOS expression in these cells. In addition, increased pro-inflammatory cytokines that are chemoattractants for neutrophils, such as IL-8 and LTB4, might also result in augmented iNOS expression in other cells such as the bronchial epithelium (13).

However, despite the biological rationale that could link neutrophilic inflammation to NO levels, FeNO values of COPD are within the normal range. One possible explanation for this controversy is that FeNO levels are normal in clinically stable COPD patients, not because there is not NO into airways, but because NO is reacting with other free radicals, such as the superoxide anion, produced by activated neutrophils and/or by peroxidase-dependent mechanisms (14) and undergoing denitrification by bacteria (15), thereby decreasing the observed exhaled levels. In patients with cystic fibrosis - a condition with a similar neutrophilic predominance and bacterial colonization as COPD - FeNO is normal or lower than in healthy control subjects.

Pulmonary Arterial Hypertension

It is known that NO is a potent vasodilator and therefore low NO levels into airway in pulmonary hypertension may have a pathological significance (16). Indeed, several studies suggest that pulmonary hypertension may be associated with low FeNO levels. For example, Cremona and colleagues (17) showed that the rate of NO production in patients with primary pulmonary hypertension was 2.85 ± 0.7 nM/min compared with 4.69 ± 0.35 nM/min in healthy individuals. FeNO has been shown to decrease in response to a decrease in pulmonary blood flow and positive correlations between blood flow and NO have been shown (17). Kharitonov and co-workers have shown that concomitant pulmonary hypertension in patients with systemic sclerosis is associated with low FeNO levels, whereas systemic sclerosis without this complication is associated with increased NO (18). In the natural history of COPD, right heart failure leading to increased pulmonary artery pressure is a common finding. Pulmonary artery hypertension, in this scenario, is likely due to a primary hypoxic vasoconstriction associated to the direct toxic effect of tobacco smoke into the intrapulmonary vessels, with abnormal production of substances that control vasoconstriction, vasodilatation, and vascular cell proliferation, ultimately leading to extensive pulmonary artery remodelling (19). Pulmonary hypertension is frequently observed in patients with COPD, especially at advanced stages, and is considered a predictor of worse outcome. NO, produced by endothelial cells, is the central stimulus for releasing and dilating pulmonary arterial vasculature. NO production is oxygen-dependent and lack of NO synthesis, under hypoxic conditions such as COPD, contributes to chronic hypoxic pulmonary vasoconstriction, leading to pulmonary artery hypertension (20). It is now appreciated that NO release is impaired in the pulmonary vasculature of COPD patients, and FeNO levels are significantly reduced in COPD associated with pulmonary hypertension. Authors found that levels of exhaled NO were positively correlated with PaO_2 and negatively correlated with $PaCO_2$, implying diminished NO production in the more hypoxic and more severe COPD (21).

Different Phenotypes of COPD

A further reason for inconsistent findings in FeNO values in COPD may relate to the different phenotypes of patents with COPD, including chronic bronchitis, emphysema and asthmatic bronchitis. In fact, although the current definition of COPD is bases on functional parameters only, clear pathophysiological differences are present among phenotypes. Delen et al. (22) reported that FeNO values in COPD with chronic bronchitis were elevated to levels comparable to those in asthma, in contrast to COPD without bronchitis, in which FeNO levels were normal. This raises the possibility that subsets of COPD with bronchitis, or perhaps eosinophils in sputum, may have different FeNO profiles. For instance, a high prevalence of iNOS-positive cells in alveolar walls in subjects with a more severe COPD is expected, but not in patients with severe emphysema who show a lower percentage of iNOS-positive alveolar macrophages than in those with milder disease (23). On the other hand, no differences in FeNO levels have been found comparing COPD patients with and without emphysema (24).

Finally, patients with alpha-1-antitrypsin (AAT) deficiency show increased FeNO levels compared to COPD patients and controls; FeNO levels have been proved to be related to the reduced concentration of plasma AAT (25). AAT deficiency is under-recognized by clinicians, with long diagnostic delays between patients' first symptom and initial diagnosis. Recent recommendations by official societies encourage testing for AAT deficiency in all symptomatic adults with spirometric evidence of COPD (26).

Heart failure

Heart failure and COPD show an important overlap in signs and symptoms, and elderly patients with dyspnoea face their physicians with the diagnostic challenge to determine whether the patient suffers from heart failure, COPD or both (27). The possibility of the concomitant presence of both conditions is underestimated in clinical practice and research. Since the presence of one syndrome in the presence of the other has important therapeutic and prognostic implications, knowledge about the concomitant prevalence is clinically relevant.

Studies dealing with FeNO values in patients with heart failure suggest that the basal production of endogenous NO in patients with heart failure is impaired and that these levels are more reduced in the most severe [(New York Heart Association (NYHA) classes III-IV)] than the less severe patients (NYHA classes I-II) (28, 29). Chronic pulmonary hypoxia could be an important cause for the reduced FeNO in heart failure patients, possibly through the inhibition of the expression of constitutive NO synthase.

Clinical Applications of FeNO in COPD Patients

Possible clinical applications of FeNO measurements in COPD patients are described bellow.

FeNO in Exacerbation of COPD

Some studies have documented that FeNO levels during COPD exacerbations were higher than those values measured during a clinically stable phase. Maziak et al. found significantly higher FeNO levels in a group of patients with exacerbated or severe COPD than in patients with stable COPD or in smokers without COPD (30). Agusti et al. showed higher NO levels during an exacerbation than in the clinically stable phase of the disease several months later, when NO levels were no longer different from control values of healthy subjects (31). Bhowmik et al. confirmed these findings in a prospective cohort study including 79 outpatients with COPD (32). Paired stable and exacerbation readings could be obtained in 67 exacerbations from 38 patients; FeNO levels during acute exacerbations were significantly higher than during a stable phase of COPD. In particular, NO is increased in exhaled breath from very early stages of the common cold, which often triggers exacerbation in COPD, during winter time. In fact, data showed that the highest FeNO levels were found during October to December.

What is the biological explanation for having increased NO production into airways during exacerbated COPD in contrast to normal NO values observed in stable phases? A possible explanation is the change in degree (more prominent) and, most of all, type of airway inflammation which may occur in exacerbated COPD patients; in particular, an increase in airway eosinophils can be found during COPD exacerbation and could cause enhanced iNOS induction with increased FeNO levels (33, 34). However, it must be underlined that, despite the increase in FeNO levels in exacerbated COPD patients, the increase is much less than those usually observed in asthmatic, even in clinically stable phase. In addition, validation studies aimed at assessing whether FeNO change in COPD may be predictive of COPD exacerbation are still missing; nor clinical studies aimed at demonstrating the use of FeNO in the clinical management of exacerbated COPD patients have been properly performed.

FeNO to predict inhaled corticosteroid response in COPD

It has been suggested that monitoring FeNO might be a useful marker of COPD patients who would benefit from corticosteroid therapy and might have a better bronchodilator response. Papi et al. reported that increased sputum eosinophils and FeNO levels occur in those COPD who showed a partial reversibility of airflow limitation after inhalation of salbutamol (35). International guidelines distinguish between nonreversible and reversible airflow limitation, by stating that reversible airflow limitation results in increased FEV_1 by >12% baseline/predicted and by >200 ml after inhalation of salbutamol (36). COPD patients with partially reversible airflow limitation characterized by an increase in FEV_1 of <12% baseline/predicted but >200 ml after bronchodilator inhalation might have different pathophysiological characteristics than COPD patients with nonreversible airflow limitation. These COPD patients share some pathologic abnormalities which are mainly evident in asthma, in particular intraluminal eosinophilia. As a consequence, FeNO concentrations in COPD might predict partially reversible airflow limitation associated with eosinophilic inflammation of the airways and may help to identify those COPD patients who could respond to pharmacologic treatment. This is in line with the data showing that the use of induced sputum eosinophilic count as the predictor is encouraging (37). In that study, 22 out of 67 patients with COPD whose induced sputum eosinophilic count was in the uppermost tertile, had significant symptomatic as well as physiological improvements with oral prednisone. On the same line, Zietkowski et al. (38) showed that the increase in post-bronchodilator FEV_1 after two months of open label treatment with inhaled budesonide 800 mg/day was strongly correlated with baseline FeNO levels in 19 ex-smoking patients with COPD. Kunisaky et al performed a prospective study in patients who were treated with inhaled corticosteroids for severe COPD; authors showed that low FeNO values at baseline were associated with a lack of significant FEV_1 responses to four weeks of ICS (39). Therefore, the main practical conclusion from these data is that FeNO might be useful in the identification of "*asthmatic features*" in those patients whose COPD has been diagnosed: these COPD patients might benefit from treatment with inhaled corticosteroids. On the contrary, those COPD patients showing normal FeNO values are probably characterized by a low degree of eosinophilic inflammation and, probably, by a lower response to corticosteroid treatment. Nevertheless - at variance with asthma - no correlation between FeNO concentrations and the percentage of sputum eosinophils has been found in COPD, despite the existence of a well known clinical relationship between airway eosinophilic inflammation and response to corticosteroids. This may be partially explained by the wide variability of eosinophil counts in sputum of COPD patients.

FeNO to assess the effects of treatment in COPD

FeNO has been used to assess airway inflammatory response to drugs for COPD, but no clear conclusions can be drawn.

Inhaled Corticosteroids
Whereas there have been no direct measurements of acute inhaled corticosteroid effects FeNO in COPD, few data are available on their

short term effect. Ferreira et al. (40) showed that the inhalation of 1,000 µg/day of beclomethasone dipropionate in stable ex-smokers with COPD reduces their elevated baseline FeNO levels in as little as 1 week. This decrease in FeNO values occurred in the absence of clinically or statistically significant changes in FEV_1.

Kunisaki et al. (39) conducted a single-arm, open-label study in ex-smokers with severe COPD, and participants spent four weeks free of any inhaled corticosteroids, followed by four weeks of fluticasone propionate, 500 µg twice daily. FeNO was measured immediately before and after the four weeks of steroid use. Authors showed a reduction in FeNO values (median FeNO change= -7 ppb). This observation is in line with that of Zietkowski et al. (38) who demonstrated a similar decrease in FeNO after 2 months of budesonide, 800 µg/day.

However, the main message which was derived from both studies is that the reduction in FeNO values was observed mainly in patients with a higher baseline FeNO levels, thus identifying COPD patients who most likely profit from inhaled corticosteroids treatment.

Theophylline

Cosio et al. (41) recruited thirty-five patients hospitalised because of exacerbation of COPD and treated according to international guidelines, were randomised to receive (or not) low dose oral theophylline (100 mg bid). Interestingly, FeNO recovery during clinical stability showed a trend, although not statistically significant, to be enhanced in patients receiving theophylline. This would be in keeping with previous studies, showing that theophylline reduces nitrative stress *in vitro* (42).

Physical Training

Impaired exercise tolerance is a common finding in patients with COPD. It has been shown that pulmonary rehabilitation programmes are likely to improve exercise capacity and health related quality of life. Clini et al. (43) assessed the effects on FeNO of an 8 week outpatient rehabilitation programme including exercise training in patients with mild to moderate COPD. Authors showed that an improvement in exercise tolerance following a multidisciplinary pulmonary rehabilitation programme including lower limb training was associated with an increase in resting FeNO. Authors suggested that the measurement of FeNO might be a useful marker for assessing the pathophysiological adaptation to training in patients with COPD. However, further prospective randomised controlled studies are needed to better define this role.

FeNO to Differentiate Asthma from COPD

One of the challenges in diagnosing asthma can be distinguishing asthma from COPD, in particular in old patients with fixed airflow obstruction. In these cases, physiological tests alone are unhelpful in discriminating those with asthma who would otherwise be classified as having COPD. Asthmatics with fixed airway obstruction are often diagnosed as having COPD, even if the differential diagnosis between asthma and COPD in patients with fixed airflow obstruction may be important as the natural history as well as the response to treatment are different. Fabbri et al. have shown that patients with historical evidence of asthma have eosinophilic airway inflammation in association with raised FeNO levels (44). In keeping with the previous observation, Di Lorenzo et al. (45) showed that, within a group of elderly patients with fixed airflow obstruction, those with asthma have distinct airway inflammation as compared with those with COPD and history of smoking-induced airway disease. These findings suggest that asthmatic airway inflammation does not change with the development of fixed airflow obstruction and thus does not become similar to the airway inflammation characteristic of COPD. Therefore, data indicate that FeNO may be useful to differentiate COPD from asthma, mainly when fixed airflow obstruction in asthma is present.

FeNO for Assessing COPD Severity and Monitoring

Several studies analysed a potential correlation between FeNO levels and severity of lung function impairment assessed by FEV_1, but no consistent results could be found. Some studies found a positive correlation between NO and FEV1, others found a negative correlation or no correlation between the two parameters (1, 3). Therefore, FeNO should not be used to assess COPD severity.

De Laurentis et al. (45) monitored FeNO levels in COPD patients during 1-year assessment in the outpatient setting. The long-term FeNO mean value was $33.9 \pm 16.4\%$ (range 8.1-83.1%), and it was significantly associated with exacerbation rate. Moreover, COPD patients with FeNO coefficient of variation >40% reported a twofold increase in exacerbation rate as compared to the COPD with FeNO coefficient of variation less than 40%, with the highest FeNO values close to the exacerbation.

The Future of FENO in COPD Patients

A possible and more interesting application of FeNO in COPD management could derive from recent discoveries confirming that – through the sampling of exhaled NO at different expiratory flow rates – it could be theoretically possible to assess separately the alveolar and bronchial components of pulmonary inflammation. On the contrary, the current single expiratory technique measure predominantly samples larger airway-derived NO and may only partially reflect peripheral inflammation (46). Whereas this is not an issue in asthma studies, it might be the missing point explaining why FeNO is almost normal in exhaled breath of COPD patients. In fact, small airways and lung parenchyma are predominant sites of inflammation in patients with COPD, whose progression is associated with accumulation of inflammatory mucous exudates in lumen and infiltration of small airway wall by inflammatory cells. Furthermore, there is a high level of expression of iNOS presence in sputum macrophages, alveolar walls, small airway epithelium and vascular smooth muscle of COPD patients (11). In patients with COPD, this may result in an increased production of NO and NO-related species in the lung periphery.

It is possible to measure exhaled NO at different flows (multiple exhalation flow technique), so that it is feasible to partition large airway-derived NO and peripheral NO derived from alveoli and probably small airways (47, 48). Mathematical models to calculate these two fractions of exhaled NO have been described by several groups (48). Using a two-compartment model as a research tool, it has been demonstrated that NO is elevated in the alveolar compartment of COPD patients and correlated with disease severity. What is more, multiple exhalation flow technique is unaffected by smoking, and therefore can be used for smoking COPD patients (49). This multiple exhalation flow technique is promising for studying COPD patients, but further studies are required to validate this potential tool for monitoring inflammation in COPD. Furthermore, at present this is technically demanding and beyond the scope of routine laboratory testing.

References

1. Corradi M, Majori M, Cacciani GC, Consigli GF, de'Munari E, Pesci A. Increased exhaled nitric oxide in patients with stable chronic obstructive pulmonary disease. Thorax. 1999 Jul;54(7):572-5.
2. Bessa V, Tseliou E, Bakakos P, Louki-

des S. Noninvasive evaluation of airway inflammation in asthmatic patients who smoke: implications for application in clinical practice. Ann Allergy Asthma Immunol. 2008 Sep;101(3):226-32; quiz 32-4, 78.

3. Montuschi P, Kharitonov SA, Barnes PJ. Exhaled carbon monoxide and nitric oxide in COPD. Chest. 2001 Aug; 120(2):496-501.

4. Hoyt JC, Robbins RA, Habib M, Springall DR, Buttery LD, Polak JM, et al. Cigarette smoke decreases inducible nitric oxide synthase in lung epithelial cells. Exp Lung Res. 2003 Jan-Feb;29(1):17-28.

5. Hogman M, Holmkvist T, Walinder R, Merilainen P, Ludviksdottir D, Hakansson L, et al. Increased nitric oxide elimination from the airways after smoking cessation. Clin Sci (Lond). 2002 Jul;103(1):15-9.

6. Michils A, Louis R, Peche R, Baldassarre S, Van Muylem A. Exhaled nitric oxide as a marker of asthma control in smoking patients. Eur Respir J. 2009 Jun;33(6):1295-301.

7. Barnes PJ. Immunology of asthma and chronic obstructive pulmonary disease. Nat Rev Immunol. 2008 Mar;8(3):183-92.

8. Malerba M, Ragnoli B, Radaeli A, Tantucci C. Usefulness of exhaled nitric oxide and sputum eosinophils in the long-term control of eosinophilic asthma. Chest. 2008 Oct;134(4):733-9.

9. Hubert D, Aubourg F, Fauroux B, Trinquart L, Sermet I, Lenoir G, et al. Exhaled nitric oxide in cystic fibrosis: relationships with airway and lung vascular impairments. Eur Respir J. 2009 Jul;34(1):117-24.

10. Silvestri M, Sabatini F, Spallarossa D, Fregonese L, Battistini E, Biraghi MG, et al. Exhaled nitric oxide levels in non-allergic and allergic mono- or polysensitised children with asthma. Thorax. 2001 Nov;56(11):857-62.

11. Ricciardolo FL, Nijkamp FP, Folkerts G. Nitric oxide synthase (NOS) as therapeutic target for asthma and chronic obstructive pulmonary disease. Curr Drug Targets. 2006 Jun;7 (6):721-35.

12. Silkoff PE, Martin D, Pak J, Westcott JY, Martin RJ. Exhaled nitric oxide correlated with induced sputum findings in COPD. Chest. 2001 Apr;119(4):1049-55.

13. Fierro IM, Nascimento-DaSilva V, Arruda MA, Freitas MS, Plotkowski MC, Cunha FQ, et al. Induction of NOS in rat blood PMN in vivo and in vitro: modulation by tyrosine kinase and involvement in bactericidal activity. J Leukoc Biol. 1999 Apr;65(4):508-14.

14. Ichinose M, Sugiura H, Yamagata S, Koarai A, Tomaki M, Ogawa H, et al. Xanthine oxidase inhibition reduces reactive nitrogen species production in COPD airways. Eur Respir J. 2004; 23(3):496.

15. Mitsui T, Kondo T. Effects of mouth cleansing on the levels of exhaled nitrous oxide in young and older adults. Sci Total Environ. 1998 Dec 11;224 (1-3):177-80.

16. Smith AP, Demoncheaux EA, Higenbottam TW. Nitric oxide gas decreases endothelin-1 mRNA in cultured pulmonary artery endothelial cells. Nitric Oxide. 2002 Mar;6(2):153-9.

17. Cremona G, Higenbottam T, Borland C, Mist B. Mixed expired nitric oxide in primary pulmonary hypertension in relation to lung diffusion capacity. QJM. 1994 Sep;87(9):547-51.

18. Kharitonov SA, Cailes JB, Black CM, du Bois RM, Barnes PJ. Decreased nitric oxide in the exhaled air of patients with systemic sclerosis with pul-

monary hypertension. Thorax. 1997 Dec;52(12):1051-5.

19. Hegewald MJ, Elliott CG. Sustained improvement with iloprost in a COPD patient with severe pulmonary hypertension. Chest. 2009 Feb;135(2):536-7.

20. Elwing J, Panos RJ. Pulmonary hypertension associated with COPD. Int J Chron Obstruct Pulmon Dis. 2008; 3(1):55-70.

21. Carratu P, Scoditti C, Maniscalco M, Seccia TM, Di Gioia G, Gadaleta F, et al. Exhaled and arterial levels of endothelin-1 are increased and correlate with pulmonary systolic pressure in COPD with pulmonary hypertension. BMC Pulm Med. 2008;8:20.

22. Delen FM, Sippel JM, Osborne ML, Law S, Thukkani N, Holden WE. Increased exhaled nitric oxide in chronic bronchitis: comparison with asthma and COPD. Chest. 2000 Mar;117(3):695-701.

23. Maestrelli P, Paska C, Saetta M, Turato G, Nowicki Y, Monti S, et al. Decreased haem oxygenase-1 and increased inducible nitric oxide synthase in the lung of severe COPD patients. Eur Respir J. 2003 Jun;21(6):971-6.

24. Boschetto P, Quintavalle S, Zeni E, Leprotti S, Potena A, Ballerin L, et al. Association between markers of emphysema and more severe chronic obstructive pulmonary disease. Thorax. 2006 Dec;61(12):1037-42.

25. Malerba M, Ragnoli B, Radaeli A. Exhaled nitric oxide levels in alpha-1-antitrypsin PiMZ subjects. J Intern Med. 2009 Mar;265(3):382-7.

26. Rahaghi F, Ortega I, Rahaghi N, Oliveira E, Ramirez J, Smolley L, et al. Physician alert suggesting alpha-1 antitrypsin deficiency testing in pulmonary function test (PFT) results. COPD. 2009 Feb;6(1):26-30.

27. Brinkley TE, Leng X, Miller ME, Kitzman DW, Pahor M, Berry MJ, et al. Chronic inflammation is associated with low physical function in older adults across multiple comorbidities. J Gerontol A Biol Sci Med Sci. 2009 Apr;64(4):455-61.

28. Agostoni P, Bussotti M. Exhaled nitric oxide and exercise performance in heart failure. Arch Physiol Biochem. 2003 Oct;111(4):293-6.

29. Bussotti M, Andreini D, Agostoni P. Exercise-induced changes in exhaled nitric oxide in heart failure. Eur J Heart Fail. 2004 Aug;6(5):551-4.

30. Maziak W, Loukides S, Culpitt S, Sullivan P, Kharitonov SA, Barnes PJ. Exhaled nitric oxide in chronic obstructive pulmonary disease. Am J Respir Crit Care Med. 1998 Mar; 157(3 Pt 1):998-1002.

31. Agusti AG, Villaverde JM, Togores B, Bosch M. Serial measurements of exhaled nitric oxide during exacerbations of chronic obstructive pulmonary disease. Eur Respir J. 1999 Sep;14(3):523-8.

32. Bhowmik A, Seemungal TA, Donaldson GC, Wedzicha JA. Effects of exacerbations and seasonality on exhaled nitric oxide in COPD. Eur Respir J. 2005 Dec;26(6):1009-15.

33. Rohde G, Borg I, Wiethege A, Kauth M, Jerzinowski S, An Duong Dinh T, et al. Inflammatory response in acute viral exacerbations of COPD. Infection. 2008 Oct;36(5):427-33.

34. Bathoorn E, Kerstjens H, Postma D, Timens W, MacNee W. Airways inflammation and treatment during acute exacerbations of COPD. Int J Chron Obstruct Pulmon Dis. 2008;3(2):217-29.

35. Papi A, Romagnoli M, Baraldo S, Braccioni F, Guzzinati I, Saetta M, et al. Partial reversibility of airflow limitation and

increased exhaled NO and sputum eosinophilia in chronic obstructive pulmonary disease. Am J Respir Crit Care Med. 2000 Nov;162(5):1773-7.

36. Miller MR, Hankinson J, Brusasco V, Burgos F, Casaburi R, Coates A, et al. Standardisation of spirometry. Eur Respir J. 2005 Aug;26(2):319-38.

37. Brightling CE, McKenna S, Hargadon B, Birring S, Green R, Siva R, et al. Sputum eosinophilia and the short term response to inhaled mometasone in chronic obstructive pulmonary disease. Thorax. 2005 Mar;60(3):193-8.

38. Zietkowski Z, Kucharewicz I, Bodzenta-Lukaszyk A. The influence of inhaled corticosteroids on exhaled nitric oxide in stable chronic obstructive pulmonary disease. Respir Med. 2005 Jul;99(7):816-24.

39. Kunisaki KM, Rice KL, Janoff EN, Rector TS, Niewoehner DE. Exhaled nitric oxide, systemic inflammation, and the spirometric response to inhaled fluticasone propionate in severe chronic obstructive pulmonary disease: a prospective study. Ther Adv Respir Dis. 2008 Apr;2(2):55-64.

40. Ferreira IM, Hazari MS, Gutierrez C, Zamel N, Chapman KR. Exhaled nitric oxide and hydrogen peroxide in patients with chronic obstructive pulmonary disease: effects of inhaled beclomethasone. Am J Respir Crit Care Med. 2001 Sep 15;164(6):1012-5.

41. Cosio BG, Iglesias A, Rios A, Noguera A, Sala E, Ito K, et al. Low-dose theophylline enhances the anti-inflammatory effects of steroids during exacerbations of COPD. Thorax. 2009 May;64(5):424-9.

42. Hirano T, Yamagata T, Gohda M, Yamagata Y, Ichikawa T, Yanagisawa S, et al. Inhibition of reactive nitrogen species production in COPD airways: comparison of inhaled corticosteroid and oral theophylline. Thorax. 2006 Sep;61(9):761-6.

43. Clini E, Bianchi L, Vitacca M, Porta R, Foglio K, Ambrosino N. Exhaled nitric oxide and exercise in stable COPD patients. Chest. 2000 Mar;117(3):702-7.

44. Fabbri LM, Romagnoli M, Corbetta L, Casoni G, Busljetic K, Turato G, et al. Differences in airway inflammation in patients with fixed airflow obstruction due to asthma or chronic obstructive pulmonary disease. Am J Respir Crit Care Med. 2003 Feb 1;167(3):418-24.

45. Di Lorenzo G, Mansueto P, Ditta V, Esposito-Pellitteri M, Lo Bianco C, Leto-Barone MS, et al. Similarity and differences in elderly patients with fixed airflow obstruction by asthma and by chronic obstructive pulmonary disease. Respir Med. 2008 Feb;102(2):232-8.

46. Barnes PJ. Emerging pharmacotherapies for COPD. Chest. 2008 Dec;134(6):1278-86.

47. Condorelli P, Shin HW, Aledia AS, Silkoff PE, George SC. A simple technique to characterize proximal and peripheral nitric oxide exchange using constant flow exhalations and an axial diffusion model. J Appl Physiol. 2007 Jan;102(1):417-25.

48. Tsoukias NM, Shin HW, Wilson AF, George SC. A single-breath technique with variable flow rate to characterize nitric oxide exchange dynamics in the lungs. J Appl Physiol. 2001 Jul;91(1):477-87.

49. Brindicci C, Ito K, Resta O, Pride NB, Barnes PJ, Kharitonov SA. Exhaled nitric oxide from lung periphery is increased in COPD. Eur Respir J. 2005 Jul;26(1):52-9.

Induced Sputum - Technical Considerations

Silvano Dragonieri • Olga Toungoussova • Andrea Zanini • Antonio Spanevello

During the last 15 years the use of sputum induction by inhalation of hypertonic saline solution to study the cellular and biochemical composition of the airways has been increased significantly. The induced sputum technique, which is inexpensive and does not require complex instruments, allows a relatively non-invasive sampling of airway content. Thus, adequate samples of lower airway secretions can be collected even from patients who are not able to produce sputum spontaneously and the features of airway inflammation in asthma, chronic obstructive pulmonary disease (COPD) and other respiratory diseases can be investigated.

The method of induced sputum induction has been shown to be reproducible, sensitive and valid (1-3). Since the first description of a standardized method (4) there has been an impressive increase of publications on induced sputum and its application to study various aspects of airway inflammation. In order to harmonize the different

Correspondence

Prof. Antonio Spanevello

Department of Respiratory Diseases, Fondazione Salvatore Maugeri, Via Roncaccio 16, 21040 Tradate (VA), Italy

e-mail: antonio.spanevello@fsm.it

techniques used worldwide a standardized methodology of sputum induction and processing has been issued in 2002 by a European Respiratory Society Task Force (5). Since that date several new methodological studies have widened our knowledge about outstanding issues such as the optimum method for inducing sputum, its homogenization and processing. The aim of this book chapter is to review the current literature and to provide an extension on the technical considerations in the field of induced sputum.

Sputum Induction

The aim of sputum induction is to collect an adequate sample of lower airway secretions in patients who are not able to produce sputum spontaneously. Sputum induction consists of inhalation of nebulized saline solution (isotonic or hypertonic) over different time periods and subsequent expectoration of secretions into a Petri-dish.

Proper facilities and instruments are needed to perform sputum induction. In particular a quiet environment with fresh sterile saline solution, an ultrasonic nebulizer, a spirometer and safety equipment (resuscitation equipment, oxygen supply and rescue medications) are required.

Safety

The induction procedure is considered to be safe (5). No fatalities or need of hospitalization in subjects undergoing sputum induction have been reported. The adverse effect, bronchoconstriction caused by the inhalation of hypertonic saline solution, can be quickly reversed by the administration of inhaled short acting β_2-agonists. Sputum induction is well-tolerated in patients with mild to moderate airflow limitation such as asthma and COPD (4, 6-10). With the precaution of using a modified procedure (11) it can also be safe in patients with moderate to severe airflow limitation (11-14) and a recent study showed that induced sputum can be safely performed in patients with an ongoing exacerbation of COPD (15). Considerable decreases in FEV_1 during the induction procedure can occur, but they can be tolerated well. Moreover, induced sputum can be safely performed by children with mild to moderate asthma (16) and one study has demonstrated that sputum induction can be performed safely following exercise-induced bronchoconstriction (17).

However, the risk of airway constriction in subjects with airways hyperresponsiveness (AHR) cannot be underestimated. Therefore, pretreatment with salbutamol 200 mg delivered via a standard metered dose inhaler is always recommended (18). Some authors have used 400 µg, arguing that breakthrough bronchospasm may occur with 200 µg but higher doses are not suggested since this may reduce the effectiveness of any additional required doses during the procedure.

Monitoring lung function is an important safety procedure. The use of a spirometer is preferred to a peak flow meter because of the higher sensitivity of FEV_1. Spirometry should be always performed before the induction procedure to determine the baseline FEV_1 before and 10 minutes after the administration of pre-induction inhaled β_2-agonist. After the beginning of the inhalation procedure, it is recommended to measure pulmonary function after 1 minute of nebulization as some subjects are very sensitive to hypertonic saline. Afterwards spirometry should be performed after each inhalation interval. The procedure should be interrupted if FEV_1 falls to >20% of the post-bronchodilator baseline value or if a patient reports breathlessness or wheeze. In such cases an additional dose of β_2-agonists should be given. It is advised to restart inhalation only after that FEV_1 has returned to 5% of post-bronchodilator baseline. At the end of the last inhalation procedure if FEV_1 has decreased to >10% of post-bronchodilator baseline an additional dose of β_2-agonist is suggested. Patients should be monitored until their FEV_1 has returned to at least 5% of the baseline value.

Concentration of Saline Solution and Duration of Inhalation

Since the early 1990s different concentrations of saline solution ranging from 0.9 to 7% have been used for sputum induction (6, 19-21). In some studies, the concentrations of saline solution were modified during induction procedure, progressively increasing from 3 to 4 or 5% (4, 22). The European Respiratory Society Task Force guidelines suggest the use of 4,5% saline solution as standard (5) (Figure 1). However, in patients with high-risk for bronchoconstriction, an alternative method with isotonic saline solution should be used (Figure 1).

Although hypertonic solutions are more effective than isotonic in

Standard Method	Alternative method
INSTRUCT PATIENTS PROPERLY	INSTRUCT PATIENTS PROPERLY
CHECK ALL THE EQUIPMENT AND SET ULTRASONIC NEBULIZER TO APPROX 1ML/MIN	CHECK ALL THE EQUIPMENT AND SET ULTRASONIC NEBULIZER TO APPROX 1ML/MIN
MEASURE PRE- BRONCHODILATOR FEV1	MEASURE PRE-BRONCHODILATOR FEV1
ADMINISTER 200 µG OF INHALED SALBUTAMOL	ADMINISTER 200µG OF INHALED SALBUTAMOL
MEASURE POST-BRONCHODILATRO FEV1 AFTER 10 MINUTES	MEASURE POST- BRONCHODILATRO FEV1 AFTER 10 MINUTES
USE EITHER A FIXED CONCENTRATION OF STERILE SALINE SOLUTION (3 OR 4,5%) OR INCREASING CONCENTRATIONS OF SALINE (3,4 AND 5%)	START WITH 0,9% STERILE SALINE SOLUTION AND INDUCE FOR 30SEC, 1 MIN AND 5 MIN. IF NO SPUTUM IS PRODUCED INCREASE TO 3% AND INDUCE FOR 30SEC, 1 MIN AND 2 MIN. IF UNSUCCESSFUL INCREASE TO 4,5% AND INDUCE FOR 30 SEC, 1 MIN, 2 MIN, 4 MIN AND 8 MIN. DO NOT INCREASE CONCENTRATIONS IF ISOTONIC SALINE IS SUCCESSFUL IN INDUCING SPUTUM
PERFORM INDUCTION IN 5- MIN INTERVALS FOR NO LONGER THAN 20 MINUTES OR AT 1,4 AND 5 MIN WITH THREE FURTHER 5-MIN PERIODS	MEASURE FEV1 AT THE END OF EACH INDUCTION INTERVAL (induction must be stopped if FEV1 falls >20% of baseline or if symptoms occur)
MEASURE FEV1 AT THE END OF EACH INDUCTION INTERVAL (induction must be stopped if FEV1 falls >20% of baseline or if symptoms occur)	IF PATIENT DOES NOT COUGH SPONTANEOUSLY, ASK THEM TO ATTEMPT TO COUGH AND SPIT AFTER THE 4 AND 8 MIN PERIODS
ASK THE PATIENT TO COUGH AND SPIT AT THE 10TH, 15TH AND 20TH MINUTE OF INDUCTION OR WHENEVER THEY GET THE URGE TO DO SO	

FIGURE 1

Standard and alternative methods for sputum induction. Reproduced after permission from European Respiratory Society Task Force. Standardized methodology of sputum induction and processing. Eur Respir J 2002;20:(Suppl.37),1s-55s.

inducing sputum (23), no difference in cellular composition of induced sputum in the comparison between isotonic and hypertonic solutions were evidenced (21, 24).

The type of the nebulizer and its output should be considered when performing sputum induction. Ultrasonic nebulizers have been shown to be more effective in producing adequate sputum samples in comparison with jet nebulizers (23). Moreover, a study showed that the comparison between sputum with a high output ultrasonic nebulizer (1.9 ml/min) and a lower output (0.7 ml/min) gives different results in terms of cell counts and fluid phase measures (25). Thus, there is a consensus that an ultrasonic nebulizer should be used and that an output of 1ml/min is enough to obtain an adequate sample (5).

The duration of inhalation is another relevant issue in sputum induction. Several studies have reported the changes of cellular and biochemical elements of induced sputum during the inhalation procedure (25-28).

According to the above, neutrophils and eosinophils prevail in sputum samples collected during the early phases of the induction, whereas lymphocyte and macrophages are prominent in samples collected during later phases. This suggests that the later expectorated samples originate from more peripheral airways.

Changes of cellular composition during the induction can introduce a bias when performing induced sputum analysis. It is important to keep the duration of inhalation constant between subjects to allow comparisons. Shorter inhalation times (15-20 minutes) appear to have similar success rate and feasibility to longer inhalation times (30 minutes)(5). For most purposes, guidelines suggest that the duration of induction phase should be between 15 and 20 minutes (5). However a recent study showed that the mean percentage of neutrophils, eosinophils, lymphocytes and epithelial cells did not change significantly in samples obtained consecutively after 5, 10 and 15 minutes and in the mixture of the three samples, suggesting that 15 minutes of induction procedure with the fixed concentration of the hypertonic saline and processing of the mixed sample can be recommended for clinical setting and clinical trials (29).

Expectoration Technique

Authors have suggested various recommendations for the expectoration during sputum induction, i.e. fasting for several hours before the procedure to avoid nausea and vomit, washing the mouth with water, blowing the nose before the induction or wearing a nose clip. These procedures however did not show clear benefits. Some protocols suggest interruption of inhalation procedure at predefined time intervals [e.g. every 5 minutes] or to stop only when a patient feels a need to cough. This does not influence the result. One study has shown that spitting saliva before the expectoration maneuver decreases the percentage of squamous cells in the whole sputum by 30% and increases the concentration of ECP in the supernatant by 80% (30). Therefore the influence of expectoration techniques on the feasibility and validity of the procedure has not been clarified yet. The consensus suggests to ask the patient to cough and produce sputum at the end of every set inhalation time or whenever a patient feels a need to do so(5). Finally some subjects, in particular those with acute asthma exacerbations or COPD, can easily produce spontaneous sputum. Spontaneously produced sputum has been shown to have a similar percentage of cell composition and fluid-phase mediators (31, 32). Nevertheless, spontaneous sputum has significantly lower cell viability compared to induced sputum (31, 32) and it has a poorer quality of samples (33). Therefore it may be relevant to perform induced sputum even in subjects who may spontaneously expectorate for a better comparison with individuals who do not produce sputum spontaneously.

Sputum Processing for Cell Cytology, Immunocytochemistry and in situ Hybridization

Entire vs. Selected Plug

Two basically different techniques of sputum processing are currently in use. In the first method all the viscid portions of sputum sample are selected with the aid of an inverted microscope (4, 34). In the second technique the analysis of sputum 'sample is performed on the whole expectorate, thus including sputum plus some saliva (34-36). Patients should be instructed to discard saliva before spitting sputum in order to reduce salivary contamination (30). The advantage of selected plug processing is the improvement of the quality of cytospin slides due to the reduced salivary contamination (34, 36, 37). The disadvantages of using selected sputum are that selecting plugs takes longer to perform and requires an inverted microscope. The advantages of using the whole sputum include its quickness to perform, however the presence of variable quantity of saliva may dilute the sputum and alter its analysis. Indeed samples processed in this way tend to contain more squamous cells, making the count of inflammatory cells more difficult to perform. Moreover, it has been shown that the cell counts reproducibility is lower if squamous cells percentage is higher than 20% of all cells (36).

Processing Phase

Processing of sputum should be performed as soon as possible and within 2 hours from the collection in order to ensure adequate cell count and staining (34, 38). If for any reason the processing is delayed, the sample can be refrigerated at 4°C for up to 8 hours without affecting cell counts (39).

Initially, when this method was just implemented, direct smears were produced and stained for cell analysis (20). However the assessment of smears is difficult and unreliable because cells are seen entrapped in mucus. Therefore it is recommended to use dithiotreitol (DTT) or its optical isomer dithioerytriol (DTE), which breaks disulphide bonds in mucin molecules and releases the cells. The use of these mucolytic agents significantly improves TCC and cytospin quality (40, 41). Homogeneization with DTT does not affect cell counts, but it may alter the levels of several fluid-phase mediators (40-42). Latest recommendations suggest that after mixing sputum with DTT or DTE the suspension should be homogenized in a shaking water bath or rocker for about 15 minutes at either 22°C or 37°C (5). Moreover, it is advisable to remove the sample periodically for its brief aspiration. After the homogenization the suspension should be carefully filtered through a 48 µm nylon gauze to remove mucus and debris. Although there is a slight decrease in total cell count, this improves the slide quality and differential cell count is unaffected (35, 43).

One part of the filtered suspension should be taken for the manual total cell count and viability assessment and the remaining part is used for preparation of cytospins. Centrifugation is required to separate sputum cells from the fluid phase. A 5-10 minutes centrifugation time at 300-1500xg centrifugal force is adequate for separating cells from supernatant (38, 41, 44). Supernatant is collected and stored at -20 to -70°C for further analysis of fluid-phase mediators.

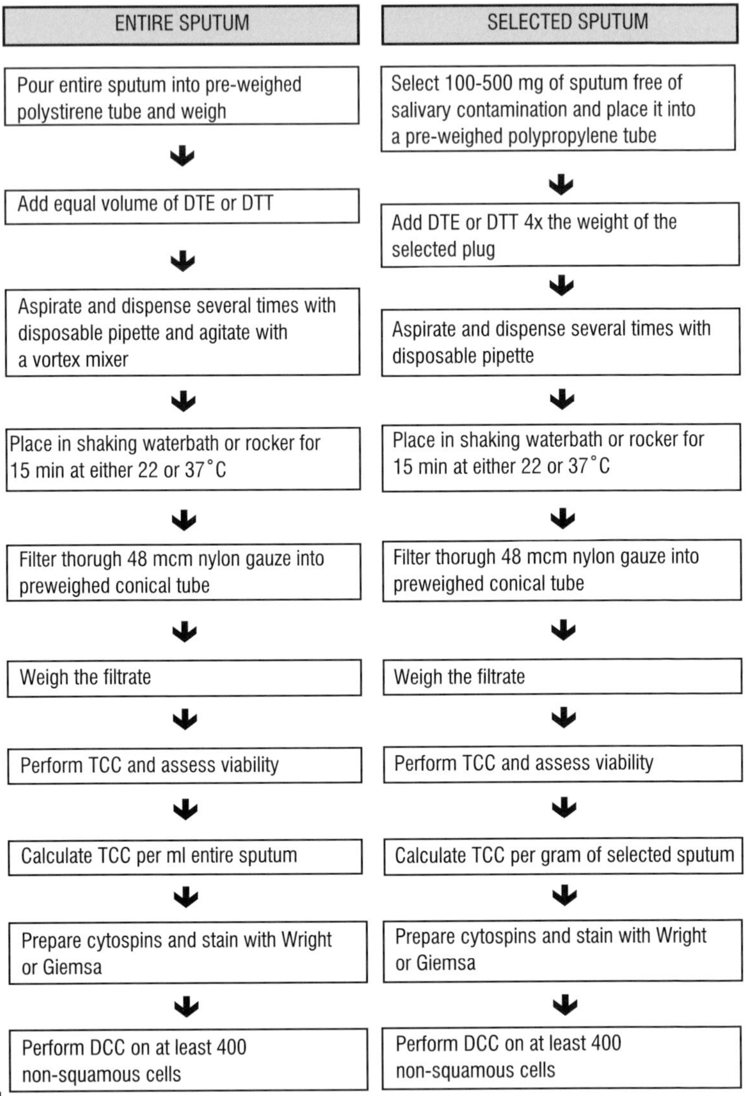

ENTIRE SPUTUM	SELECTED SPUTUM
Pour entire sputum into pre-weighed polystirene tube and weigh	Select 100-500 mg of sputum free of salivary contamination and place it into a pre-weighed polypropylene tube
⬇	⬇
Add equal volume of DTE or DTT	Add DTE or DTT 4x the weight of the selected plug
⬇	⬇
Aspirate and dispense several times with disposable pipette and agitate with a vortex mixer	Aspirate and dispense several times with disposable pipette
⬇	⬇
Place in shaking waterbath or rocker for 15 min at either 22 or 37°C	Place in shaking waterbath or rocker for 15 min at either 22 or 37°C
⬇	⬇
Filter thorugh 48 mcm nylon gauze into preweighed conical tube	Filter thorugh 48 mcm nylon gauze into preweighed conical tube
⬇	⬇
Weigh the filtrate	Weigh the filtrate
⬇	⬇
Perform TCC and assess viability	Perform TCC and assess viability
⬇	⬇
Calculate TCC per ml entire sputum	Calculate TCC per gram of selected sputum
⬇	⬇
Prepare cytospins and stain with Wright or Giemsa	Prepare cytospins and stain with Wright or Giemsa
⬇	⬇
Perform DCC on at least 400 non-squamous cells	Perform DCC on at least 400 non-squamous cells

FIGURE 2

Sputum processing methods for entire and selected sputum. Reproduced after permission from European Respiratory Society Task Force. Standardized methodology of sputum induction and processing. Eur Respir J 2002;20:(Suppl.37),1s-55s. DTE: dithioerythriol; DTT: dithiotreitol; TCC: total cell count; DCC: differential cell count

Cell Counts, Cytospin Preparation and Staining

Cytology is the main component of sputum analysis and it has to be performed in any sputum assessment, even if the aim of the study is to detect fluid phase mediators.

First of all, total cell count (TCC) and cell viability are required. TCC is manually performed by using a haemocytometer counting chamber and cell viability is assessed by a Trypan blue exclusion method (38, 44). A cell viability of less than 40% may influence the d-ifferential cell count. It is recommended to perform TCC and viability before centrifugation, since a cell reduction after centrifugation has been shown (45, 46).

The optimum number of cells for obtaining adequate cytospins ranges from 40 to 60x 10^3 (38, 47). After centrifugation, cell pellet should be resuspended in phospate buffered saline solution and cell concentration should be adjusted to 1.0 to 1.6 cells/ml^{-1} (48). A new method to improve cytospin quality has been suggested by the use of sterile minimum essential medium (MEM), filtered through three types of net filters and separated from the residual debris by Percoll gradient centrifugation (49). This method is more time consuming than the usual one and it may cause some total cell loss but it could be potentially useful for samples with relevant contamination by squamous cells and debris and when sputum cells are used for more sophisticated techniques (49).

Authors have used cytocentrifugation speeds ranging 10-51xg for 6 minutes (38, 47). Sputum lymphocytes can be lost at lower speeds (50, 51), therefore cytocentrifugation speed should be taken into account when investigating this cell type.

Cytospins for differential cell count (DCC) should be stained with Giemsa or Wright's method. At least 400 non-squamous cells should to be counted to determine the percentage of macrophages, neutrophils, eosinophils, lymphocytes and bronchial epithelial cells. The percentage of squamous cells should always be reported separately.

Finally, one study has compared 3 methods for DCC in induced sputum. Samples were smeared without treatment with DTT (technique A), after treatment with DTT (technique B) and after treatment with DTT and cytospin (technique C). All the three techniques are good indicators of airway inflammation (52), The technique C is recommended for research projects and techniques A and B, which are faster and less costly, could be implemented in clinical practice (52).

Quality Control

Sputum induction, sputum processing and analysis should be performed by qualified and well trained personnel, following a standard operative procedure (S.O.P.). A monthly quality control should be performed to ensure an adequate slide reading and equipment calibration. This is extremely important in order to avoid legal implications, especially when using slide reading to monitor patient treatment, as incorrect results can lead to wrong diagnosis and treatment.

Immunochemistry and In Situ Hybridization of Sputum Specimens

The application of techniques such as immunocytochemistry and in-situ hybridization (ISH) are not as common as Wright or Giemsa, but they widen the opportunities for further research and diagnosis.

Immunocytochemistry can be performed by using different methods, the most recommended being the alkaline phospatase/anti alkaline phospatase technique (APAAP) (53-55). In this technique, cytospin samples are incubated with monoclonal antibodies to develop an antigen/antibody complex. After overnight incubation at 4°C secondary antibodies are applied and the antigen/antibody complex is visualized using the alkaline phospatase linked substrate. The cytoplasm of positive cells stains red or blue.

Sputum preparation with mucus and/or large number of squamous cells should not be used as such slides make immunocytochemistry very hard to interpret. Moreover, negative controls should always be included in order to help excluding false positives. For many cytokines which are hardly detected by immunocytochemistry, an ISH is required. ISH uses radioactive non non-radioactive antisense cRNA probes that detect intracellular mRNA.

Hybridization can be performed according to standard protocols (56). This technique requires special care to avoid RNA degradation and combination with RNAses. After hybridization slides should be high stringency washed and a sense probe should be used as control. As for immunocytochemistry, mucus and squamous cells should be avoided and negative controls should be used.

References

1. Spanevello A, Migliori GB, Sharara A, Ballardini L, Bridge P, Pisati P, et al. Induced sputum to assess airway inflammation: a study of reproducibility. Clin Exp Allergy. 1997 Oct;27(10):1138-44.

2. in 't Veen JC, de Gouw HW, Smits HH, Sont JK, Hiemstra PS, Sterk PJ, et al. Repeatability of cellular and soluble markers of inflammation in induced sputum from patients with asthma. Eur Respir J. 1996 Dec;9(12):2441-7.

3. Kips JC, Fahy JV, Hargreave FE, Ind PW, in't Veen JC. Methods for sputum induction and analysis of induced sputum: a method for assessing airway inflammation in asthma. Eur Respir J Suppl. 1998 Mar;26:9S-12S.

4. Pin I, Gibson PG, Kolendowicz R, Girgis-Gabardo A, Denburg JA, Hargreave FE, et al. Use of induced sputum cell counts to investigate airway inflammation in asthma. Thorax. 1992 Jan;47(1):25-9.

5. Djukanovic R, Sterk PJ, Fahy JV, Hargreave FE. Standardised methodology of sputum induction and processing. Eur Respir J Suppl. 2002 Sep;37:1s-2s.

6. Wong HH, Fahy JV. Safety of one method of sputum induction in asthmatic subjects. Am J Respir Crit Care Med. 1997 Jul;156(1):299-303.

7. de la Fuente PT, Romagnoli M, Godard P, Bousquet J, Chanez P. Safety of inducing sputum in patients with asthma of varying severity. Am J Respir Crit Care Med. 1998 Apr;157(4 Pt 1):1127-30.

8. Hunter CJ, Ward R, Woltmann G, Wardlaw AJ, Pavord ID. The safety and success rate of sputum induction using a low output ultrasonic nebuliser. Respir Med. 1999 May;93(5):345-8.

9. Grootendorst DC, van den Bos JW, Romeijn JJ, Veselic-Charvat M, Duiverman EJ, Vrijlandt EJ, et al. Induced sputum in adolescents with severe stable asthma. Safety and the relationship of cell counts and eosinophil cationic protein to clinical severity. Eur Respir J. 1999 Mar;13(3):647-53.

10. Vlachos-Mayer H, Leigh R, Sharon RF, Hussack P, Hargreave FE. Success and safety of sputum induction in the clinical setting. Eur Respir J. 2000 Nov;16(5):997-1000.

11. Pizzichini MM, Pizzichini E, Clelland L, Efthimiadis A, Mahony J, Dolovich J, et al. Sputum in severe exacerbations of asthma: kinetics of inflammatory indices after prednisone treatment. Am J Respir Crit Care Med. 1997 May;155(5):1501-8.

12. Pizzichini E, Pizzichini MM, Gibson P, Parameswaran K, Gleich GJ, Berman L, et al. Sputum eosinophilia predicts benefit from prednisone in smokers with chronic obstructive bronchitis. Am J Respir Crit Care Med. 1998 Nov;158(5 Pt 1):1511-7.

13. Pizzichini MM, Pizzichini E, Clelland L, Efthimiadis A, Pavord I, Dolovich J, et al. Prednisone-dependent asthma: inflammatory indices in induced sputum. Eur Respir J. 1999 Jan;13(1):15-21.

14. Wilson AM, Leigh R, Hargreave FE, Pizzichini MM, Pizzichini E. Safety of sputum induction in moderate-to-severe smoking-related chronic obstructive pulmonary disease. COPD. 2006 Jun;3(2):89-93.

15. Bathoorn E, Liesker J, Postma D, Koeter G, van Oosterhout AJ, Kerstjens

HA. Safety of sputum induction during exacerbations of COPD. Chest. 2007 Feb;131(2):432-8.

16. Covar RA, Spahn JD, Martin RJ, Silkoff PE, Sundstrom DA, Murphy J, et al. Safety and application of induced sputum analysis in childhood asthma. J Allergy Clin Immunol. 2004 Sep;114(3):575-82.

17. Carlsten C, Aitken ML, Hallstrand TS. Safety of sputum induction with hypertonic saline solution in exercise-induced bronchoconstriction. Chest. 2007 May;131(5):1339-44.

18. Boulet LP, Turcotte H, Tennina S. Comparative efficacy of salbutamol, ipratropium, and cromoglycate in the prevention of bronchospasm induced by exercise and hyperosmolar challenges. J Allergy Clin Immunol. 1989 May;83(5):882-7.

19. Pavia D, Thomson ML, Clarke SW. Enhanced clearance of secretions from the human lung after the administration of hypertonic saline aerosol. Am Rev Respir Dis. 1978 Feb;117(2): 199-203.

20. Iredale MJ, Wanklyn SA, Phillips IP, Krausz T, Ind PW. Non-invasive assessment of bronchial inflammation in asthma: no correlation between eosinophilia of induced sputum and bronchial responsiveness to inhaled hypertonic saline. Clin Exp Allergy. 1994 Oct;24(10):940-5.

21. Bacci E, Cianchetti S, Paggiaro PL, Carnevali S, Bancalari L, Dente FL, et al. Comparison between hypertonic and isotonic saline-induced sputum in the evaluation of airway inflammation in subjects with moderate asthma. Clin Exp Allergy. 1996 Dec;26(12):1395-400.

22. Bacci E, Cianchetti S, Ruocco L, Bartoli ML, Carnevali S, Dente FL, et al. Comparison between eosinophilic markers in induced sputum and blood in asthmatic patients. Clin Exp Allergy. 1998 Oct;28(10):1237-43.

23. Popov TA, Pizzichini MM, Pizzichini E, Kolendowicz R, Punthakee Z, Dolovich J, et al. Some technical factors influencing the induction of sputum for cell analysis. Eur Respir J. 1995 Apr;8(4): 559-65.

24. Cataldo D, Foidart JM, Lau L, Bartsch P, Djukanovic R, Louis R. Induced sputum: comparison between isotonic and hypertonic saline solution inhalation in patients with asthma. Chest. 2001 Dec;120(6):1815-21.

25. Belda J, Hussack P, Dolovich M, Efthimiadis A, Hargreave FE. Sputum induction: effect of nebulizer output and inhalation time on cell counts and fluid-phase measures. Clin Exp Allergy. 2001 Nov;31(11):1740-4.

26. Holz O, Jorres RA, Koschyk S, Speckin P, Welker L, Magnussen H. Changes in sputum composition during sputum induction in healthy and asthmatic subjects. Clin Exp Allergy. 1998 Mar;28(3):284-92.

27. Richter K, Holz O, Jorres RA, Mucke M, Magnussen H. Sequentially induced sputum in patients with asthma or chronic obstructive pulmonary disease. Eur Respir J. 1999 Sep;14(3):697-701.

28. Gershman NH, Liu H, Wong HH, Liu JT, Fahy JV. Fractional analysis of sequential induced sputum samples during sputum induction: evidence that different lung compartments are sampled at different time points. J Allergy Clin Immunol. 1999 Aug;104(2 Pt 1):322-8.

29. Toungoussova O, Migliori GB, Foschino Barbaro MP, Esposito LM, Dragonieri S, Carpagnano GE, et al. Changes in sputum composition during 15 min of sputum induction in healthy subjects and patients with asthma and chronic obstructive pulmonary disease. Respir Med. 2007 Jul;101(7):1543-8.

30. Gershman NH, Wong HH, Liu JT, Mahlmeister MJ, Fahy JV. Comparison of two methods of collecting induced sputum in asthmatic subjects. Eur Respir J. 1996 Dec;9(12):2448-53.

31. Bhowmik A, Seemungal TA, Sapsford RJ, Devalia JL, Wedzicha JA. Comparison of spontaneous and induced sputum for investigation of airway inflammation in chronic obstructive pulmonary disease. Thorax. 1998 Nov;53(11):953-6.

32. Pizzichini MM, Popov TA, Efthimiadis A, Hussack P, Evans S, Pizzichini E, et al. Spontaneous and induced sputum to measure indices of airway inflammation in asthma. Am J Respir Crit Care Med. 1996 Oct;154(4 Pt 1):866-9.

33. Bartoli ML, Bacci E, Carnevali S, Cianchetti S, Dente FL, Di Franco A, et al. Quality evaluation of samples obtained by spontaneous or induced sputum: comparison between two methods of processing and relationship with clinical and functional findings. J Asthma. 2002 Sep;39(6):479-86.

34. Pizzichini E, Pizzichini MM, Efthimiadis A, Hargreave FE, Dolovich J. Measurement of inflammatory indices in induced sputum: effects of selection of sputum to minimize salivary contamination. Eur Respir J. 1996 Jun;9(6):1174-80.

35. Efthimiadis A, Popov T, Kolendowicz R, Dolovich J, Hargreave FE. Increasing the yield of sputum cells for examination. Am J Respir Crit Care Med. 1994;149:A949.

36. Efthimiadis A, Pizzichini MMM, Kolendowicz R, Weston S, Dolovich J, Hargreave FE. The influence of cell viability and squamous epithelial cell contamination on the reliability of sputum differential cell counts. Am J Respir Crit Care Med. 1995;151:A384.

37. Pavord ID, Pizzichini MM, Pizzichini E, Hargreave FE. The use of induced sputum to investigate airway inflammation. Thorax. 1997 Jun;52(6):498-501.

38. Fahy JV, Liu J, Wong H, Boushey HA. Cellular and biochemical analysis of induced sputum from asthmatic and from healthy subjects. Am Rev Respir Dis. 1993 May;147(5):1126-31.

39. Efthimiadis A, Jayaram L, Weston S, Carruthers S, Hargreave FE. Induced sputum: time from expectoration to processing. Eur Respir J. 2002 Apr;19(4):706-8.

40. Efthimiadis A, Pizzichini MM, Pizzichini E, Dolovich J, Hargreave FE. Induced sputum cell and fluid-phase indices of inflammation: comparison of treatment with dithiothreitol vs phosphate-buffered saline. Eur Respir J. 1997 Jun;10(6):1336-40.

41. Louis R, Shute J, Goldring K, Perks B, Lau LC, Radermecker M, et al. The effect of processing on inflammatory markers in induced sputum. Eur Respir J. 1999 Mar;13(3):660-7.

42. Woolhouse IS, Bayley DL, Stockley RA. Effect of sputum processing with dithiothreitol on the detection of inflammatory mediators in chronic bron-

chitis and bronchiectasis. Thorax. 2002 Aug;57(8):667-71.

43. Efthimiadis A, Weston S, Carruthers S, Hussack P, Hargreave FE. Induced sputum: effect of filtration on the total and differential cell counts. Am J Respir Crit Care Med. 2000;161:A853.

44. Pizzichini E, Pizzichini MM, Efthimiadis A, Evans S, Morris MM, Squillace D, et al. Indices of airway inflammation in induced sputum: reproducibility and validity of cell and fluid-phase measurements. Am J Respir Crit Care Med. 1996 Aug;154(2 Pt 1):308-17.

45. Rerecich T, Gauvreau GM, Kelly MM, Hargreave FE, O'Byrne PM. Optimization of sputum fluid phase measurements. . Am J Respir Crit Care Med. 1999;159:A849.

46. Efthimiadis A, Hussack P, Weston S, Carruthers S, Hargreave FE. Induced sputum: effect of centrifugation on the total and differential cell counts. Eur Respir J. 2000;16:Suppl 31, 251s.

47. Popov T, Gottschalk R, Kolendowicz R, Dolovich J, Powers P, Hargreave FE. The evaluation of a cell dispersion method of sputum examination. Clin Exp Allergy. 1994 Aug;24(8):778-83.

48. Spanevello A, Beghe B, Bianchi A, Migliori GB, Ambrosetti M, Neri M, et al. Comparison of two methods of processing induced sputum: selected versus entire sputum. Am J Respir Crit Care Med. 1998 Feb;157(2):665-8.

49. Ronchi MC, Galli G, Zonefrati R, Tanini A, Scano G, Duranti R. Sputum processing: a new method to improve cytospin quality. Clin Exp Allergy. 2002 May;32(5):674-80.

50. Fleury-Feith J, Escudier E, Pocholle MJ, Carre C, Bernaudin JF. The effects of cytocentrifugation on differential cell counts in samples obtained by bronchoalveolar lavage. Acta Cytol. 1987 Sep-Oct;31(5):606-10.

51. Mordelet-Dambrine M, Arnoux A, Stanislas-Leguern G, Sandron D, Chretien J, Huchon G. Processing of lung lavage fluid causes variability in bronchoalveolar cell count. Am Rev Respir Dis. 1984 Aug;130(2):305-6.

52. Saraiva-Romanholo BM, Barnabe V, Carvalho AL, Martins MA, Saldiva PH, Nunes Mdo P. Comparison of three methods for differential cell count in induced sputum. Chest. 2003 Sep; 124(3):1060-6.

53. Gauvreau GM, Lee JM, Watson RM, Irani AM, Schwartz LB, O'Byrne PM. Increased numbers of both airway basophils and mast cells in sputum after allergen inhalation challenge of atopic asthmatics. Am J Respir Crit Care Med. 2000 May;161(5):1473-8.

54. Brandtzaeg P. The increasing power of immunohistochemistry and immunocytochemistry. J Immunol Methods. 1998 Jul 1;216(1-2):49-67.

55. Frew AJ, Kay AB. The relationship between infiltrating CD4+ lymphocytes, activated eosinophils, and the magnitude of the allergen-induced late phase cutaneous reaction in man. J Immunol. 1988 Dec 15;141(12):4158-64.

56. Hamid Q, Wharton J, Terenghi G, Hassall CJ, Aimi J, Taylor KM, et al. Localization of atrial natriuretic peptide mRNA and immunoreactivity in the rat heart and human atrial appendage. Proc Natl Acad Sci U S A. 1987 Oct; 84(19):6760-4.

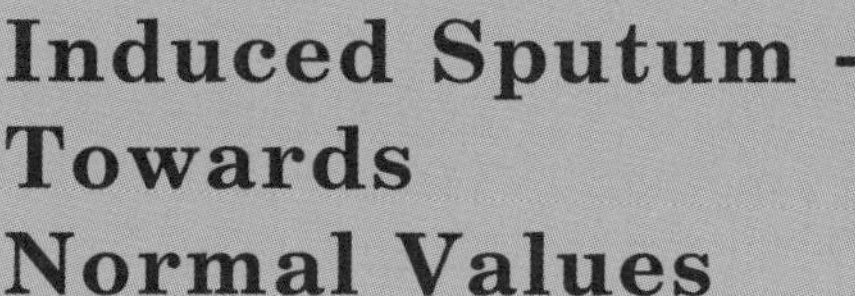

Induced Sputum - Towards Normal Values

Renaud Louis • *Laurent Godinas* • *Florence Schleich*

nduced sputum is a non invasive technique to collect airway cells and lining fluid. Since its first description in the early nineties as a diagnostic tool to spot Pneumocystis carinii in AIDS patients (1), the technique has been abundantly employed as a research tool in chronic airway diseases and in particular in asthma and COPD. It soon appears that induced sputum read-outs had the potential to be used in order to monitor airway inflammation in clinical practice. However such an application obviously first requires to determine whether the technique is sufficiently reliable and what can be considered as an abnormal value.

Success Rate of the Procedure

When considering the utility of a new investigation technique, it is always of paramount importance to assess the success rate of the pro-

Correspondence ———————————————————————————————————
Prof. Renaud Louis
Department of Pneumology, CHU Liege, GIGA Research Group Infection, Inflammation and Immunity, University of Liege, Belgium
e-mail: R.Louis@chu.ulg.ac.be

cedure. As far as induced sputum is concerned the success rate is defined by an induction that ultimately gives a countable cytospin. In healthy subjects it is around 80% (2, 3), while it reaches 90% in mild to moderate asthma (4, 5). The success rate in severe asthma is somewhat less only approaching 70% (6, 7). Series in COPD are more limited. Rytila et al reported that 96% (26/27) of patients were able to produce an adequate sample (8). Sputum induction is recognized to be more difficult in children with a reported success rate of 56% on a series of 114 healthy children whose mean age was 11 years (9).

Cell Counts in Healthy Subjects

As the technique is non-invasive it has been applied to a large series of healthy subjects in order to derive reference values. There are at least three detailed published studies that investigated the sputum cell counts in a large number of healthy subjects (Table 1). All these three studies selected non smoking subjects who denied any respiratory symptoms by the time of the sputum induction. They all had normal spirometric values and no bronchial hyperresponsiveness to methacholine. All these investigators used the "plug" method to process the sputum. The first one conducted by Belda et al in Canada looked at subjects recruited through local advertisement (2). It showed that the average total cell counts were around 4. 10^6/ml of sputum and that macrophages and neutrophils accounted for most of the cells since they made up together more than 95% of the cells recovered. Spanevello et al made a very similar finding on a series of 96 healthy subjects derived from northern Italy (3), although the proportion of neutrophils appears to be less and that of macrophages greater than in Belda's study. The percentages of macrophages and neutrophils appeared to be normally distributed while the total cell counts and the percentage of eosinophils, lymphocytes and epithelial cells followed a non Gaussian distribution. The third study by Thomas et al was conducted in UK and recruited 66 healthy subjects. Here the percentage of neutrophils was the highest of the three studies with a clear positive correlation between the age and the percentage of neutrophils (10).

Our own experience (Godinas) on a series of 113 healthy subjects, including 24 current smokers, shows that the total number of cells was slightly lower averaging 1. 10^6 cells/g of sputum. The lower total cell counts may be explained by the fact that we used the "whole sample" thereby diluting the cells in airway lining fluid and saliva. We confirm that macrophage and neutrophils were the two prominent cell types. Interestingly, we found a greater percentage of columnar epithelial cells than in the three other studies that used the "plug" method (Table 1).

When deriving the upper limit of the 90% reference interval (mean + 1.7 SD), abnormally high neutrophil count ranges from 49% according to Spanevello to 93% according to Thomas, most of the authors setting the threshold between 61% and 76% (Table 2). Furthermore, in keeping

TABLE 1

REFERENCE VALUES FOR TOTAL AND DIFFERENTIAL CELL COUNTS IN HEALTHY SUBJECTS

Authors	N	Procedure	Cell count	Mean	SD
Belda	96	Plug	Total (10^6/ml)	4.13	4.81
			Macrophages (%)	58.8	21
			Neutrophils (%)	37.5	20.1
			Eosinophils (%)	0.4	0.9
			Lymphocytes (%)	1	1.1
			Epithelial cells (%)	1.6	3.9
Spanevello	96	Plug	Total (10^6/ml)	2.70	2.50
			Macrophages (%)	69.2	13
			Neutrophils (%)	27.3	13
			Eosinophils (%)	0.6	0.8
			Lymphocytes (%)	1	1.2
			Epithelial cells (%)	1.5	1.8
Thomas	66	Plug	Total (10^6/ml)	2.1	2.36
			Macrophages (%)	49	25.2
			Neutrophils (%)	47	27
			Eosinophils (%)	0.3	0.6
			Lymphocytes (%)	1	1.4
			Epithelial cells (%)	2.5	3.2
Godinas	113	Whole	Total (10^6/g)	0.97	1.3
			Macrophages (%)	50.6	22.2
			Neutrophils (%)	34.9	24.3
			Eosinophils (%)	0.4	1.3
			Lymphocytes (%)	2.8	2.4
			Epithelial cells (%)	10.9	13.4

TABLE 2

REFERENCE VALUES FOR THE PERCENTAGE OF SPUTUM NEUTROPHILS

	N	Mean age	Mean	SD	Upper limit of 90% reference interval +
Belda	96	?	37.5	20.1	71%
Spanevello	96	38	27.3	13	49%
Green	34	34	30.8	19	65%
Simpson	42	?	?	?	61%*
Thomas	66	44	47	27	93%
Godinas	113	37	34.9	24.3	76%

+ two tailed test
* 95% percentile

to what found by Thomas et al, the influence of age on sputum neutrophil counts was critical in our series, with an abnormal threshold of 64% in subjects younger than 40 years while only percentage >81% should be considered as abnormal in those older than 40 years.

However, irrespective of the age, the range is surprisingly wide between the studies and the explanation for this is not clear at present. It is recognized that the number of neutrophils may rise rapidly in the sputum as a consequence of airways irritation(11) or exposure to various pollutants (12-14). Thus, it is conceivable that ambient atmospheric pollution or the type of job of the volunteers may be important. Some studies reported greater percentage of neutrophils in healthy smokers as compared to healthy non smokers (15), but this is not our experience as long the smoking subjects deny chronic respiratory symptoms. Whichever the reason, it calls for caution in the interpretation of what is considered as a neutrophilic phenotype. Indeed this phenotype can only be defined in comparison to what is observed in healthy subjects.

The percentage of sputum eosinophils in healthy subjects remains very low, usually less than 2% in all studies. As opposed to what has been found for neutrophils, there is much less variation according to the centres with respect to the eosinophil percentage. The abnormal threshold ranges from 1% according to Simpson et al. (16) to 2.6% according to our own reference values (Table 3). Thomas established that the age was not influencing the eosinophil counts. Belda et al found that both the female gender and the atopic status were associated with a slightly increased sputum eosinophil count which remained on average less than 1% in healthy subjects. From all these studies and to give a safe margin in the cell counting, it has been accepted that an abnormal sputum eosinophil count is $\geq 3\%$.

Comparison with Bal and Bronchial Biopsies

Compared to BAL, sputum displays greater cell density and a different cytological profile. The proportion of granulocytes is much greater in sputum while the mononuclear cell fraction, and the lymphocyte count in particular, is less prominent (17-21). Comparison of bronchial biopsies and sputum in the same subject showed that sputum eosinophils reflects airway wall eosinophil content while this did not hold true for the neutrophils (17, 19). The latter are present in greater number in airway lumen and therefore in sputum than in airway wall. Conversely, the lymphocytes, which are prominent in the bronchial mucosa, are rare in sputum samples and not correlated with the biopsy content (17, 19). Although being rare, sputum lymphocytes are still in sufficient quantities to allow for a phenotypic characterisation using flow cytometry. CD3 represents the majority of

TABLE 3

REFERENCE VALUE FOR THE PERCENTAGE OF SPUTUM EOSINOPHILS

	N	Mean age	Mean	SD	Upper limit of 95% reference interval+
Belda	96	?	0.4	0.9	2.2%
Spanevello	96	38	0.6	0.8	2.2%
Green	34	34	?	?	1.9%
Simpson	42	?	?	?	1%*
Thomas	66	44	0.3	0.5	1.3%
Godinas	113	37	0.4	1.3	2.6%

+ one tailed test
* 95% percentile

lymphocytes recovered from sputum averaging approximately 90% of lymphocytes. CD4 are the dominant T cells representing from 50 to 75% of T cells according to a study (22).

Asthmatics with Abnormal Cell Counts

The proportion of asthmatics with raised sputum eosinophil counts has been analysed in several studies. We found that 69% of newly diagnosed non smoking mild to moderate corticoid naive asthmatics exhibited sputum eosinophilia >2% (4). This also means that approximately one third of untreated asthmatics did not have raised sputum eosinophil count. This finding is important to bear in mind in view of the negative predictive value of non eosinophilic asthma on the short term response to inhaled corticosteroids (23). Gibson et al found that only 41% of non smoking asthmatics had a sputum eosinophil counts >2.5% (24). In a series of 259 patients, Green et al found that 52% of asthmatics had a sputum eosinophil percentage greater than 1.9% (25). In a new series of almost 300 patients coming from our asthma clinic, the proportion of patients with sputum eosinophil count >3% in steroid naive patients was 44%. When considering asthmatics already receiving regular treatment with inhaled corticosteroids the proportion of patients with raised sputum eosinophil counts slightly decreases with the dose of corticosteroids to 36% for those receiving moderate dose of inhaled corticosteroids and then rises again to 45% in those more severe patients receiving high dose of inhaled corticosteroids (Figure 1). As far as neutrophils are concerned we defined an abnormally high sputum neutrophil count as a percentage >76% (> mean + 1.7 SD of our reference value found in healthy subjects matched for the age. By selecting this threshold we found that neutrophilic asthma only accounts for approximately 20% of steroid naive patients. It was observed in 6% of patients receiving low dose of corticosteroids, but rose to almost 20% in those receiving moderate to high doses of corticosteroids (Figure 1).

COPD with Abnormal Cell Counts

COPD has traditionally been seen as a neutrophilic disease, based on higher sputum neutrophil counts as compared to healthy subjects. However many early studies did not match COPD and control

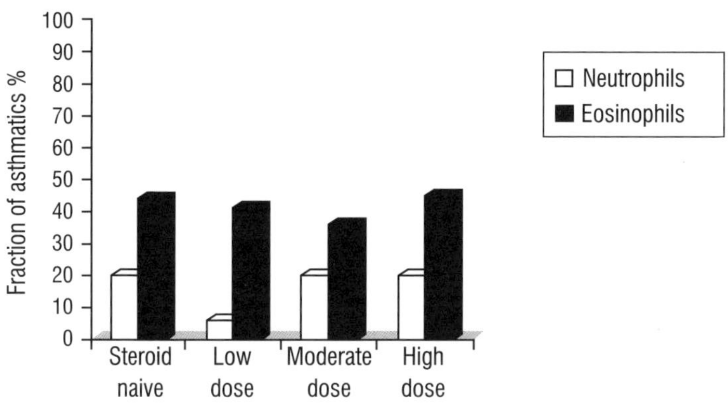

FIGURE 1

Fraction of asthmatics seen in daily parctice (N=295) with significant sputum neutrophilia (> 76%) or eosinophilia (>3%)

subjects for age, with control subjects being generally younger. Therefore most of the early studies did not account for the influence of the age on neutrophil counts and overestimate the intensity of neutrophilic inflammation in COPD. If we apply our reference value for healthy subjects greater than 40 years, it would appear that only 34% (32/94) of our stable COPD actually exhibit raised sputum neutrophil counts that is a sputum percentage of neutrophils greater than 81%. This figure may seem surprisingly low but it is still twice as much as the fraction of eosinophilic COPD in our experience. Indeed on a series of 94 COPD patients the fraction of eosinophilic COPD was 18%. On the other hand, Brightling et al found even greater proportion of eosinophilic COPD with 22 subjects out of 67 (33%) having a percentage of sputum eosinophil count >4.5%. This was confirmed by Siva et al who found that 28% COPD (23 patients out of 82) had a sputum percentage of eosinophils greater than 3%.

Does a Normal Sputum Cell Count Value Predict Response to Treatment?

It seems that asthmatics with normal sputum eosinophil counts do not benefit from a short term treatment with moderate dose of inhaled corticosteroids neither in term of symptoms and quality of life nor in term of lung function including airway hyperresponsiveness(26-28). It seems to be particularly the case for those with normal eosinophils and high sputum neutrophil counts(25). However, no long term studies in those patients looking at severe exacerbations as an outcome have been performed so far.

Does the Patient Benefit from a Return Towards a Normal Sputum Cell Count?

This question has been answered regarding the sputum eosinophil counts. It is well recognized that inhaled and oral corticosteroids are able to strongly reduce the extent of sputum eosinophil count (29, 30). As described in details in another chapter of this book, targeting a sputum eosinophilia lower than 2-3% by adjusting the dose of corticosteroids leads to significant reduction of severe exacerbation and hospitalization in both moderate to severe asthma (31, 32) and COPD (33). No studies with comparable design have been undertaken with drugs lowering the sputum neutrophils counts so far, although some drugs like theophylline and clarithromycin were reported to attenuate slightly the intensity of neutrophilic inflammation in COPD (34) and asthmatic (35) patients.

Is there any Reference Value for Biochemical Markers?

The studies looking at biochemical compounds have been much less than those looking at cell counts. The number of potentially measurable mediators/proteins is impressively high and preclude establishment of reference values for each of them. There are however some important points to bear in mind when interpreting values of biochemical compounds measured in the fluid phase of the sputum. First, the value of the mediator/protein is critically depending on the processing technique. The plug method will give much greater concentration than the method using the whole sample (36). Second, the use of a mucolytic agent for homogenising the sample and improving the quality of cytospins may profoundly alter the level of some mediators.

For example, using DTE may rise the recovered amount of ECP and tryptase (37) whereas it may reduce that of MPO (38).

Conclusion

Much work has been done to validate the cell counts in induced sputum. It stands clear that the percentages of eosinophils and neutrophils are valuable and robust parameters that can be taken into consideration in phenotyping the airway diseases and in particular asthma and COPD.

References

1. Bigby TD, Margolskee D, Curtis JL, Michael PF, Sheppard D, Hadley WK, et al. The usefulness of induced sputum in the diagnosis of Pneumocystis carinii pneumonia in patients with the acquired immunodeficiency syndrome. Am Rev Respir Dis. 1986 Apr;133(4):515-8.
2. Belda J, Leigh R, Parameswaran K, O'Byrne PM, Sears MR, Hargreave FE. Induced sputum cell counts in healthy adults. Am J Respir Crit Care Med. 2000 Feb;161(2 Pt 1):475-8.
3. Spanevello A, Confalonieri M, Sulotto F, Romano F, Balzano G, Migliori GB, et al. Induced sputum cellularity. Reference values and distribution in normal volunteers. Am J Respir Crit Care Med. 2000 Sep;162(3 Pt 1):1172-4.
4. Louis R, Sele J, Henket M, Cataldo D, Bettiol J, Seiden L, et al. Sputum eosinophil count in a large population of patients with mild to moderate steroid-naive asthma: distribution and relationship with methacholine bronchial hyperresponsiveness. Allergy. 2002 Oct;57(10):907-12.
5. Vlachos-Mayer H, Leigh R, Sharon RF, Hussack P, Hargreave FE. Success and safety of sputum induction in the clinical setting. Eur Respir J. 2000 Nov;16(5):997-1000.
6. de la Fuente PT, Romagnoli M, Godard P, Bousquet J, Chanez P. Safety of inducing sputum in patients with asthma of varying severity. Am J Respir Crit Care Med. 1998 Apr;157 (4 Pt 1):1127-30.
7. ten Brinke A, de Lange C, Zwinderman AH, Rabe KF, Sterk PJ, Bel EH. Sputum induction in severe asthma by a standardized protocol: predictors of excessive bronchoconstriction. Am J Respir Crit Care Med. 2001 Sep 1;164(5):749-53.
8. Rytila PH, Lindqvist AE, Laitinen LA. Safety of sputum induction in chronic obstructive pulmonary disease. Eur Respir J. 2000 Jun;15(6):1116-9.
9. Kulkarni N, Pierse N, Rushton L, Grigg J. Carbon in airway macrophages and lung function in children. N Engl J Med. 2006 Jul 6;355(1):21-30.
10. Thomas RA, Green RH, Brightling CE, Birring SS, Parker D, Wardlaw AJ, et

al. The influence of age on induced sputum differential cell counts in normal subjects. Chest. 2004 Dec;126(6):1811-4.

11. Holz O, Richter K, Jorres RA, Speckin P, Mucke M, Magnussen H. Changes in sputum composition between two inductions performed on consecutive days. Thorax. 1998 Feb;53(2):83-6.

12. Nightingale JA, Rogers DF, Hart LA, Kharitonov SA, Chung KF, Barnes PJ. Effect of inhaled endotoxin on induced sputum in normal, atopic, and atopic asthmatic subjects. Thorax. 1998 Jul;53(7):563-71.

13. Nightingale JA, Maggs R, Cullinan P, Donnelly LE, Rogers DF, Kinnersley R, et al. Airway inflammation after controlled exposure to diesel exhaust particulates. Am J Respir Crit Care Med. 2000 Jul;162(1):161-6.

14. Michel O, Nagy AM, Schroeven M, Duchateau J, Neve J, Fondu P, et al. Dose-response relationship to inhaled endotoxin in normal subjects. Am J Respir Crit Care Med. 1997 Oct;156(4 Pt 1):1157-64.

15. Keatings VM, Barnes PJ. Granulocyte activation markers in induced sputum: comparison between chronic obstructive pulmonary disease, asthma, and normal subjects. Am J Respir Crit Care Med. 1997 Feb;155(2):449-53.

16. Simpson JL, Scott R, Boyle MJ, Gibson PG. Inflammatory subtypes in asthma: assessment and identification using induced sputum. Respirology. 2006 Jan;11(1):54-61.

17. Grootendorst DC, Sont JK, Willems LN, Kluin-Nelemans JC, Van Krieken JH, Veselic-Charvat M, et al. Comparison of inflammatory cell counts in asthma: induced sputum vs bronchoalveolar lavage and bronchial biopsies. Clin Exp Allergy. 1997 Jul;27(7):769-79.

18. Keatings VM, Evans DJ, O'Connor BJ, Barnes PJ. Cellular profiles in asthmatic airways: a comparison of induced sputum, bronchial washings, and bronchoalveolar lavage fluid. Thorax. 1997 Apr;52(4):372-4.

19. Maestrelli P, Saetta M, Di Stefano A, Calcagni PG, Turato G, Ruggieri MP, et al. Comparison of leukocyte counts in sputum, bronchial biopsies, and bronchoalveolar lavage. Am J Respir Crit Care Med. 1995 Dec;152(6 Pt 1):1926-31.

20. Pizzichini E, Pizzichini MM, Kidney JC, Efthimiadis A, Hussack P, Popov T, et al. Induced sputum, bronchoalveolar lavage and blood from mild asthmatics: inflammatory cells, lymphocyte subsets and soluble markers compared. Eur Respir J. 1998 Apr;11(4):828-34.

21. Fahy JV, Wong H, Liu J, Boushey HA. Comparison of samples collected by sputum induction and bronchoscopy from asthmatic and healthy subjects. Am J Respir Crit Care Med. 1995 Jul;152(1):53-8.

22. Louis R, Shute J, Biagi S, Stanciu L, Marrelli F, Tenor H, et al. Cell infiltration, ICAM-1 expression, and eosinophil chemotactic activity in asthmatic sputum. Am J Respir Crit Care Med. 1997 Feb;155(2):466-72.

23. Haldar P, Pavord ID. Noneosinophilic asthma: a distinct clinical and pathologic phenotype. J Allergy Clin Immunol. 2007 May;119(5):1043-52; quiz 53-4.

24. Gibson PG, Simpson JL, Saltos N. Heterogeneity of airway inflammation in persistent asthma: evidence of neutrophilic inflammation and increased sputum interleukin-8. Chest. 2001 May;119(5):1329-36.

25. Green RH, Brightling CE, Woltmann G, Parker D, Wardlaw AJ, Pavord ID. Analysis of induced sputum in adults with asthma: identification of subgroup with isolated sputum neutrophilia and poor response to inhaled corticosteroids. Thorax. 2002 Oct;57(10): 875-9.

26. Bacci E, Cianchetti S, Bartoli M, Dente FL, Di Franco A, Vagaggini B, et al. Low sputum eosinophils predict the lack of response to beclomethasone in symptomatic asthmatic patients. Chest. 2006 Mar;129(3):565-72.

27. Berry M, Morgan A, Shaw DE, Parker D, Green R, Brightling C, et al. Pathological features and inhaled corticosteroid response of eosinophilic and non-eosinophilic asthma. Thorax. 2007 Dec;62(12):1043-9.

28. Pavord ID, Brightling CE, Woltmann G, Wardlaw AJ. Non-eosinophilic corticosteroid unresponsive asthma. Lancet. 1999 Jun 26;353(9171): 2213-4.

29. Claman DM, Boushey HA, Liu J, Wong H, Fahy JV. Analysis of induced sputum to examine the effects of prednisone on airway inflammation in asthmatic subjects. J Allergy Clin Immunol. 1994 Nov;94(5):861-9.

30. Lim S, Jatakanon A, John M, Gilbey T, O'Connor B J, Chung KF, et al. Effect of inhaled budesonide on lung function and airway inflammation. Assessment by various inflammatory markers in mild asthma. Am J Respir Crit Care Med. 1999 Jan;159(1):22-30.

31. Green RH, Brightling CE, McKenna S, Hargadon B, Parker D, Bradding P, et al. Asthma exacerbations and sputum eosinophil counts: a randomised controlled trial. Lancet. 2002 Nov 30;360(9347):1715-21.

32. Jayaram L, Pizzichini MM, Cook RJ, Boulet LP, Lemiere C, Pizzichini E, et al. Determining asthma treatment by monitoring sputum cell counts: effect on exacerbations. Eur Respir J. 2006 Mar;27(3):483-94.

33. Siva R, Green RH, Brightling CE, Shelley M, Hargadon B, McKenna S, et al. Eosinophilic airway inflammation and exacerbations of COPD: a randomised controlled trial. Eur Respir J. 2007 May;29(5):906-13.

34. Culpitt SV, de Matos C, Russell RE, Donnelly LE, Rogers DF, Barnes PJ. Effect of theophylline on induced sputum inflammatory indices and neutrophil chemotaxis in chronic obstructive pulmonary disease. Am J Respir Crit Care Med. 2002 May 15;165(10): 1371-6.

35. Simpson JL, Powell H, Boyle MJ, Scott RJ, Gibson PG. Clarithromycin targets neutrophilic airway inflammation in refractory asthma. Am J Respir Crit Care Med. 2008 Jan 15;177(2):148-55.

36. Spanevello A, Beghe B, Bianchi A, Migliori GB, Ambrosetti M, Neri M, et al. Comparison of two methods of processing induced sputum: selected versus entire sputum. Am J Respir Crit Care Med. 1998 Feb;157(2):665-8.

37. Louis R, Shute J, Goldring K, Perks B,

Lau LC, Radermecker M, et al. The effect of processing on inflammatory markers in induced sputum. Eur Respir J. 1999 Mar;13(3):660-7.

38. Woolhouse IS, Bayley DL, Stockley RA. Effect of sputum processing with dithiothreitol on the detection of inflammatory mediators in chronic bronchitis and bronchiectasis. Thorax. 2002 Aug;57(8):667-71.

Induced Sputum in Asthma: Application in Clinical Practice

Ian D. Pavord
Neil Martin

Although airway inflammation is thought to be an important component of asthma it is not routinely assessed in clinical practice. However, over the last 15-20 years there has been an explosion of interest in the potential clinical application of non-invasive measures of airway inflammation and this situation may change. In this chapter we review the use of induced sputum as a means of assessing airway inflammation and speculate on the potential clinical value of this assessment in asthma.

Induced sputum and sputum differential inflammatory cell counting can be used to determine the characteristics and intensity of the lower airway inflammatory response (Table 1). It has notable advantages over exhaled nitric oxide (FeNO), which provides only limited information on the nature of the inflammatory response. The main limitation of induced sputum is that results are not available immedi-

Correspondence

Prof. Ian D. Pavord
Institute for Lung Health, Department of Respiratory medicine, Allergy and Thoracic Surgery, Glenfield Hospital, University of Leicester Hospitals NHS Trust, Groby Road, Leicester, LE3 9QP, UK
e-mail: ian.pavord@uhl-tr.nhs.uk

CELL TYPES AND MOLECULAR MARKERS THAT HAVE BEEN SUCCESSFULLY MEASURED IN INDUCED SPUTUM

Cells	Effector Mediators	Cellular Markers	Cytokines/ chemokines
eosinophils	leukotrienes	eosinophilic	Interleukin-8
neutrophils	$C/D/E_4$	cationic	
macrophages	prostaglandin	protein	
lymphocytes	D_2	neutrophil	
epithelial	histamine	elastase	
Mast cells			

ately, limiting the application of the technique in asthma monitoring. FeNO has the advantage of being simple to measure and provides an immediate result. The different strengths and weaknesses of the techniques suggests that they may find different roles, with FeNO being used mainly in primary care to facilitate diagnosis and to titrate corticosteroid therapy and induced sputum used in secondary and tertiary care, where more detailed information on the type of lower airway inflammation is necessary.

Sputum differential cell counts have been shown to correlate closely with bronchial wash cell counts (1), less closely with bronchoalveolar lavage counts (1, 2), and not at all with biopsy cell counts (3). This may reflect sampling of different airway compartments by the different techniques and the fact that some cell types (notably eosinophils and neutrophils) are not tissue dwelling.

Normal ranges have been published for a large adult population (4-6) (Table 2). Age has been shown to influence differential sputum neutrophil counts, with the higher values occurring in the older age groups (6). Sputum differential eosinophils, macrophage and neutrophil counts and the sputum supernatant concentration of eosinophilic cationic protein, cysteinyl-leukotrienes, prostanoids and IL-8 can be measured repeatably in asthma (7-9) (Table 2). The differential lymphocyte and epithelial cell count and the total cell count are less repeatable (8). Spontaneous and induced sputum have similar cell and molecular characteristics and they can be used interchangeably in asthma; there is no evidence that pre-treatment with salbutamol or a prior methacholine inhalation test influences sputum cell counts.

TABLE 2

NORMAL RANGES AND WITHIN SUBJECT REPEATABILITY OF INDUCED SPUTUM CELL COUNTS IN ADULTS.

*Figures represent mean (SD). Repeatability expressed as intra-class correlation coefficient (within subject SD or *log within subject SD). Repeatability was assessed over 2-days (in't Veen et al), 6-days (Pizzichini et al) and 1-week (Spanevello et al). #Within subject log standard deviation of sputum eosinophil count overly influenced by small absolute differences in normals; in subjects with asthma it was 0.25.*

	Normal ranges			Repeatability		
Author	Belda	Spanevello	Thomas	Pizzichini	in't Veen	Spanevello
Number (male)	96 (54)	96 (46)	66 (24)	39 (20)	21 (10)	88 (44)
Characteristics	Healthy	Healthy	Healthy	Asthma (19) Healthy (10), Smokers (10)	Asthma	Asthma (53) Healthy (19) Rhinitis (16)
Mean age	Not recorded	Not recorded	46 (25)	39	24 (4)	38
TCC ($\times 10^6$/g)	4.1 (4.8)	2.7 (2.5)	2.1 (2.4)	0.35		0.44
Eosinophils (%)	0.4 (0.9)	0.6 (0.8)	0.3 (0.6)	0.94 (0.75*)#	0.85 (6.2)	0.84 (0.17*)
Neutrophils (%)	37.5 (20.1)	27.3 (13.0)	47.0 (27.0)	0.81 (14.0)	0.57 (15.5)	0.75
Macrophages (%)	58.8 (21.0)	69.2 (13.0)	49.0 (25.2)	0.71	0.64 (7.7)	0.76
Lymphocytes (%)	1.0 (1.1)	1.0 (1.2)	1.0 (1.4)	0.25	0.76 (3.9)	0.39
Epithelial cells (%)	1.6 (3.9)	1.5 (1.8)	2.5 (3.2)		0.64 (7.7)	0.56

The sputum eosinophil count is responsive in that it increases when asthma worsens after allergen challenge and following relevant occupational exposures (10, 11), and decreases when asthma improves with inhaled corticosteroid treatment (12). Sputum and bronchoscopy studies before and after treatment with corticosteroids (12, 13) and anti IL-5 (14, 15) suggest that the sputum eosinophil count is more responsive than tissue eosinophil counts. Based on what is known about the responsiveness and repeatability of the sputum eosinophil count, a two-fold change is regarded as clinically significant (16).

Induced Sputum Findings in Asthma

Clinically relevant patterns of airway inflammation include neutrophilic, eosinophilic and mixed eosinophilic and neutrophilic (Figure 1). The latter pattern is most commonly seen in COPD, refractory asthma and in exacerbations of airway disease. A sputum neutrophilia with a raised total cell count suggests infective bronchitis, COPD and bronchiectasis; a neutrophilia with a normal total cell count is more non-specific but is commonly seen in chronic cough and non-eosinophilic asthma. A significant minority of patients with airway disease have paucigranulocytic sputum characterised by normal sputum eosinophil and neutrophil counts (Figure 1).

A raised sputum eosinophil count is the most characteristic finding in patients with asthma. 60-80% of patients with symptomatic untreated asthma and up to 50% of patients taking inhaled corticosteroids have a sputum eosinophil count above the normal range. A minority of patients with asthma of all severity grades have consistently non-eosinophilic sputum; many have a sputum neutrophilia. A raised sputum eosinophil count is not exclusive to asthma: 30-40% of patients with cough and a similar proportion of patients with COPD have a sputum eosinophilia. Roughly a half of patients with cough and a sputum eosinophilia have evidence of variable airflow obstruction and/or airway hyperresponsiveness and meet diagnostic criteria for cough variant asthma. The remainder consistently do not and are classified as having eosinophilic bronchitis. Patients with COPD and a sputum eosinophilia may have more asthma like features such as bronchodilator reversibility, atopy and airway hyperresponsiveness but there is too much overlap in the presence of these features to make it possible to reliably predict pathology on the basis of these tests.

	Normal eosinophil count (<1.9%)	Raised eosinophil count
Normal neutrophil count (<61%)	**Paucigranulocytic** Well controlled or intermittent asthma Consider alternative diagnosis	**Eosinophilic** Asthma Eosinophilic bronchitis
Raised neutrophil count	**Neutrophilic** Acute infection (viral or bacterial) Chronic infection (chlamydia, adenovirus) Smoking and COPD Environmental pollutants (ozone, NO_2) Occupational antigens Endotoxin exposure Obesity Chronic cough syndromes	**Mixed granulocytic** Exacerbations Refractory asthma COPD

FIGURE 1

Classification based on induced sputum patterns of cellular inflammation in airway disease

New Insights into the Importance of Airway Inflammation in Asthma

The development of a non-invasive technique to assess airway inflammation has made it possible to relate the presence of airway inflammation to objective measures of disordered airway function in large and more heterogeneous populations. These studies have suggested a complex relationship between airway inflammation and the pattern and severity of airway dysfunction (17-19). Clinicians and researchers interested in using measures of airway inflammation need to be aware of this relationship in order to fully appreciate the added value such measures provide. A number of key observations are particularly important.

Firstly, the pattern of airway inflammation is not closely related to either the pattern or the severity of the airway dysfunction or symptoms. A raised sputum eosinophil count is seen in 60-80% of corticosteroid naive patients with asthma and in 50% of corticosteroid treated patients with symptomatic asthma (20). There is at best a weak correlation between the presence of eosinophilic airway inflammation and the severity of symptoms or disordered airway function

(18). Thus, little can be deduced about the presence, nature and severity of airway inflammation from a standard clinical assessment (21).

This observation is important as it strongly implies that there is not a close causal link between eosinophilic airway inflammation and the airway dysfunction that underlies many of the day-to-day clinical manifestations of asthma. Further support for this view is provided by studies showing that treatment with anti-IL-5 markedly reduced eosinophilic airway inflammation, but does not affect asthma symptoms, lung function or airway responsiveness (15, 22). A comparative bronchial biopsy study of asthma and eosinophilic bronchitis has shown that infiltration of the airway smooth muscle with mast cell is only seen in asthma (23). Moreover, the extent of infiltration is closely related to airway hyperresponsiveness implying that it is the interaction between mast cells and airway smooth muscle that of fundamental importance in the genesis of airway hyperresponsiveness.

Secondly, the presence of eosinophilic airway inflammation is more closely associated with a positive response to corticosteroids than other clinical measures and is seen irrespective of the pattern of airway disease in which eosinophilic airway inflammation occurs (Figure 3) (12, 24-27). Thus, if the clinical question were whether a patient with symptoms suggesting asthma should receive corticosteroid treatment (as it often is), then the identification of eosinophilic airway inflammation would be a better basis for making this decision than the findings of other tests.

Thirdly, the sputum eosinophil count is a better marker for titrating corticosteroid therapy than standard clinical measures. Studies in asthma (28, 29) have shown that a management strategy which uses the the sputum eosinophil count to guide corticosteroid treatment results in a lower frequency of exacerbations and more economical use of corticosteroids than management guided by traditional clinical measures (Figure 2) . The findings of these studies, together with evidence that a sputum eosinophilia is an important and independent predictor of the occurrence of an asthma exacerbation following corticosteroid withdrawal (30, 31), suggest that eosinophilic airway inflammation is a more valid surrogate marker of preventable exacerbation risk than other currently available markers.

Fourthly, there is a clear and consistent positive correlation between a raised sputum neutrophil count and the presence of fixed airflow obstruction as reflected by a reduced post-bronchodilator FEV_1 and FEV_1/FVC. This is seen in patients with asthma (32) and COPD

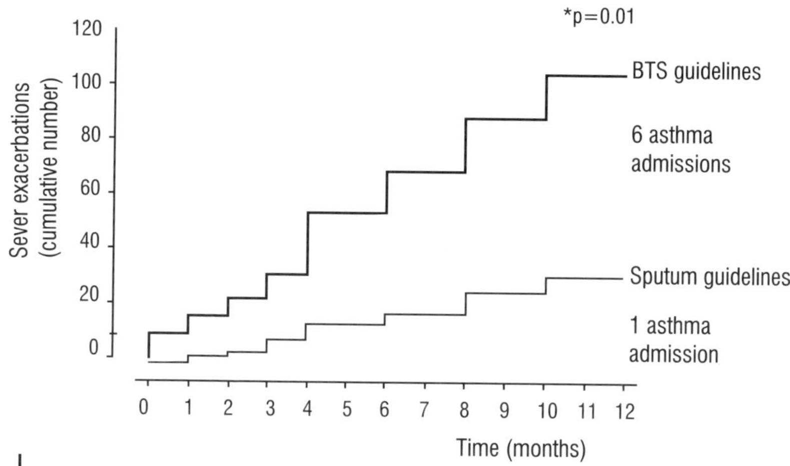

FIGURE 2

Comparison of effects of two treatment strategies on rates of severe exacerbations of asthma. One strategy (BTS guidelines) utilised standard guidelines of the British Thoracic Society (BTS)) and the other (sputum guidelines) adjusted the anti-inflammatory treatment with corticosteroids based on the sputum eosinophil counts (Reproduced after permission from Reference 6).

(33). In COPD a raised sputum neutrophil count is associated with longitudinal decline in FEV_1 (34). These findings raise the possibility of a common mechanism for the development of fixed airflow obstruction involving neutrophilic airway inflammation. Much more information is required before we can be sure that there is a causal link between neutrophilic airway inflammation and fixed airflow obstruction. In particular, there is a need for longitudinal studies evaluating the effect of reducing neutrophilic airway inflammation. Nevertheless, there is sufficient evidence to speculate that a raised sputum neutrophil count is a useful biomarker of risk of subsequent decline in lung function.

The new understanding of the importance of airway inflammation in airway disease has opened the way for a new approach to the management of airways disease in clinical practice (inflammometry), where assessment of airway inflammation is used to identify risk of future adverse outcome and likely response to treatment.

Potential Clinical Role of Inflammometry

Role in diagnosis

None of the currently available diagnostic tests are sufficiently sensitive to rule out asthma (35, 36) with the result that treatment trials are often instigated without good evidence of the condition. One study has shown that out of 263 subjects referred to a tertiary referral centre with suspected asthma, 160 received an alternative diagnosis (37). Many of these had received prolonged treatment with potentially toxic therapy before the correct diagnosis was reached. Even in tertiary referral centres the diagnosis of refractory asthma can be difficult to make with certainty (38). The presence of sputum eosinophilia in untreated asthma is sufficiently common to suggest that these findings may have a role in the diagnosis of asthma. Hunter et al (36) showed that the sensitivity of a sputum eosinophil count outside the normal range in identifying asthma (defined as consistent symptoms with objective evidence of abnormal variable airflow obstruction) was around 80%, significantly better than PEF amplitude % mean and the acute bronchodilator response, and approaching the sensitivity and specificity of measurement of airway responsiveness. Smith et al. (35) have reported similar findings; in this study a high exhaled nitric oxide concentration achieved a similarly high diagnostic accuracy.

Arguably it matters more to patients what can be done to help them than the diagnostic label attached to them. Thus, testing strategies that identify patients who are going to respond well to corticosteroid and provide guidance on the dosing of corticosteroids might be particularly helpful. There is now compelling evidence that the presence of sputum eosinophilia predicts corticosteroid responsiveness. This was first clearly demonstrated by Morrow-Brown in the 1950's who showed that patients with airway disease and a sputum eosinophilia responded to corticosteroid treatment whereas those without a sputum eosinophilia did not (39). It has since been shown that patients with non-eosinophilic asthma respond less well to inhaled budesonide than a group with more typical sputum features (12, 27). This is also the case with longer-term corticosteroid treatment in patients with more severe asthma(29). A sputum eosinophilia (40) is a predictor of a steroid response irrespective of the clinical context: patients with chronic cough respond well to inhaled corticosteroids if there is a sputum eosinophilia (25, 41) and patients with

COPD with a sputum eosinophilia respond better to systemic and inhaled corticosteroids than those without (24, 26, 42).

Role in monitoring asthma

Once a decision is made to start corticosteroid treatment the next question is how best to titrate this therapy. Traditionally dose titration is done by assessing the clinical response to treatment and attempting to define the lowest dose of inhaled corticosteroid that maintains this. Many patients do very well with this approach (43) but there is evidence that the use of the induced sputum eosinophil count to titrate therapy results in a lower exacerbation frequency with no overall increase in treatment (Figure 2) (28, 29).

The benefit of sputum eosinophil directed management is much more clearly seen in patients with more severe asthma (28). Patients taking long acting β_2-agonists do particularly well and it is possible that the increased dissociation between eosinophilic airway inflammation and symptoms seen after treatment with long acting β_2-agonists (44) is an important determinate of this. Whether inflammation guided management offers advantages to symptom guided management in patients with less severe asthma is uncertain. Experience with FeNO as the biomarker in this sort of population has been mixed (40, 45, 46) although in one study equally good asthma control was achieved with FeNO guided management with a 45% lower daily dose of inhaled corticosteroids (40).

The identification of severe asthma phenotypes and phenotype specific management

Why does inflammation guided management work so much better in patients with severe asthma? One possibility is that the phenotypic diversity is greater in patients with severe asthma and non-invasive measures of airway inflammation facilitate identification of this diversity allowing appropriate targeting of treatment. We have recently explored the phenotypes of severe asthma using a multidimensional analysis technique called cluster analysis (47). Figure 3 shows the outcome of this analysis in 2 populations: a population of adults with mainly mild to moderate asthma recruited from primary care; and a population recruited from secondary care who met American Thoracic Society criteria (48) for refractory asthma. The cluster analysis identified 2 clusters unique to refractory asthma which were characterised by marked discrepancy between the day-to-day clinical expression of their disease and eosinophilic airway inflammation. Traditional symptom guided management would lead to over- or under-treatment of these phenotypes, leading to poor outcomes. Retrospective analysis of an earlier study (29) showed that inflammation guided asthma management allowed these phenotypes to be identified and facilitated appropriate targeting of treatment. In the inflammation predominant cluster, the main benefit of this approach was a reduction in severe asthma exacerbations whereas in the symptom-predominant cluster excess corticosteroid treatment was avoided and more fruitful management approaches were explored at an earlier stage.

Identification of different inflammatory phenotypes of asthma may be particularly important in the development of new highly selective immunomodulatory agents. Mepolizumab, a monoclonal antibody to IL-5, is an effective inhibitor of eosinophilic airway inflammation, but its preclinical development was delayed after disappointing findings on asthma symptoms and lung function (15, 49). However, patients participating in these studies were selected on the basis of physiological findings rather than the presence of eosinophilic airway inflammation and the outcomes measures chosen are not closely linked to eosinophilic airway inflammation. Recent trials done in patients selected by inflammatory phenotype have shown much more encouraging results against asthma exacerbations, an outcome measure particularly relevant to that phenotype (50, 51).

Identification of the symptom predominant, non-eosinophilic cluster may also allow appropriate targeting of new treatments. Treatments directed against airway smooth muscle such as bronchial thermoplasty may be particularly helpful. Many patients in this cluster have sputum evidence of neutrophilic airway inflammation and anti-neutrophil strategies may be of particular value in this sub-group. In support of this, Simpson et al have shown that long-term treatment with clarithromycin in patients with refractory asthma was particularly beneficial in patients with non-eosinophilic asthma (52).

Future Directions

There is an urgent need for a non-invasive technique capable of providing accurate information on the characteristics of the lower airway inflammatory response from an easily accessible sample. The technique should be capable of providing an immediate result and

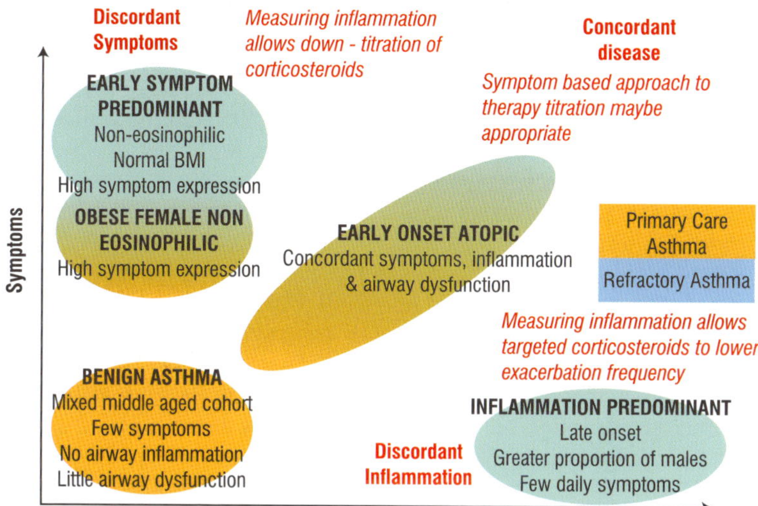

FIGURE 3

A summary of phenotypes identified using cluster analysis in primary and secondary care asthma populations. The clusters are plotted according to their relative expression of symptoms and inflammation as these are the two clinically pertinent and modifiable dimensions of the disease. The plot highlights greater discordance to be a feature of secondary care asthma. Although reasons for this dissociation are unclear, the utilisation of measures of airway inflammation in these subgroups is clinically informative [Adapted after permission from Haldar et al. (47)].

be useable in acute as well as outpatient settings. Whether FeNO or exhaled breath condensate analysis as they currently stand are ideal for this purpose is doubtful. Refinements of breath analysis, or perhaps identification of novel biomarkers in urine or blood are perhaps most likely to advance this area. Work already done with induced sputum provides a strong scientific rationale for the use of these markers as a means of defining risk and likely treatment response.

References

1. Keatings VM, Evans DJ, O'Connor BJ, Barnes PJ. Cellular profiles in asthmatic airways: a comparison of induced sputum, bronchial washings,

and bronchoalveolar lavage fluid. Thorax. 1997 Apr;52(4):372-4.

2. Pizzichini E, Pizzichini MM, Kidney JC, Efthimiadis A, Hussack P, Popov T, et al. Induced sputum, bronchoalveolar lavage and blood from mild asthmatics: inflammatory cells, lymphocyte subsets and soluble markers compared. Eur Respir J. 1998 Apr;11(4):828-34.

3. Maestrelli P, Saetta M, Di Stefano A, Calcagni PG, Turato G, Ruggieri MP, et al. Comparison of leukocyte counts in sputum, bronchial biopsies, and bronchoalveolar lavage. Am J Respir Crit Care Med. 1995 Dec;152(6 Pt 1):1926-31.

4. Belda J, Leigh R, Parameswaran K, O'Byrne PM, Sears MR, Hargreave FE. Induced sputum cell counts in healthy adults. Am J Respir Crit Care Med. 2000 Feb;161(2 Pt 1):475-8.

5. Spanevello A, Confalonieri M, Sulotto F, Romano F, Balzano G, Migliori GB, et al. Induced sputum cellularity. Reference values and distribution in normal volunteers. Am J Respir Crit Care Med. 2000 Sep;162(3 Pt 1):1172-4.

6. Thomas RA, Green RH, Brightling CE, Birring SS, Parker D, Wardlaw AJ, et al. The influence of age on induced sputum differential cell counts in normal subjects. Chest. 2004 Dec;126(6):1811-4.

7. in 't Veen JC, de Gouw HW, Smits HH, Sont JK, Hiemstra PS, Sterk PJ, et al. Repeatability of cellular and soluble markers of inflammation in induced sputum from patients with asthma. Eur Respir J. 1996 Dec;9(12):2441-7.

8. Pizzichini E, Pizzichini MM, Efthimiadis A, Evans S, Morris MM, Squillace D, et al. Indices of airway inflammation in induced sputum: reproducibility and validity of cell and fluid-phase measurements. Am J Respir Crit Care Med. 1996 Aug;154(2 Pt 1):308-17.

9. Pavord ID, Ward R, Woltmann G, Wardlaw AJ, Sheller JR, Dworski R. Induced sputum eicosanoid concentrations in asthma. Am J Respir Crit Care Med. 1999 Dec;160(6):1905-9.

10. Lemiere C, Pizzichini MM, Balkissoon R, Clelland L, Efthimiadis A, O'Shaughnessy D, et al. Diagnosing occupational asthma: use of induced sputum. Eur Respir J. 1999 Mar;13(3):482-8.

11. Pizzichini MM, Kidney JC, Wong BJ, Morris MM, Efthimiadis A, Dolovich J, et al. Effect of salmeterol compared with beclomethasone on allergen-induced asthmatic and inflammatory responses. Eur Respir J. 1996 Mar;9(3):449-55.

12. Pavord ID, Brightling CE, Woltmann G, Wardlaw AJ. Non-eosinophilic corticosteroid unresponsive asthma. Lancet. 1999 Jun 26;353(9171):2213-4.

13. Bentley AM, Hamid Q, Robinson DS, Schotman E, Meng Q, Assoufi B, et al. Prednisolone treatment in asthma. Reduction in the numbers of eosinophils, T cells, tryptase-only positive mast cells, and modulation of IL-4, IL-5, and interferon-gamma cytokine gene expression within the bronchial mucosa. Am J Respir Crit Care Med. 1996 Feb;153(2):551-6.

14. Flood-Page P, Menzies-Gow A, Phipps S, Ying S, Wangoo A, Ludwig MS, et al. Anti-IL-5 treatment reduces deposition of ECM proteins in the bronchial subepithelial basement membrane of mild atopic asthmatics.

J Clin Invest. 2003 Oct;112(7):1029-36.

15. Leckie MJ, ten Brinke A, Khan J, Diamant Z, O'Connor BJ, Walls CM, et al. Effects of an interleukin-5 blocking monoclonal antibody on eosinophils, airway hyper-responsiveness, and the late asthmatic response. Lancet. 2000 Dec 23-30;356(9248):2144-8.

16. Pavord ID, Sterk PJ, Hargreave FE, Kips JC, Inman MD, Louis R, et al. Clinical applications of assessment of airway inflammation using induced sputum. Eur Respir J Suppl. 2002 Sep;37:40s-3s.

17. Green RH, Brightling CE, Woltmann G, Parker D, Wardlaw AJ, Pavord ID. Analysis of induced sputum in adults with asthma: identification of subgroup with isolated sputum neutrophilia and poor response to inhaled corticosteroids. Thorax. 2002 Oct;57(10):875-9.

18. Rosi E, Ronchi MC, Grazzini M, Duranti R, Scano G. Sputum analysis, bronchial hyperresponsiveness, and airway function in asthma: results of a factor analysis. J Allergy Clin Immunol. 1999 Feb;103(2 Pt 1):232-7.

19. Crimi E, Spanevello A, Neri M, Ind PW, Rossi GA, Brusasco V. Dissociation between airway inflammation and airway hyperresponsiveness in allergic asthma. Am J Respir Crit Care Med. 1998 Jan;157(1):4-9.

20. Gibson PG, Fujimura M, Niimi A. Eosinophilic bronchitis: clinical manifestations and implications for treatment. Thorax. 2002 Feb;57(2):178-82.

21. Parameswaran K, Pizzichini E, Pizzichini MM, Hussack P, Efthimiadis A, Hargreave FE. Clinical judgement of airway inflammation versus sputum cell counts in patients with asthma. Eur Respir J. 2000 Mar;15(3):486-90.

22. Kips JC, O'Connor BJ, Langley SJ, Woodcock A, Kerstjens HA, Postma DS, et al. Effect of SCH55700, a humanized anti-human interleukin-5 antibody, in severe persistent asthma: a pilot study. Am J Respir Crit Care Med. 2003 Jun 15;167(12):1655-9.

23. Brightling CE, Bradding P, Symon FA, Holgate ST, Wardlaw AJ, Pavord ID. Mast-cell infiltration of airway smooth muscle in asthma. N Engl J Med. 2002 May 30;346(22):1699-705.

24. Brightling CE, Monteiro W, Ward R, Parker D, Morgan MD, Wardlaw AJ, et al. Sputum eosinophilia and short-term response to prednisolone in chronic obstructive pulmonary disease: a randomised controlled trial. Lancet. 2000 Oct 28;356(9240):1480-5.

25. Brightling CE, Ward R, Wardlaw AJ, Pavord ID. Airway inflammation, airway responsiveness and cough before and after inhaled budesonide in patients with eosinophilic bronchitis. Eur Respir J. 2000 Apr;15(4):682-6.

26. Pizzichini E, Pizzichini MM, Gibson P, Parameswaran K, Gleich GJ, Berman L, et al. Sputum eosinophilia predicts benefit from prednisone in smokers with chronic obstructive bronchitis. Am J Respir Crit Care Med. 1998 Nov;158(5 Pt 1):1511-7.

27. Berry M, Morgan A, Shaw DE, Parker D, Green R, Brightling C, et al. Pathological features and inhaled corticosteroid response of eosinophilic and non-eosinophilic asthma. Thorax. 2007 Dec;62(12):1043-9.

28. Jayaram L, Pizzichini MM, Cook RJ, Boulet LP, Lemiere C, Pizzichini E, et

al. Determining asthma treatment by monitoring sputum cell counts: effect on exacerbations. Eur Respir J. 2006 Mar;27(3):483-94.

29. Green RH, Brightling CE, McKenna S, Hargadon B, Parker D, Bradding P, et al. Asthma exacerbations and sputum eosinophil counts: a randomised controlled trial. Lancet. 2002 Nov 30;360 (9347):1715-21.

30. Jatakanon A, Lim S, Barnes PJ. Changes in sputum eosinophils predict loss of asthma control. Am J Respir Crit Care Med. 2000 Jan;161 (1):64-72.

31. Leuppi JD, Salome CM, Jenkins CR, Anderson SD, Xuan W, Marks GB, et al. Predictive markers of asthma exacerbation during stepwise dose reduction of inhaled corticosteroids. Am J Respir Crit Care Med. 2001 Feb;163 (2):406-12.

32. Shaw DE, Berry MA, Hargadon B, McKenna S, Shelley MJ, Green RH, et al. Association between neutrophilic airway inflammation and airflow limitation in adults with asthma. Chest. 2007 Dec;132(6):1871-5.

33. Keatings VM, Collins PD, Scott DM, Barnes PJ. Differences in interleukin-8 and tumor necrosis factor-alpha in induced sputum from patients with chronic obstructive pulmonary disease or asthma. Am J Respir Crit Care Med. 1996 Feb;153(2):530-4.

34. Stanescu D, Sanna A, Veriter C, Kostianev S, Calcagni PG, Fabbri LM, et al. Airways obstruction, chronic expectoration, and rapid decline of FEV1 in smokers are associated with increased levels of sputum neutrophils. Thorax. 1996 Mar;51(3):267-71.

35. Smith AD, Cowan JO, Filsell S, McLachlan C, Monti-Sheehan G, Jackson P, et al. Diagnosing asthma: comparisons between exhaled nitric oxide measurements and conventional tests. Am J Respir Crit Care Med. 2004 Feb 15;169(4):473-8.

36. Hunter CJ, Brightling CE, Woltmann G, Wardlaw AJ, Pavord ID. A comparison of the validity of different diagnostic tests in adults with asthma. Chest. 2002 Apr;121(4):1051-7.

37. Joyce DP, Chapman KR, Kesten S. Prior diagnosis and treatment of patients with normal results of methacholine challenge and unexplained respiratory symptoms. Chest. 1996 Mar;109(3):697-701.

38. Robinson DS, Campbell DA, Durham SR, Pfeffer J, Barnes PJ, Chung KF. Systematic assessment of difficult-to-treat asthma. Eur Respir J. 2003 Sep; 22(3):478-83.

39. Brown HM. Treatment of chronic asthma with prednisolone; significance of eosinophils in the sputum. Lancet. 1958 Dec 13;2(7059):1245-7.

40. Smith AD, Cowan JO, Brassett KP, Herbison GP, Taylor DR. Use of exhaled nitric oxide measurements to guide treatment in chronic asthma. N Engl J Med. 2005 May 26;352(21): 2163-73.

41. Pizzichini MM, Pizzichini E, Parameswaran K, Clelland L, Efthimiadis A, Dolovich J, et al. Nonasthmatic chronic cough: No effect of treatment with an inhaled corticosteroid in patients without sputum eosinophilia. Can Respir J. 1999 Jul-Aug;6(4):323-30.

42. Brightling CE, McKenna S, Hargadon B, Birring S, Green R, Siva R, et al.

Sputum eosinophilia and the short term response to inhaled mometasone in chronic obstructive pulmonary disease. Thorax. 2005 Mar;60(3):193-8.

43. Bateman ED, Boushey HA, Bousquet J, Busse WW, Clark TJ, Pauwels RA, et al. Can guideline-defined asthma control be achieved? The Gaining Optimal Asthma ControL study. Am J Respir Crit Care Med. 2004 Oct 15; 170(8):836-44.

44. McIvor RA, Pizzichini E, Turner MO, Hussack P, Hargreave FE, Sears MR. Potential masking effects of salmeterol on airway inflammation in asthma. Am J Respir Crit Care Med. 1998 Sep;158(3):924-30.

45. Shaw DE, Berry MA, Thomas M, Green RH, Brightling CE, Wardlaw AJ, et al. The use of exhaled nitric oxide to guide asthma management: a randomized controlled trial. Am J Respir Crit Care Med. 2007 Aug 1;176(3):231-7.

46. Szefler SJ, Mitchell H, Sorkness CA, Gergen PJ, O'Connor GT, Morgan WJ, et al. Management of asthma based on exhaled nitric oxide in addition to guideline-based treatment for inner-city adolescents and young adults: a randomised controlled trial. Lancet. 2008 Sep 20;372(9643):1065-72.

47. Haldar P, Pavord ID, Shaw DE, Berry MA, Thomas M, Brightling CE, et al. Cluster analysis and clinical asthma phenotypes. Am J Respir Crit Care Med. 2008 Aug 1;178(3):218-24.

48. Proceedings of the ATS workshop on refractory asthma: current understanding, recommendations, and unanswered questions. American Thoracic Society. Am J Respir Crit Care Med. 2000 Dec;162(6):2341-51.

49. Flood-Page P, Swenson C, Faiferman I, Matthews J, Williams M, Brannick L, et al. A study to evaluate safety and efficacy of mepolizumab in patients with moderate persistent asthma. Am J Respir Crit Care Med. 2007 Dec 1;176(11):1062-71.

50. Haldar P, Brightling CE, Hargadon B, Gupta S, Monteiro W, Sousa A, et al. Mepolizumab and exacerbations of refractory eosinophilic asthma. N Engl J Med. 2009 Mar 5;360(10):973-84.

51. Nair P, Pizzichini MM, Kjarsgaard M, Inman MD, Efthimiadis A, Pizzichini E, et al. Mepolizumab for prednisone-dependent asthma with sputum eosinophilia. N Engl J Med. 2009 Mar 5;360(10):985-93.

52. Simpson JL, Powell H, Boyle MJ, Scott RJ, Gibson PG. Clarithromycin targets neutrophilic airway inflammation in refractory asthma. Am J Respir Crit Care Med. 2008 Jan 15; 177(2):148-55.

Induced Sputum in COPD: Application in Clinical Practice

Nikoletta Rovina • Georgios Hillas • Petros Bakakos

Induced sputum is a semi-invasive well-tolerated procedure, providing information about cells, mediators, and markers of oxidative/nitrative stress (Figure 1, Table 1). Many patients with COPD produce suitable sputum spontaneously; however, spontaneous sputum may contain a high proportion of dead cells (1), which can potentially give misleading cell counts and mediator measurements (2, 3). Thus, induced sputum has usually been the procedure of choice (Table 2). Some differences in methodology still exist between various research groups. An important question, therefore, is whether these differences in methodology influence the validity and reliability of induced sputum in the assessment of airway inflammation. Standardization of the technique is important for reducing the high variability in the biomarkers.

It should be recognized that "sputum" obtained after inhaling nebulized hypertonic saline may have a different composition than mucus, may be more similar to a washing of proximal airways, and may

Correspondence

Dr. Petros Bakakos
11 Kononos St, Athens 11634, Greece
e-mail: petros44@hotmail.com

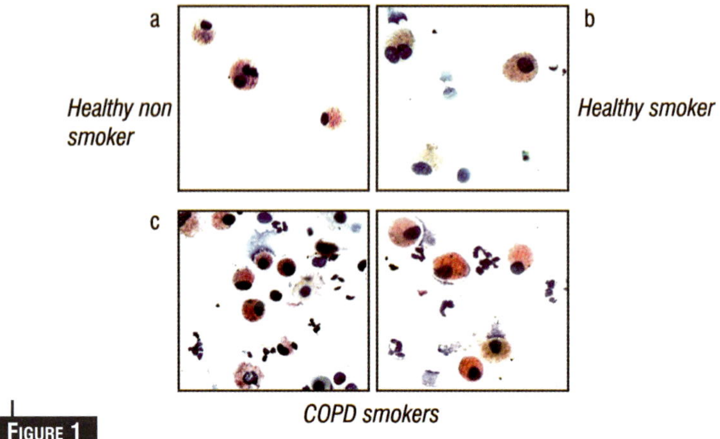

Induced sputum obtained from (a) healthy non smokers, (b) healthy smokers and (c) COPD patients. Images are shown at magnification x 400 (Reproduced after permission from Reference 27).

not reflect the inflammatory process in the lung periphery. The procedure is well-tolerated by patients with severe disease (FEV_1 greater than 30% predicted), and is safe even during exacerbations. Details of the safety precautions and methods are outlined in the European Respiratory Society guidelines (4, 5).

The widespread application of induced sputum in a variety of airway diseases, such as COPD, and across the spectrum of disease severity has given an insight into the relationship between airway function and airway inflammation, proposed new possible disease phenotypes, defined which of these phenotypes respond to current therapy, and perhaps most importantly provided a tool to guide the clinical management of patients with airway disease (6, 7).

Clinical Applications

Sputum induction is considered to be a technique whose value is not restricted to sputum cell counts, as inflammatory mediators can also be measured in the supernatants. Additionally, despite the predominating sputum neutrophilia, there is increasing evidence that the presence of sputum eosinophilia predicts an objective response to

TABLE 1

CELLS AND MEDIATORS ASSAYED IN INDUCED SPUTUM

Cell counts
- Eosinophils
- Neutrophils
- Lymphocytes (and subsets)
- Macrophages
- Epithelial cells

Mediators
- Histamine
- Tryptase
- ECP
- MPO
- CysLTs
- LTB4
- Cytokines and growth factors
- Substance P, neurokinin A

Serum proteins
- Albumin
- Transferin
- Alpha2 macroglobulin

Leptin

Surfactant phospholipids and proteins

Indices of tissue remodeling
- Mettaloproteases and TIMPs
- Hyalorunan

Viruses

Bacteria

Oxidative stress
- 8-iso-PGF (2alpha)
- Glutathione and glutathione peroxidase

Inhaled particles

steroid treatment in patients with COPD. However none of the measurable biomarkers in sputum supernatants is considered applicable in clinical practice and none has been related to disease severity or progression.

COMPARISON OF THE ADVANTAGES AND DISADVANTAGES OF BRONCHOSCOPY AND INDUCED SPUTUM

	Advantages	**Disadvantages**
Bronchoscopy	• Allows biopsy and BAL: samples can be obtained from mucosal tissue, and cells and mediators from the airway lumen	• Requires trained personnel and expensive equipment • Invasive
	• Provides information on structural changes (relating to epithelium, basement membrane and laminae)	• There is mixing of content from alveolar and bronchial compartments
	• Can be followed by immunohistochemistry, in situ hybridization, or electron microscopy	• Can be contaminated with blood
	• Allows the use of bronchial wash (cells for in vitro study)	• Biopsy samples can only be obtained from the larger airways and cell count reproducibility is low
Induced sputum	• Relatively non invasive	• Risk of bronchoconstriction
	• Allows samples to be obtained from several proximal airways	• Success rate around 80%
	• Can be undertaken repeatedly	• Processing methods fairly laborious
	• Safe even in cases of severe disease	• Results not available immediately
	• No expensive equipment required	
	• Allows study of large patient populations	

BAL: bronchoalveolar lavage

Sputum Cell Counts

There is a different pattern of inflammatory cells in COPD patients compared to healthy subjects. An increase in the number of total inflammatory cells, primarily in the percentage of neutrophils and sometimes of eosinophils is observed (8-10). CD8$^+$ T lymphocyte subpopulations are also increased in induced sputum of COPD patients (11).

Neutrophils have been studied most extensively, and are increased in number also compared to matched smokers with normal lung function (12). The raised sputum neutrophil count is related to reduced FEV_1 and the increased rate of decline in FEV_1, suggesting that neutrophilic airway inflammation is functionally important (13).

Several studies have reported the effects of drugs on sputum neutrophils. Sputum induction provides an excellent tool to assess the effect of current and novel therapies on neutrophilic inflammation. Confalonieri et al. (14) studied the effects of a two-month treatment with inhaled beclomethasone dipropionate (1,500 µg/day) on bronchial inflammation in patients with stable, mild to moderate COPD, using sputum induction. They found that the number of neutrophils in induced sputum samples decreased after treatment. Moreover, a short course of oral steroid treatment has been demonstrated to improve pulmonary function in some patients with COPD, but not all (15). Most studies however, have shown no change in inflammatory cells with inhaled or oral corticosteroids (16-18); however, a reduction with oral theophylline has been reported (19).

Up to 40% of COPD patients have a sputum eosinophil count of at least 3% (9, 10). There is increasing evidence that the presence of sputum eosinophilia predicts an objective response to oral (9, 20) and inhaled corticosteroid treatment in COPD (10). Brightling et al. (9) reported that the response in terms of lung function, health status and exercise tolerance to a 2-week course of oral prednisolone increased as the baseline sputum eosinophil count increased, and was associated with a marked treatment-induced fall in the sputum eosinophil count, but no change in sputum markers of neutrophilic inflammation. This finding suggests that eosinophilic airway inflammation is functionally important in a subgroup of COPD patients. Thus, the beneficial effects of corticosteroids are partly due to modification of this aspect of the complex airway inflammation. Siva et al. (21) showed that a management approach over a 12-month period with the additional aim of reducing the sputum eosinophil count <3% using corticosteroids was associated with a 62% reduction in severe exacerbations of COPD requiring hospitalization when compared to traditional symptom-based management. Fujimoto et al. (15) investigated the influence of corticosteroids in the reversibility of eosinophilic inflammation in patients with pulmonary emphysema. They found that the reversibility of airway obstruction following treatment could be correlated with the eosinophil count in the induced sputum, and that the treatment significantly reduced eosinophil count and eosinophilic mediators. In addition, patients who did not show improvement in FEV_1 had lower baseline eosinophil counts. Based on these reports, a measurement of sputum eosinophil counts can be used to identify COPD patients with corticosteroid responsive disease and to guide treatment.

Inflammatory Mediators in Supernatant

Many mediators have been reported to be increased in the supernatant of induced sputum of patients with COPD. Most of them show a greater increase in COPD than in normal smokers, with a further increase during exacerbations. Sputum concentrations of inflammatory mediators are generally unaffected by corticosteroids, but reduced by theophylline (16-19).

Sputum IL-8 and TNF-α have been studied more extensively. IL-8 is increased in induced sputum of COPD patients compared with smokers, is related to disease severity, and is further increased with exacerbations (12, 22, 23). Increased concentrations of TNF-α and soluble TNF receptors are found in sputum of patients with COPD compared with normal smokers (24).

TNF-α, IL-8, and IL-6 concentrations have been reported higher in patients with more severe COPD compared with those with less severe COPD (25). Broekhuizen et al. reported that leptin is detectable in induced sputum of COPD patients and is correlated with other inflammatory markers, including TNF-α and C-reactive protein (26). In a recent study, it was demonstrated that in patients with COPD, increased levels of IL-18 in induced sputum were associated with airflow limitation (27), suggesting its potential role as a marker of disease severity.

MMP-8 and MMP-9 (13, 28, 29), MMP-12(30), neutrophil elastase (31) and many other proteases have been found in increased concentrations in sputum of COPD patients.

Sputum markers of structural changes in the airways have been difficult to identify. Dentener et al. (32) has recently reported that hyaluronan, a component of extracellular matrix, has been found in higher concentrations in sputum of COPD patients compared to normal smokers and non-smokers, especially in those patients with the most severe disease. This might indicate increased breakdown of extracellular matrix in COPD.

Boschetto et al. (33) found no differences in the concentrations of tachykinins, substance P and neurokinin A between patients with COPD, normal smokers and non-smokers, although there was a reduction in tachykinins during exacerbations of COPD. Patients with bronchitis type of COPD have raised vascular endothelial growth factor (VEGF) levels in induced sputum, whereas patients with emphysema have lower levels compared to normal controls (34). This might point at a stage- or subtype-dependent expression of VEGF in COPD (35) which is measurable in induced sputum.

The detection of elevated levels of particular sputum chemokines and cytokines in individual patients may provide a rationale for specific therapies.

Disadvantages of Sputum Induction in COPD

Induced sputum is sampled predominantly from large airways and may not reflect the peripheral inflammation that may be important for clinical outcomes in COPD (36). The reducing and denaturant effects of DTT diminish the detectable levels of mediators such as TNF-α, LTB4 and myeloperoxidase (MPO). IL-1β, IL-6, IL-8, secretory leukocyte protease inhibitor (SLPI) and neutrophil elastase are unaffected (36). There is also a problem with proteases in causing decreased detectable levels of IL-5 and it has been shown that IL-5 levels can be significantly increased by adding protease inhibitors (37, 38). In a recent study, Erin et al. (39) showed that after protease inhibition and optimized dialysis of sputum supernatants containing DTT, an increase in the levels of some chemokines and cytokines was detected. Accordingly, they suggested that the technique of optimized dialysis and protease inhibition should be used to partially overcome the denaturant effects of DTT and the proteolytic effect of proteases so as to identify particular cytokines and chemokines.

References

1. Pizzichini MM, Popov TA, Efthimiadis A, Hussack P, Evans S, Pizzichini E, et al. Spontaneous and induced sputum to measure indices of airway inflammation in asthma. Am J Respir Crit Care Med. 1996 Oct;154(4 Pt 1):866-9.

2. Tsoumakidou M, Tzanakis N, Siafakas NM. Induced sputum in the investigation of airway inflammation of COPD. Respir Med. 2003 Aug;97(8):863-71.

3. Bhowmik A, Seemungal TA, Sapsford RJ, Devalia JL, Wedzicha JA. Comparison of spontaneous and induced sputum for investigation of airway inflammation in chronic obstructive pulmonary disease. Thorax. 1998 Nov;53(11):953-6.

4. Pizzichini E, Pizzichini MM, Leigh R, Djukanovic R, Sterk PJ. Safety of sputum induction. Eur Respir J Suppl. 2002 Sep;37:9s-18s.

5. Efthimiadis A, Spanevello A, Hamid Q, Kelly MM, Linden M, Louis R, et al. Methods of sputum processing for cell counts, immunocytochemistry and in situ hybridisation. Eur Respir J Suppl. 2002 Sep;37:19s-23s.

6. Donaldson GC, Seemungal TA, Patel IS, Bhowmik A, Wilkinson TM, Hurst JR, et al. Airway and systemic inflammation and decline in lung function in patients with COPD. Chest. 2005 Oct;128(4):1995-2004.

7. Leigh R, Pizzichini MM, Morris MM, Maltais F, Hargreave FE, Pizzichini E. Stable COPD: predicting benefit from high-dose inhaled corticosteroid treatment. Eur Respir J. 2006 May;27(5):964-71.

8. Stanescu D, Sanna A, Veriter C, Kostianev S, Calcagni PG, Fabbri LM, et al. Airways obstruction, chronic expectoration, and rapid decline of FEV1 in smokers are associated with increased levels of sputum neutrophils. Thorax. 1996 Mar;51(3):267-71.

9. Brightling CE, Monteiro W, Ward R, Parker D, Morgan MD, Wardlaw AJ, et al. Sputum eosinophilia and short-term response to prednisolone in chronic obstructive pulmonary disease: a randomised controlled trial. Lancet. 2000 Oct 28;356(9240):1480-5.

10. Brightling CE, McKenna S, Hargadon B, Birring S, Green R, Siva R, et al. Sputum eosinophilia and the short term response to inhaled mometasone in chronic obstructive pulmonary disease. Thorax. 2005 Mar;60(3):193-8.

11. Tzanakis N, Chrysofakis G, Tsoumakidou M, Kyriakou D, Tsiligianni J, Bouros D, et al. Induced sputum CD8+ T-lymphocyte subpopulations in chronic obstructive pulmonary disease. Respir Med. 2004 Jan;98(1):57-65.

12. Keatings VM, Collins PD, Scott DM, Barnes PJ. Differences in interleukin-8 and tumor necrosis factor-alpha in induced sputum from patients with chronic obstructive pulmonary disease or asthma. Am J Respir Crit Care Med. 1996 Feb;153(2):530-4.

13. Beeh KM, Beier J, Kornmann O, Buhl R. Sputum matrix metalloproteinase-9, tissue inhibitor of metalloprotinease-1, and their molar ratio in patients with chronic obstructive pulmonary disease, idiopathic pulmonary fibrosis and healthy subjects. Respir Med. 2003 Jun;97(6):634-9.

14. Confalonieri M, Mainardi E, Della Porta R, Bernorio S, Gandola L, Beghe B, et al. Inhaled corticosteroids reduce neutrophilic bronchial inflammation in patients with chronic obstructive pulmonary disease. Thorax. 1998 Jul;53(7):583-5.

15. Fujimoto K, Kubo K, Yamamoto H, Ya-

maguchi S, Matsuzawa Y. Eosinophilic inflammation in the airway is related to glucocorticoid reversibility in patients with pulmonary emphysema. Chest. 1999 Mar;115(3):697-702.

16. Keatings VM, Jatakanon A, Worsdell YM, Barnes PJ. Effects of inhaled and oral glucocorticoids on inflammatory indices in asthma and COPD. Am J Respir Crit Care Med. 1997 Feb;155 (2):542-8.

17. Culpitt SV, Maziak W, Loukidis S, Nightingale JA, Matthews JL, Barnes PJ. Effect of high dose inhaled steroid on cells, cytokines, and proteases in induced sputum in chronic obstructive pulmonary disease. Am J Respir Crit Care Med. 1999 Nov;160(5 Pt 1): 1635-9.

18. Loppow D, Schleiss MB, Kanniess F, Taube C, Jorres RA, Magnussen H. In patients with chronic bronchitis a four week trial with inhaled steroids does not attenuate airway inflammation. Respir Med. 2001 Feb;95(2):115-21.

19. Culpitt SV, de Matos C, Russell RE, Donnelly LE, Rogers DF, Barnes PJ. Effect of theophylline on induced sputum inflammatory indices and neutrophil chemotaxis in chronic obstructive pulmonary disease. Am J Respir Crit Care Med. 2002 May 15;165(10): 1371-6.

20. Pizzichini E, Pizzichini MM, Gibson P, Parameswaran K, Gleich GJ, Berman L, et al. Sputum eosinophilia predicts benefit from prednisone in smokers with chronic obstructive bronchitis. Am J Respir Crit Care Med. 1998 Nov; 158(5 Pt 1):1511-7.

21. Siva R, Green RH, Brightling CE, Shelley M, Hargadon B, McKenna S, et al. Eosinophilic airway inflammation and exacerbations of COPD: a randomised controlled trial. Eur Respir J. 2007 May;29(5):906-13.

22. Yamamoto C, Yoneda T, Yoshikawa M, Fu A, Tokuyama T, Tsukaguchi K, et al. Airway inflammation in COPD assessed by sputum levels of interleukin-8. Chest. 1997 Aug;112(2): 505-10.

23. Aaron SD, Angel JB, Lunau M, Wright K, Fex C, Le Saux N, et al. Granulocyte inflammatory markers and airway infection during acute exacerbation of chronic obstructive pulmonary disease. Am J Respir Crit Care Med. 2001 Feb;163(2):349-55.

24. Vernooy JH, Kucukaycan M, Jacobs JA, Chavannes NH, Buurman WA, Dentener MA, et al. Local and systemic inflammation in patients with chronic obstructive pulmonary disease: soluble tumor necrosis factor receptors are increased in sputum. Am J Respir Crit Care Med. 2002 Nov 1;166(9):1218-24.

25. Hacievliyagil SS, Gunen H, Mutlu LC, Karabulut AB, Temel I. Association between cytokines in induced sputum and severity of chronic obstructive pulmonary disease. Respir Med. 2006 May;100(5):846-54.

26. Broekhuizen R, Vernooy JH, Schols AM, Dentener MA, Wouters EF. Leptin as local inflammatory marker in COPD. Respir Med. 2005 Jan;99(1):70-4.

27. Rovina N, Dima E, Gerassimou C, Kollintza A, Gratziou C, Roussos C. Interleukin-18 in induced sputum: association with lung function in chronic obstructive pulmonary disease. Respir Med. 2009 Jul;103(7):1056-62.

28. Vernooy JH, Lindeman JH, Jacobs JA, Hanemaaijer R, Wouters EF. Increased

activity of matrix metalloproteinase-8 and matrix metalloproteinase-9 in induced sputum from patients with COPD. Chest. 2004 Dec;126(6):1802-10.

29. Culpitt SV, Rogers DF, Traves SL, Barnes PJ, Donnelly LE. Sputum matrix metalloproteases: comparison between chronic obstructive pulmonary disease and asthma. Respir Med. 2005 Jun;99(6):703-10.

30. Demedts IK, Morel-Montero A, Lebecque S, Pacheco Y, Cataldo D, Joos GF, et al. Elevated MMP-12 protein levels in induced sputum from patients with COPD. Thorax. 2006 Mar;61(3):196-201.

31. Hill AT, Bayley D, Stockley RA. The interrelationship of sputum inflammatory markers in patients with chronic bronchitis. Am J Respir Crit Care Med. 1999 Sep;160(3):893-8.

32. Dentener MA, Vernooy JH, Hendriks S, Wouters EF. Enhanced levels of hyaluronan in lungs of patients with COPD: relationship with lung function and local inflammation. Thorax. 2005 Feb;60(2):114-9.

33. Boschetto P, Miotto D, Bononi I, Faggian D, Plebani M, Papi A, et al. Sputum substance P and neurokinin A are reduced during exacerbations of chronic obstructive pulmonary disease. Pulm Pharmacol Ther. 2005;18(3): 199-205.

34. Kanazawa H. Role of vascular endothelial growth factor in the pathogenesis of chronic obstructive pulmonary disease. Med Sci Monit. 2007 Nov;13(11):RA189-95.

35. Rovina N, Papapetropoulos A, Kollintza A, Michailidou M, Simoes DC, Roussos C, et al. Vascular endothelial growth factor: an angiogenic factor reflecting airway inflammation in healthy smokers and in patients with bronchitis type of chronic obstructive pulmonary disease? Respir Res. 2007;8:53.

36. Holz O, Richter K, Jorres RA, Speckin P, Mucke M, Magnussen H. Changes in sputum composition between two inductions performed on consecutive days. Thorax. 1998 Feb;53(2):83-6.

37. Nightingale JA, Rogers DF, Barnes PJ. Effect of repeated sputum induction on cell counts in normal volunteers. Thorax. 1998 Feb;53(2):87-90.

38. Kelly MM, Keatings V, Leigh R, Peterson C, Shute J, Venge P, et al. Analysis of fluid-phase mediators. Eur Respir J Suppl. 2002 Sep;37:24s-39s.

39. Erin EM, Barnes PJ, Hansel TT. Optimizing sputum methodology. Clin Exp Allergy. 2002 May;32(5):653-7.

Exhaled Breath Condensate- Technical Considerations

Ildikó Horváth

György Losonczy

Exhaled breath collection during tidal breathing represents the least invasive approach for sampling the respiratory system. Collection of exhaled breath condensate (EBC) simply means capture of exhaled breath by a cooling chamber during tidal breathing. Although the first publication appeared around 30 years ago, intensive work using this matrix for the assessment of respiratory biomarkers has only been performed in recent years. The number of international publications using this technique is around 800 at the time of writing the chapter and only small part of them has addressed technical questions. Exhaled molecules may be captured by other techniques, i.e. on warmed filters. Samples obtained by these means however are not considered as EBC.

EBC contains several components. Water represents large part of the sample (approximately 99%) and only a small fraction is de-

Correspondence ——

Dr. Ildikó Horváth

Semmelweis University, Department of Pulmonology, Budapest, Dios arok 1/C,
125 Hungary
e-mail: hildiko@pulm.sote.hu, hildiko@elet2.sote.hu

rived from respiratory droplets containing nonvolatile molecules. Different volatiles are also present in the sample (1). The mechanisms by which airway/alveolar lining fluid (ALF) substances or those from the mucus layer are removed from the surfaces and added to EBC samples are not clear. Furthermore, although the technique of EBC collection seems to be trivial, there are several important methodological considerations. The European Respiratory Society/American Thoracic Society Taskforce Report on Exhaled Breath Condensate published in 2005 represents an expert consensus on technical issues of sample collection and mediator determination, highlighting open areas and need for further research (1). This chapter follows the structure of the Report and concentrates on those areas where relevant information has been gathered since its publication.

Mode of EBC Collection

EBC collection is generally performed by asking the subject for tidal breathing through a mouthpiece that allows inhalation of room air and exhalation through a cooling chamber. For EBC collection no resistance is applied against expiration. Generally 1-2 ml of EBC is collected over a 10 min sampling period. Inhalation may vary between nasal and oral breathing. During nasal inhalation inhaled air is humidified in the upper airways and mediators released in the upper airways are more likely added to the sample. Although nasal inhalation is the most natural, one has to consider that the same mediators that are relevant in the lung are produced in the upper airways and sinuses and during nasal inhalation they are swiped down to the lower airways and may be added to EBC samples. This process may be of special importance in cases of upper airway diseases (rhinitis, sinusitis, etc). It has been demonstrated that in healthy subjects there is no difference in concentration of adenosine, thromboxane B_2 (TxB_2) and pH between samples collected with nasal or oral inhalation in orally exhaled breath samples (2, 3). In allergic rhinitis however increased concentration of adenosine can be found in samples collected with nasal inhalation than in those collected via oral inhalation (4). But even if the subject is asked for oral inhalation, mediators from the upper airways may enter the sample because the soft palate is not closed during tidal breathing. This issue cannot be solved even with the use of a noseclip. Increased concentrations of H_2O_2, interleukin (IL)-6, IL-4, leukotriene B_4 (LTB_4) and decreased pH have also been described in orally collected EBC samples from patients with upper airway disease (5-7). The latter data however can be explained both by direct mediator addition from the upper airways and also by low grade lower airway inflammation accompanying upper airway diseases. Another approach to assess the upper airway mediator content in health and disease is condensate collection when breath is exhaled through the nose and comparison of data with those obtained from orally exhaled samples (8-10).

Oropharyngeal mediator uptake is an important issue. Although there are studies demonstrating the protein and electrolyte content of EBC differs from that of saliva (11, 12) this information does not rule out the potential influence of the oral cavity on mediator content of EBC. In a few studies EBC samples obtained through a tracheotomy tube were compared to those collected through the mouth (2, 3). Concentrations of adenosine, thromboxane B_2 (TxB_2) and pH were similar between the two types of samples. Concentration of ammonia however was found to be pronouncedly lower in samples obtained through tracheotomies than in EBCs collected through the mouth (2, 12). Furthermore there are evolving data showing that oral bacterial flora plays an important part in EBC nitrite level (13-15). According to some data oral contribution to EBC is responsible for its LTB_4 concentration (16) but others found LTB_4 even in EBC samples obtained directly from the trachea (17). Periodontitis, gingivitis, or other oral inflammatory diseases may also be important determinants of certain mediators found in EBC, however there are no data available on this topic.

Salivary traps are used to avoid salivary contamination and detection of salivary amylase is a frequently used method to exclude saliva contamination in EBC. However, a negative signal does not completely exclude contribution from the mouth.

EBC collection can be performed under special conditions including mechanical ventilation. Condensers can be connected to the outgoing limb of most respirators but the humidification system may influence EBC content. Similarly special considerations are required when trying to collect EBC samples from infants. In this case different masks can be tried and relatively low sample volume is expected. Since general recommendations cannot be properly used for these occasions more cautions sample collecting procedure and data interpretation are required.

Condensing Equipments

Several different devices have been designed for EBC collection including tubing of different materials (Teflon, polypropylene tubing), double-wall glass chambers or big bag like collecting systems (1, 18-20). Cooling is achieved either by covering the collecting surface by pre-chilled material (ice, dry ice, metal or air) or continuously cooling the surrounding of the collecting surface. Condensing temperature around 0°C can be kept using wet (salty) ice, resulting liquid phase EBC. At lower temperatures achieved using dry ice, liquid nitrogen, placing cooling sleeve to required temperature or cooling air to pre-set temperature EBC is collected as frozen material. There are different commercially available devices available including (RTube, Respiratory Research Inc., Charlottesville, VA) (Ecoscreen, Jaeger, Germany), Anacon (Biostec, Spain) and the TURBO-DECC (ItalChill, Parma, Italy). Comparison studies between different commercially available devices demonstrated that they are not interchangeable when measuring pH, leukotrienes or proteins (21-24). The observed differences may be linked with differing collecting surface material and/or collecting temperature.

Efficiency, Duration and Temperature of Condensation

Roughly, 1-3 mL of EBC can be collected from resting adult subjects during tidal breathing for 10 minutes. Calculating from estimated water loss the currently available condensing devices collect approximately 40-60% of total expiratory water vapor regardless if they are connected to a mouth piece or a tracheal tube (25-27). No difference was found in the efficiency of water vapor extraction between healthy subjects and patients with chronic obstructive pulmonary disease (COPD) (26). No major difference was found in sample volume between the different devices (21, 23).

Time for EBC collection is 8-15 minutes in most studies, however in a few studies very short (3 min) or rather prolonged (60 min) collection time was used (3, 28). Comparison of collection times was performed regarding pH, showing no difference in EBC pH between samples collected for 3 min or 30 min (3). Definition of collection time is a very simple approach; however, it does not take into account that the volume of expired air can be very different between subjects when using this approach. It was previously shown that beside EBC volume total protein and urea content of the samples were also related to total expired volume (26). Therefore, another mode of normalization, collection of EBC samples for fixed expired volume (usually 100 L) has also been used (26, 29).

Environmental Conditions, Ambient Air

Components of environmental air may influence EBC composition by directly appearing in EBC samples; by influencing ALF constituents and causing secondary changes in EBC sample constituents. Environmental NO reduces exhaled H_2O_2 concentration (30) and human skin keratins can be recovered from EBC samples suggesting that they can be inhaled and then exhaled to the samples (31). Potential interaction of EBC samples with environmental gases should be considered when leaving samples at room temperature after collection. It has been shown that EBC pH changes rapidly with decrease in EBC partial concentration of carbon dioxide (32). Finally, velocity, temperature and humidity of inhaled air may all influence the volume and content of EBC, as it has been shown (33, 34). Rapid uptake of environmental volatiles and appearance in EBC samples was demonstrated for toluene (35).

Breathing Pattern and Flow - Dependency of EBC Mediator Concentrations

Subjects are asked for performing tidal breathing during EBC collection. It is difficult to do so having a mouthpiece between the lips resulting in usually a higher than tidal volume per each breath. Potential flow dependency was tested for some biomarkers including adenosine, H_2O_2, malondialdehyde (MDA) and pH. Exhalation flow rate influences the level of exhaled H_2O_2; at higher flows exhaled H_2O_2 concentration is lower suggesting that its major part is added to EBC at the level of conductive airways (36).

EBC volume does not depend on lung function parameters including forced expiratory volume in one second and forced vital capacity (FVC) either in normal subjects or in patients with COPD. There are data that reveal no change in EBC pH and adenosine after acute airway obstruction induced by metacholine (3, 37).

Circadian Rhythm, Food and Drink, Smoking

A circadian rhythm has been demonstrated for EBC H_2O_2 level (34, 38). Circadian changes were - at least partly - explained by food and/or drink intake. No circadian rhythm was identified for pH (3). No prospective studies are available to show or rule out any diurnal variation of EBC volume or other mediators present in EBC. Smoking (both chronic and acute smoke exposure) has considerable effect on H_2O_2, isoprostane, nitrite and nitrotyrosine levels measured in EBC, but not on ATP (39-44).

Safety

Collection of EBC is safe. Collection is performed during tidal breathing therefore it does not have any influence on lung function or mediator levels. It can be repeated several times with short intervals (minutes) between measurements. Even if some people tend to hyperventilate especially at the beginning of EBC collection, this has not led to any adverse event. Care must be taken to potential infections. The possibility that the collecting system transmits microbes to subsequent users seems real. This risk can be minimised by using disposable mouthpieces and tubing between the mouth and condenser and a one-way valve to avoid inhaling from the condenser. The use of disposable condensers is an alternative approach.

Disinfection of reusable condensers must be carried out with special caution, since some residual disinfection agents (i.e. those work with formaldehyde) may destroy mediators collected in the disinfected collection tubes, and residual contamination from the cleaning process may affect subsequent sample analysis.

Dilution Factor

The volume of EBC is a reproducible characteristic of EBC, but mediator levels are more variable than EBC volume even if reference techniques are used for biomarker determination. Two components seem to have importance in determining variability: potential changes in dilution (for non-volatiles) and large same sample variability of some of the assay techniques used. The importance of a dilution factor is based on the assumption that the ratio of liberated solutes to exhaled water vapor is unpredictable and can change, therefore a "dilution factor" should be determined from each EBC sample by determining the concentration of a constituent of EBC, which has a well known concentration in sera and diffuses through the cell membranes, but is not produced in the alveoli or airways. Using a dilution factor has been proposed to provide a better mean of data normalization and also a required approach for the calculation of ALF mediator concentration from EBC results. Exhaled ions, urea, protein concentration or conductance of lyophilized samples have been suggested as potential dilution factors (1). The simplest of these is the measurement of conductivity of lyophilized samples (45). One study however found only a small inter-day intra-subject variability in the concentration of sodium and chloride concentrations in EBC samples from healthy subjects and patients with CF, suggesting that variable dilution is not likely a major cause of variable biomarker levels (46). Estimated dilution of EBC using conductivity as a dilution marker is between 5,000 and 25,000. Use of mass spectrometry enables investigators to assess biomarker of interest together with a dilution factor (47, 48). Although determination of a dilution factor has been helpful in assessing ALF concentration of different biomarkers detected in EBC it has not yet been convincingly demonstrated that better reproducibility can be achieved by normalizing EBC data with a dilution factor. Although dilution may be a factor influencing EBC data, it is unlikely that changes in mediator levels observed in different airway diseases can be completely explained by changes in droplet release or formation. Furthermore, it is important to note that this approach cannot be used for volatile compounds in EBC, for which other aspects need to be considered.

Technical Issues of Biomarker Determination in EBC

Several mediators found in EBC have been determined by enzyme immuno assay (ELISA). In most cases values are in the lower range of detection of the ELISA, where the intra- and inter-assay variability of methods is large and interpretation of data is somewhat difficult (49). To overcome this difficulty, lyophilization and vacuum- evaporation or chemical extraction has been used by some investigators however reproducibility of recovery is a constant problem of these approaches. Levels are fully in the range of available assays when total protein, nitrate, pH and ammonia are measured or highly sensitive analytical methods. In this respect very careful handling of samples are required because not only the signal but all the noise (any potential contamination) as well.

Many times EBC samples are stored before measurement. The general advice is to store samples at the lowest possible temperature (mostly at -70°C). It is advisable to test the stability of mediators at the storage temperature if not published previously. Assays should be performed within the time period that the biomarker is known to be stable. The concentration of H_2O_2 is known to decrease causing detectable change in its level after a few days. Cysteinyl-leukotrienes (cys-LTs) are also unstable compounds in most biological fluids, although data on their stability in EBC is not available. On the other hand pH has been reported to be stable up to 2 yrs of storage. These are only examples from the biomarkers measured in EBC but in principle the stability of any biomarker needs to be considered.

Conclusions

In summary there are several technical aspects that have substantial influence on EBC content. Therefore for each individual biomarker measurement appropriate care needs to be taken to appropriately assess any potential influence and apply the most suitable sampling settings. This can ensure better reproducibility and more comparable values between different laboratories (50) and facilitate that EBC biomarkers will be properly placed between other non-invasive sampling methods.

References

1. Horvath I, Hunt J, Barnes PJ, Alving K, Antczak A, Baraldi E, et al. Exhaled breath condensate: methodological recommendations and unresolved questions. Eur Respir J. 2005 Sep; 26(3): 523-48.
2. Vass G, Huszar E, Barat E, Valyon M, Kiss D, Penzes I, et al. Comparison of nasal and oral inhalation during exhaled breath condensate collection. Am J Respir Crit Care Med. 2003 Mar 15; 167(6):850-5.
3. Vaughan J, Ngamtrakulpanit L, Pajewski TN, Turner R, Nguyen TA, Smith A, et al. Exhaled breath condensate pH is a robust and reproducible assay of airway acidity. Eur Respir J. 2003 Dec; 22(6): 889-94.
4. Vass G, Huszar E, Augusztinovicz M, Baktai G, Barat E, Herjavecz I, et al.

The effect of allergic rhinitis on adenosine concentration in exhaled breath condensate. Clin Exp Allergy. 2006 Jun;36(6):742-7.

5. Sandrini A, Ferreira IM, Jardim JR, Zamel N, Chapman KR. Effect of nasal triamcinolone acetonide on lower airway inflammatory markers in patients with allergic rhinitis. J Allergy Clin Immunol. 2003 Feb;111(2):313-20.

6. Carpagnano GE, Carratu P, Gelardi M, Spanevello A, Di Gioia G, Condreva T, et al. Increased IL-6 and IL-4 in exhaled breath condensate of patients with nasal polyposis. Monaldi Arch Chest Dis. 2009 Mar;71(1):3-7.

7. Tanou K, Koutsokera A, Kiropoulos TS, Maniati M, Papaioannou AI, Georga K, et al. Inflammatory and oxidative stress biomarkers in allergic rhinitis: the effect of smoking. Clin Exp Allergy. 2009 Mar;39(3):345-53.

8. Latzin P, Beck J, Bartenstein A, Griese M. Comparison of exhaled breath condensate from nasal and oral collection. Eur J Med Res. 2003 Nov 12;8(11):505-10.

9. Profita M, La Grutta S, Carpagnano E, Riccobono L, Di Giorgi R, Bonanno A, et al. Noninvasive methods for the detection of upper and lower airway inflammation in atopic children. J Allergy Clin Immunol. 2006 Nov;118(5):1068-74.

10. Svensson S, Hellgren J. pH in nasal exhaled breath condensate in healthy adults. Rhinology. 2007 Sep;45(3):214-7.

11. Griese M, Noss J, von Bredow C. Protein pattern of exhaled breath conden-sate and saliva. Proteomics. 2002 Jun;2(6):690-6.

12. Effros RM, Hoagland KW, Bosbous M, Castillo D, Foss B, Dunning M, et al. Dilution of respiratory solutes in exhaled condensates. Am J Respir Crit Care Med. 2002 Mar 1;165(5):663-9.

13. Marteus H, Tornberg DC, Weitzberg E, Schedin U, Alving K. Origin of nitrite and nitrate in nasal and exhaled breath condensate and relation to nitric oxide formation. Thorax. 2005 Mar;60(3):219-25.

14. Horvath I. The exhaled biomarker puzzle: bacteria play their card in the exhaled nitric oxide-exhaled breath condensate nitrite game. Thorax. 2005 Mar;60(3):179-80.

15. Zetterquist W, Marteus H, Kalm-Stephens P, Nas E, Nordvall L, Johannesson M, et al. Oral bacteria--the missing link to ambiguous findings of exhaled nitrogen oxides in cystic fibrosis. Respir Med. 2009 Feb;103(2):187-93.

16. Gaber F, Acevedo F, Delin I, Sundblad BM, Palmberg L, Larsson K, et al. Saliva is one likely source of leukotriene B_4 in exhaled breath condensate. Eur Respir J. 2006 Dec;28(6):1229-35.

17. Moloney ED, Mumby SE, Gajdocsi R, Cranshaw JH, Kharitonov SA, Quinlan GJ, et al. Exhaled breath condensate detects markers of pulmonary inflammation after cardiothoracic surgery. Am J Respir Crit Care Med. 2004 Jan 1;169(1):64-9.

18. Kietzmann D, Kahl R, Muller M, Burchardi H, Kettler D. Hydrogen peroxide in expired breath condensate of patients with acute respiratory failure

and with ARDS. Intensive Care Med. 1993;19(2):78-81.

19. Horvath I, Donnelly LE, Kiss A, Kharitonov SA, Lim S, Chung KF, et al. Combined use of exhaled hydrogen peroxide and nitric oxide in monitoring asthma. Am J Respir Crit Care Med. 1998 Oct;158(4):1042-6.

20. Goldoni M, Caglieri A, Andreoli R, et al. Influence of condensation temperature on selected exhaled breath parameters. BMC Pulm Med 2005;5:10.

21. Soyer OU, Dizdar EA, Keskin O, Lilly C, Kalayci O. Comparison of two methods for exhaled breath condensate collection. Allergy. 2006 Aug; 61(8):1016-8.

22. Prieto L, Ferrer A, Palop J, Domenech J, Llusar R, Rojas R. Differences in exhaled breath condensate pH measurements between samples obtained with two commercial devices. Respir Med. 2007 Aug;101(8): 1715-20.

23. Czebe K, Barta I, Antus B, Valyon M, Horvath I, Kullmann T. Influence of condensing equipment and temperature on exhaled breath condensate pH, total protein and leukotriene concentrations. Respir Med. 2008 May; 102(5):720-5.

24. Goldoni M, Caglieri A, Andreoli R, Poli D, Manini P, Vettori MV, et al. Influence of condensation temperature on selected exhaled breath parameters. BMC Pulm Med. 2005;5:10.

25. Smith CM, Anderson SD. Hyperosmolarity as the stimulus to asthma induced by hyperventilation? J Allergy Clin Immunol. 1986 May;77(5):729-36.

26. Gessner C, Kuhn H, Seyfarth HJ, Pankau H, Winkler J, Schauer J, et al. Factors influencing breath condensate volume. Pneumologie. 2001 Sep;55 (9):414-9.

27. Sznajder JI, Fraiman A, Hall JB, Sanders W, Schmidt G, Crawford G, et al. Increased hydrogen peroxide in the expired breath of patients with acute hypoxemic respiratory failure. Chest. 1989 Sep;96(3):606-12.

28. Scheideler L, Manke HG, Schwulera U, Inacker O, Hammerle H. Detection of nonvolatile macromolecules in breath. A possible diagnostic tool? Am Rev Respir Dis. 1993 Sep;148(3): 778-84.

29. Reinhold P, Jaeger J, Schroeder C. Evaluation of methodological and biological influences on the collection and composition of exhaled breath condensate. Biomarkers. 2006 Mar-Apr;11(2):118-42.

30. Latzin P, Griese M. Exhaled hydrogen peroxide, nitrite and nitric oxide in healthy children: decrease of hydrogen peroxide by atmospheric nitric oxide. Eur J Med Res. 2002 Aug 30; 7(8):353-8.

31. Hoffmann HJ, Tabaksblat LM, Enghild JJ, Dahl R. Human skin keratins are the major proteins in exhaled breath condensate. Eur Respir J. 2008 Feb;31(2):380-4.

32. Kullmann T, Barta I, Lazar Z, Szili B, Barat E, Valyon M, et al. Exhaled breath condensate pH standardised for CO2 partial pressure. Eur Respir J. 2007 Mar;29(3):496-501.

33. Kullmann T, Barta I, Antus B, Valyon M, Horvath I. Environmental temperature and relative humidity influence exhaled breath condensate pH. Eur Respir J. 2008 Feb;31(2):474-5.

34. Knobloch H, Becher G, Decker M, Reinhold P. Evaluation of H_2O_2 and pH in exhaled breath condensate samples: methodical and physiological aspects. Biomarkers. 2008 May;13(3): 319-41.

35. Maniscalco M, De Laurentiis G, Pentella C, Mormile M, Sanduzzi A, Carratu P, et al. Exhaled breath condensate as matrix for toluene detection: a preliminary study. Biomarkers. 2006 May-Jun;11(3):233-40.

36. Schleiss MB, Holz O, Behnke M, Richter K, Magnussen H, Jorres RA. The concentration of hydrogen peroxide in exhaled air depends on expiratory flow rate. Eur Respir J. 2000 Dec;16(6):1115-8.

37. Csoma Z, Huszar E, Vizi E, Vass G, Szabo Z, Herjavecz I, et al. Adenosine level in exhaled breath increases during exercise-induced bronchoconstriction. Eur Respir J. 2005 May; 25(5): 873-8.

38. Nowak D, Kalucka S, Bialasiewicz P, Krol M. Exhalation of H_2O_2 and thiobarbituric acid reactive substances (TBARs) by healthy subjects. Free Radic Biol Med. 2001 Jan 15;30(2): 178-86.

39. Guatura SB, Martinez JA, Santos Bueno PC, Santos ML. Increased exhalation of hydrogen peroxide in healthy subjects following cigarette consumption. Sao Paulo Med J. 2000 Jul 6;118(4):93-8.

40. Nowak D, Antczak A, Krol M, Pietras T, Shariati B, Bialasiewicz P, et al. Increased content of hydrogen peroxide in the expired breath of cigarette smokers. Eur Respir J. 1996 Apr;9(4): 652-7.

41. Balint B, Donnelly LE, Hanazawa T, Kharitonov SA, Barnes PJ. Increased nitric oxide metabolites in exhaled breath condensate after exposure to tobacco smoke. Thorax. 2001 Jun; 56(6):456-61.

42. Montuschi P, Collins JV, Ciabattoni G, Lazzeri N, Corradi M, Kharitonov SA, et al. Exhaled 8-isoprostane as an in vivo biomarker of lung oxidative stress in patients with COPD and healthy smokers. Am J Respir Crit Care Med. 2000 Sep;162(3 Pt 1):1175-7.

43. Garey KW, Neuhauser MM, Robbins RA, Danziger LH, Rubinstein I. Markers of inflammation in exhaled breath condensate of young healthy smokers. Chest. 2004 Jan;125(1):22-6.

44. Lazar Z, Huszar E, Kullmann T, Barta I, Antus B, Bikov A, et al. Adenosine triphosphate in exhaled breath condensate of healthy subjects and patients with chronic obstructive pulmonary disease. Inflamm Res. 2008 Aug;57 (8):367-73.

45. Effros RM, Biller J, Foss B, Hoagland K, Dunning MB, Castillo D, et al. A simple method for estimating respiratory solute dilution in exhaled breath condensates. Am J Respir Crit Care Med. 2003 Dec 15;168(12): 1500-5.

46. Zacharasiewicz A, Wilson N, Lex C, Li A, Kemp M, Donovan J, et al. Repeatability of sodium and chloride in exhaled breath condensates. Pediatr Pulmonol. 2004 Mar;37(3):273-5.

47. Esther CR, Jr., Jasin HM, Collins LB, Swenberg JA, Boysen G. A mass spectrometric method to simultaneously measure a biomarker and dilution marker in exhaled breath con-

densate. Rapid Commun Mass Spectrom. 2008;22(5):701-5.

48. Esther CR, Jr., Boysen G, Olsen BM, Collins LB, Ghio AJ, Swenberg JW, et al. Mass spectrometric analysis of biomarkers and dilution markers in exhaled breath condensate reveals elevated purines in asthma and cystic fibrosis. Am J Physiol Lung Cell Mol Physiol. 2009 Jun;296(6): L987-93.

49. Horvath I, Lazar Z, Gyulai N, Kollai M, Losonczy G. Exhaled biomarkers in lung cancer. Eur Respir J. 2009 Jul; 34(1):261-75.

50. Koutsokera A, Loukides S, Gourgoulianis KI, Kostikas K. Biomarkers in the exhaled breath condensate of healthy adults: mapping the path towards reference values. Curr Med Chem. 2008;15(6):620-30.

Exhaled Breath Condensate- Towards Normal Values

Angela Koutsokera • *Stelios Loukides* • *Konstantinos Kostikas*

The need for non-invasive assessment of airway inflammation is imperative, since inflammatory airway diseases, such as asthma and chronic obstructive pulmonary disease (COPD), are characterized by variation in their clinical presentation throughout their course. Exhaled breath condensate (EBC) collection represents a rather appealing method that can be used to conveniently and noninvasively collect a wide range of volatile and non-volatile molecules from the respiratory tract, without affecting airway function or inflammation.

EBC has the potential of providing information on the physiology of the respiratory system and on pathophysiological pathways, yet it is currently used only as a research tool, due to the lack of appropriate standardization and the absence of reference values. This chapter focuses mainly on the presentation of normal values of the most widely studied EBC markers as reported by investigators that have used healthy subjects either as controls or as their

Correspondence ————————————————————————————

Konstantinos Kostikas
Stamouli 3, Karditsa 43100, Greece
e-mail: ktk@otenet.gr

main study population. Different subpopulations and the effect of various demographic factors on healthy subjects are also reported, in an effort to provide conclusions that may lead to the establishment of reference values. Two recent consensus statements have highlighted the necessity for better standardization of EBC collection and the assessment of mediators (1, 2).

Biomarkers Detected in EBC

EBC is currently a research tool and new molecules are continuously added in the list of substances that can be detected in it. The most studied biomarkers up-to-date are hydrogen peroxide, NO-related products, arachidonic acid metabolites (eicosanoids) and pH, and these are presented below. The levels of those biomarkers in healthy non-smokers and their detectability are reported in Tables 1 to 5. More elegant approaches, including metabonomic analysis have additionally been used recently and De Laurentiis et al. have demonstrated that this technique allows a clear-cut separation between healthy subjects and patients with airway disease (3). However, the present chapter will focus on the mostly studied biomarkers in EBC in the current literature.

A. Hydrogen peroxide (H_2O_2)

H_2O_2 is a product of oxidative stress that is volatile and unstable, thus it should be rapidly stored after collection at -70°C, so that frozen samples can be safely analyzed (4). H_2O_2 has been measured spectrophotometrically (5, 6) or spectrofluorimetrically (7-9), as well as by flow injection analysis with fluorescence detection (10, 11), by a chemiluminescent method (12, 13), and with a commercially available amperometric biosensor (Ecocheck, Jaeger, Germany) (14-16).

EBC H_2O_2 of normal subjects: In some of the early studies H_2O_2 was undetectable in a large number of normal subjects (17, 18). The development of more sensitive techniques has improved H_2O_2 detection in EBC, with the lower limit of detection (LOD) being as low as 0.040 μm with flow injection analysis with fluorescence (10). The upper limits of EBC H_2O_2 values of normal subjects do not exceed 0.9 μM in the existing studies and this is in agreement with the ATS/ERS Task Force (1).

TABLE 1

LEVELS OF H_2O_2 MEASURED IN HEALTHY NON-SMOKERS (NOTE: WHERE HEALTHY EX-SMOKERS WERE USED A COMMENT IS ADDED)

	Study	Normal Values	Subjects (n)	Methodology	Comments
H_2O_2	Antczak et al. (17)	*0.11 µM	1	Custom built, FA	LOD: 0.1 µM, undetectable in 9 subjects
	Antczak et al. (19)	*0.03 ± 0.02 µM	10	Custom built, FA	LOD: 83 µM
	Chow et al. (20)	†5.89 (3.99-8.69) µM	26	Ecoscreen, CA	46% ex smokers
	Corradi et al. (21)	$0.44 (0.12-0.89) µM	8	Ecoscreen, FA	
	Emelyanov et al. (22)	*0.024 ± 0.016 µM	17	Glass condenser, CA	
	Fireman et al. (23)	0µM	10	Custom built, CA	
	Ganas et al. (24)	†0.3 (0.2-0.4) µM	10	Custom built, CA	LOD: 0.1 µM
	Gerritsen et al. (14)	*0.0333 ± 0.0039 µM	10	Ecoscreen, Ecocheck	LOD: 0.049 µM, extrapolation if below LOD
	Gerritsen et al. (25)	#0.00 (0.00-0.00) µM	15	Custom built, CA	LOD: 0.11 µM, extrapolation if below LOD
	Guatura et al. (26)	*0.74 (0.24) µM	10	Custom built, CA	
	Ho et al. (27)	0.090 µM	14	Custom built, FA	
	Horvath et al. (28)	§0.27 ± 0.04 µM	35	Glass condenser, CA	LOD: 0.1 µM
	Kwiatkowska et al. (29)	*0.2 ± 0.1µM	17	Custom built, CA	LOD: 83nM
	Kostikas et al. (30)	*0.19 ± 0.06 µM	10	Glass condenser, CA	LOD: 0.1 µM
	Loukides et al. (31)	§0.26 ± 0.04 µM	25	Glass condenser, CA	LOD: 0.1 µM
	Loukides et al. (32)	†0.2 (0.16-0.24) µM	15	Glass condenser, CA	LOD: 0.1 µM
	Luczynska et al. (33)	*0.25 ± 0.17 µM	27	Custom built, FA	LOD:0.083 µM
	Majewska et al. (34)	*0.16 ± 0.06 µM	20	Custom built, FA	LOD:0.083 µM

continued

TABLE 1

Levels of H_2O_2 Measured in Healthy Non-Smokers (Note: Where Healthy Ex-Smokers Were Used a Comment is Added) *(continued)*

Study		Normal Values	Subjects (n)	Methodology	Comments
H_2O_2	Nowak et al. (9)	*0.19 ± 0.20 µM	40	Custom built, FA	LOD: 0.083 µM
	Nowak et al. (35)	*0.05 ± 0.07 µM	17	Custom built, FA	LOD: 0.083 µM
	Petrosyan et al. (36)	*0.34 ± 0.4 uM non obese			
		1.2 ± 0.9uM obese	10		
			9	Ecoscreen, CA	LOD: 0.31 µM
	Rysz et al. (37)	§0.16 ± 0.13 µM	40	Custom built, FA	LOD: 0.083 µM
	Svensson et al. (10)	*0.48 ± 0.32 µM	19	Ecoscreen, FI-FD	LOD: 0.040 µM
	Szkudlarek et al. (38)	*0.28 ± 0.17 µM	41	Custom built, FA	LOD: 0.083 µM
	Ueno et al. (39)	*0.59 ± 0.03 µmol/L	58	Ecoscreen, FA	
	Valenzuela et al. (40)	*0.53 ± 0.55 µM	26	Custom built, spectrophotometry	
	Zappacosta et al. (13)	$0.17 (0.1-0.6) µM	20	Custom built, Chemiluminescence	

All units were converted to µM. **Symbols:** *Mean ± SD, †Mean (95% CI), §Mean ± SEM, #Median (25th, 75th percentile), $Median (ranges), Median, £ranges.

Abbreviations: FA=fluorimetric assay, CA=colorimetric assay, LOD=lower limit of detection, FI-CL=flow injection chemiluminescence, FI-FD=flow injection fluorescence detection.

B. NO-related products

Exhaled NO is one of the most extensively studied markers of airway inflammation, especially in asthma (41). NO is a free radical due to its unpaired electron and it may react with oxygen to yield nitrogen oxides (NOx) or with superoxide anion to yield peroxynitrite, a highly reactive substance that may lead to the production of NO-derived products (2, 42, 43). Thus, NO synthesis and release in the respiratory system has been assessed indirectly by quantifying nitrite/nitrate, nitrotyrosine and S-nitrosothiols in EBC (Table 2). In a recent study, Osoata et al. measured peroxynitrite using oxidation of 2',7'-dichlorofluorescein in EBC (44).

1. Nitrite/nitrate (NO_2-/NO_3-, NO_x) are produced by the reaction of NO with oxygen and by the decomposition of peroxynitrite. Nitrite/nitrate detection in EBC has been performed with colorimetric and fluorimetric assays, with the latter being more sensitive (45-47). Some studies have also used chemiluminescence (48, 49) and ion chromatography followed by conductivity measurement (50). Nitrate is commonly measured indirectly after conversion to nitrite following incubation with nitrate reductase (24, 51). A recent study suggested that there is a possibility of using polyurethane foam and 3-hydroxy-7,8-benzo-1,2,4-tetrahydroquinoline for nitrite determination by means of diffuse reflectance spectroscopy (52).

EBC nitrite/nitrate of normal subjects: Great discrepancy exists in the normal values of nitrite/nitrate, as shown in Table 2. These discrepancies may be due to the different assays used for the measurements of NO_2- and NO_3-, the efficacy of the method used for the reduction of nitrite to nitrate, and the fact that the contamination of samples is difficult to avoid since NO_x are widely present in laboratory environment (1). The significant day-to-day variability of EBC NOx measurements needs also to be considered in clinical studies (53). Data NO_x measurements must be carefully interpreted and no normal values can be extracted from the existing studies.

2. S-Nitrosothiols (RSNOs) are produced by the interaction of peroxynitrite with thiol-containing macromolecules, such as cysteine and glutathione, which act as antioxidants and limit the nitrosative stress potential of NO and NO-related products (54, 55). RSNOs have been determined in EBC with a colorimetric assay (56).

EBC nitrosothiols of healthy subjects: Based on the few studies available, the upper limit of normal values may be considered at approximately 940 nM.

TABLE 2

Levels of No-Related Products Measured in Healthy Non-Smokers (Note: Where Healthy Ex-Smokers Were Used a Comment is Added)

NO products	Study	Normal values	Subjects (n)	Methodology	Comments
NO_2-/NO_3-	Balint et al. (58)	§21.9 ± 3.2 µM	14	Ecoscreen, FA	LOD: 0.1 Mm
	Balint et al. (51)	€16.0(1.6) 12.56-19.50 µM	14	Ecoscreen, FA	
	Brindicci et al. (62)	§17.7±2.1 µM	10	Ecoscreen, CA	
	Chow et al. (20)	*28.72±17.11 µM	26	Ecoscreen, FA	LOD: 4µg/ml, 46% ex smokers
	Ganas et al. (24)	†0.63 (0.20-0.41) µM	10	Glass condenser, CA	
	Kostikas et al.(30)	*0.30±0.10 µM	10	Glass condenser, CA	
	Liu et al. (63)	$9.89 (3.73-28.58) µM	15	Glass condenser, FA	
	Rolla et al. (64)	¥9.4(4.6-10.9) µM	12	R Tube, Ion chromatography	Modified technique
Nitrate (NO_3-)	Ueno et al. (39)	*0.78 ±0.18 µmol/L	58	Ecoscreen, FA	
	Brindicci et al.	§37.3±9.8 nM	10	Ecoscreen, FA	
	Corradi et al. (50)	$9.6 (2.6-119.4) µM	15	Glass condenser, Ion chromatography	LOD: 2 Mµ
	Cruz et al. (65)	$18-29 years: 10.56 (1.90-67.80)µM 30-39 years: 13.52 (3.29-39.00)µM 40-49 years: 10.04 (2.26-34.30)µM	75	Ecoscreen, CA	Assay sensitivity: 2.5µmol/l. Age groups studied

continued

TABLE 2

LEVELS OF NO-RELATED PRODUCTS MEASURED IN HEALTHY NON-SMOKERS (NOTE: WHERE HEALTHY EX-SMOKERS WERE USED A COMMENT IS ADDED) *(continued)*

NO products	Study	Normal values	Subjects (n)	Methodology	Comments
		50-59 years: 12.39 (2.57-47.47)µM 60-80 years: 10.82 (3.05-35.79)µM			
	Effros et al. (66)	§4.3±1.0 µM	15	Glass condenser, CA	
	Hunt et al. (67)	§5.27±0.51 µM	15	Custom built, chemilu-minescence	
	Nguyen et al. (48)	¥2.6 (1.1-5.0) µM	17	Rtube, chemiluminescence	
	Petrosyan et al. (36)	* 14.4±5.9 µM non obese 10.5±5.1 µM obese	10 9	Ecoscreen, Ion chromatography	LOD: 2µM
Nitrite (NO_2-)	Balint et al.(58)	§3.2±0.5 µM	14	Ecoscreen, FA	LOD: 0.1 Mµ
	Balint et al.(51)	€3.2 (0.5) 2.25-4.4 µM	14	Ecoscreen, FA	
	Corradi et al.(56)	§0.45±0.06 µM	10	Glass condenser, CA	
	Cruz et al.(65)	$18-29years: 5.77 (2.42-15.32)µM 30-39years: 4.28 (1.04-25.34)µM			

continued

TABLE 2

LEVELS OF NO-RELATED PRODUCTS MEASURED IN HEALTHY NON-SMOKERS (NOTE: WHERE HEALTHY EX-SMOKERS WERE USED A COMMENT IS ADDED) *(continued)*

NO products	Study	Normal values	Subjects (n)	Methodology	Comments
		40-49years: 5.18 (1.88-22.77)µM 50-59years: 4.85 (1.03-19.54)µM 60-80years: 3.21 (1.70-26.36)µM	75	Ecoscreen, CA	Assay sensitivity: 1µmol/l. Age groups studied
	Effros et al. (66)	§0.76±0.14 µM	14	Glass condenser, CA	
	Garey et al. (68)	*0.016156±0.007029 µM	9	Custom built, CA	
	Gessner et al. (69)	$3.32 (1.62-6.77) µM	17	Ecosceen, CA	LOD: 0.2 µM
	Hauswirth et al. (70)	∞ 0.71 ± 1.06 umol/L,	243	Rtube, measured as NO	
	Ho et al. (71)	$0.33 (0-2.10) µM	12	Custom built, CA	LOD: 0.5 µM
	Hunt et al. (72)	$0.55 (0.33, 2.51) µM	19	Custom built, chemiluminescence	
	Hunt et al. (67)	§0.78±0.072 µM	15	Custom built, CA	
	Nguyen et al. (48)	¥1.03 (0.56-1.4) µM	17	Rtube, chemilumi-nescence	LOD: 0.1 µM
	Rolla et al. (64)	¥0.90(0.72-1.17) µM	12	R Tube, Ion chromato-graphy	Modified technique

continued

TABLE 2

Levels of No-Related Products Measured in Healthy Non-Smokers (Note: Where Healthy Ex-Smokers Were Used a Comment is Added) *(continued)*

NO products	Study	Normal values	Subjects (n)	Methodology	Comments
Nitrosothiols	Balint et al.(51)	€500 (200) 20-940 nM	14	Ecoscreen, FA	
	Corradi et al.(56)	§110±20 nM	10	Glass condenser, CA	LOD: 25 nM
Nitrotyrosine	Balint et al.(58)	§27.8±3.5 nM	14	Ecoscreen, EIA	LOD: 17.2 nM
	Balint et al.(51)	€27.8±3.5 nM	14	Ecoscreen, EIA	LOD: 17.2 nM
	Brindicci et al.(62)	§7.2±0.8 ng/mL	10	Ecoscreen, EIA	
	Chow et al.(20)	†0.39(0.13-1.18) ng/ml	26	Ecoscreen, EIA	LOD: 4ng/ml, 46% ex smokers
	Celio et al. (60)	$1.46 (0.78-3.61) nM	14	Ecoscreen, GC-NICI-MS	LOD: 0.22 nM (GC-NICI-MS),
		1.22 (<0.2-2.65) nM	10	Ecoscreen, HPLC	0.2 Nm (HPLC)
	Hanazawa et al.(59)	§27.8±3.5 nM	15	Ecoscreen, EIA	LOD: 17.2 nM
	Lärstad et al.(61)	¥0.031 (0.014, 0.053) nM	10	Ecoscreen, GC-tandem-MS	LOD: 0.0056 nM
Peroxynitrite	Osoaka et al.(44)	*2.0±1.1nmol/L	8	Ecoscreen, fluorescence	Sensitivity >0.008µmol/L

Units of nitrate/nitrite and nitrosothiols were converted to Mm, and units of nitrotyrosine to Nm.

Symbols: *Mean ± SD, †Mean (95% CI), §Mean ± SEM, €Mean (SEM) 95% confidence intervals, ¥Median (25th, 75th percentile), $Median (range), ∞ Geometric mean (SD)

Abbreviations: FA=fluorimetric assay, CA=colorimetric assay, LOD=lower limit of detection, EIA=enzyme immunoassay, HPLC=high performance liquid chromatography, LC-MS/MS= liquid chromatography and mass spectrometry, GC-tandem-MS=gas chromatography/tandem mass spectrometry; GC-NICI-MS=gas chromatography-negative ion chemical ionization-mass spectrometry, DCD-HF=2',7'-dichlorofluorescein.

3. Nitrotyrosine is produced by the reaction of peroxynitrite with tyrosine residues of proteins. An alternative source of nitrotyrosine formation is the nitration of proteins by myeloperoxidase, an enzyme of neutrophils that uses H_2O_2 (43, 57). Initially, nitrotyrosine levels were assessed with an enzyme immunoassay (EIA) (51, 58, 59), whereas later studies using high performance liquid chromatography (HPLC) and mass spectrometry (MS) provided better sensitivity (60, 61).

EBC nitrotyrosine of healthy subjects: The upper limit of normal in the studies using EIA was approximately 62 nM (14 ng/ml) (51, 58). However, studies using HPLC or MS provided lower levels of nitrotyrosine, with the upper limits of normal reaching 3.6 nM (60). The discrepancy of the results of these studies along with the few available data on reproducibility(58), warrant further studies for the standardization of nitrotyrosine measurements and the establishment of normal values.

C. Arachidonic acid metabolites (eicosanoids):

Eicosanoids represent a heterogeneous family of C20 unsaturated fatty acids derivatives. Arachidonic acid is released from cell walls by phospholipase A_2 (73) through the actions of cyclooxygenase or lipoxygenase and leads to the production of prostanoids and leukotrienes, whereas the effect of free radicals yields the isoprostanes (74, 75). Major studies on prostanoids and leukotrienes are presented in Table 3, whereas 8-isoprostane studies are summarized in Table 4.

1. Prostanoids are synthesized via the cyclooxygenase pathway and include prostaglandines and thromboxanes. Prostaglandin E_2 (PGE$_2$) levels have been determined in EBC samples by EIA (76-78) and radioimmunoassays (RIA) (79). Thromboxane A_2 (TXA$_2$) is rapidly converted to TXB$_2$, a chemically stable compound and EBC TXB$_2$ levels have been determined by EIA (80).

EBC prostaglandins and thromboxanes of healthy subjects: Different levels of PGE$_2$ have been reported for healthy non-smokers. The upper limit of normal was 21 pg/ml in one study (77), whereas it exceeded 75 pg/ml in another (78), not differing from patients with asthma. TXB$_2$ levels were undetectable in healthy non-smokers in one study (78), whereas the upper limits of normal reached 75 pg/mL in two other studies (80, 81).

TABLE 3

LEVELS OF PROSTANOIDS AND LEUKOTRIENES MEASURED IN HEALTHY NON-SMOKERS (NOTE: WHERE HEALTHY EX-SMOKERS WERE USED A COMMENT IS ADDED)

	Study	Normal values	Subjects (n)	Methodology (collection device, measurement)	Comments
PGE2	Kostikas et al.(77)	*11.7±4 pg/ml	10	Glass condenser, EIA	LOD: 8 pg/ml
	Montuschi et al.(78)	€45.6±3.9 (37.0-54.1) pg/ml	12	Ecoscreen, EIA	LOD: 30 pg/ml
	Tufvesson et al.(93)	£3-6 pg/ml	12	Ecoscreen, EIA	LOD: 2 pg/ml
TXB2	Huszar et al.(80)	$14 (5-44) pg/ml	4	Ecoscreen, EIA, RIA	LOD: 13 pg/ml, undetectable in 6
	Montuschi et al.(78)	Undetectable		Ecoscreen, EIA	LOD: 10 pg/ml, undetectable in 12
	Vass et al.(81)	*30.9±19.6 pg/ml	25	Ecoscreen, RIA	With noseclip
		24.9±18.9 pg/ml			Without noseclip
LTB4	Antczak et al. (83)	§64.6±11.66 pg/ml	15	Custom built, EIA	LOD: 4.43 pg/ml
	Antczak et al.(76)	§64.6±11.6 pg/ml	16	Custom built, EIA	LOD: 4.43 pg/ml
	Biernacki et al. (90)	*7.7±0.5 pg/ml	12	EcoScreen, EIA	LOD: 5 pg/ml
	Borrill et al.(103)	∞32.7±3.1pg/ml	10	EcoScreen, EIA	LOD: 13pg/ml
	Cap et al.(88)	¥79 (71-90) pg/ml	50	EcoScreen, GC/MS	LOD: 1 pg/ml
	Carpagnano et al.(84)	§6.8±0.7 pg/ml	15	Ecoscreen, EIA	LOD: 3 pg/ml
	Carpagnano et al.(85)	§6.1±0.3 pg/ml	14	Ecoscreen, EIA	LOD: 3 pg/ml
	Corhay et al.(104)	§34.3 ± 3.3 pg/mL	24	Ecosceen, EIA	LOD: 13pg/ml. All ex smokers.
	Corradi et al.(21)	£0.0-10.3 pg/ml	22	Ecoscreen, EIA	Groups according to genotypes
	Gaber et al. (92)	£28-100 pg/ml	4	Silicon-coated glass condenser, EIA	LOD: 3.9 pg/ml, Undetectable in 98 samples obtained from 34 subjects

continued

TABLE 3

LEVELS OF PROSTANOIDS AND LEUKOTRIENES MEASURED IN HEALTHY NON-SMOKERS (NOTE: WHERE HEALTHY EX-SMOKERS WERE USED A COMMENT IS ADDED) *(continued)*

Study	Normal values	Subjects (n)	Methodology (collection device, measurement)	Comments
Hanazawa et al.(59)	§63.1±17.3 pg/ml	15	Ecoscreen, EIA	LOD: 4.4 pg/ml
Hoffmeyer et al.(105)	£frozen immediately 29.8(23.9-36.2) Not frozen immediately 24.2(14.5-36.4)	16	Ecoscreen, EIA	LOQ: 11.7pg/ml. Argon gas deaeration. 255 Samples from 16 subjects.
Ko et al.(106)	¥5.80(5.29-7.54)pg/ml	14	Ecoscreen, high sensitivity EIA	LOD: 4pg/MI
Lehtonen et al.(107)	§15.4±2.9pg/ml	15	Ecoscreen, EIA	LOD: 1.95pg/ml, quit smoking at lease 5 years ago
Makinen et al.(108)	§3.1±0.5 pg/ml	14	Ecoscreen, EIA	
Montuschi et al.(78)	€38.8±1.8(34.9-42.7) pg	12	Ecoscreen, EIA	LOD: 4 pg/ml
Montuschi et al. (91)	Undetectable		Ecoscreen, LC/MS	LOD: 100 pg/ml, Undetectable in 2
Pelclova et al.(109)	‡29.4±7.8pg/ml	25	Ecoscreen, LC-ESI-MS	LOD: 1 pg/ml, 8 smokers
Piotrowski et al.(110)	*20.09±4.85 pg/ml	13	Ecoscreen, EIA	LOD: 4.43pg/mL, Undetectable in 4
Tanou et al.(111)	¥55.2±17.7 pg/ml	15	Ecoscreen, EIA	
Tufvesson et al.(93)	§3.8 ±0.6 pg/ml	12	Ecoscreen, EIA	LOD: 6 pg/ml

continued

TABLE 3

LEVELS OF PROSTANOIDS AND LEUKOTRIENES MEASURED IN HEALTHY NON-SMOKERS (NOTE: WHERE HEALTHY EX-SMOKERS WERE USED A COMMENT IS ADDED) *(continued)*

Study	Normal values	Subjects (n)	Methodology (collection device, measurement)	Comments
Cys-LTs Antczak et al. (76)	§19.4±2.7 pg/ml	16	Custom built, EIA	LOD: 13 pg/ml
Czebe et al.(112)	*65.8±17.0pg/ml	12	Ecoscreen, EIA	No cys-LT detected in samples collected with RTube or with Anacon.
Bucchioni et al.(87)	*26.3±2.2 pg/ml	9	Ecoscreen, EIA	LOD: 13 pg/ml
Hanazawa et al.(59)	§15.5±0.2 pg/ml	15	Ecoscreen, EIA	LOD: 15 pg/ml
Makinen et al.(108)	§12.2±1.7 pg/ml	14	Ecoscreen, EIA	
Piotrowski et al.(110)	*6.5±0 pg/ml		Ecoscreen, EIA	LOD: 13pg/mL, Undetectable in all 17
Samitas et al.(113)	§17.5±1.2pg/ml	13	Ecoscreen, EIA	LOD : 13pg/ml, Undetectable in 6
Soyer et al.(94)	¥205.4 (65.5-472.3) pg/ml 21.6 (11.87-152.2) pg/ml	30	Ecoscreen, EIA Rtube, EIA	
Tufvesson et al.(93)	£2-20 pg/ml	12	Ecoscreen, EIA	LOD: 13 pg/ml

Symbols: *Mean ± SD, †Mean (95% CI), §Mean ± SEM, €Mean ± SEM (95% CI), ¥Median (25th, 75th percentile), $Median (range), £range, ‡ mean±u_c, £=measurement above the limit of quantification (LOQ) with 95% confidence intervals, ∞ Geometric mean (SD)
Abbreviations: LOD=lower limit of detection, EIA=enzyme immunoassay, RIA=radioimmunoassay, LC-MS= liquid chromatography/mass spectrometry, GC-MS=gas chromatography/mass spectrometry, LC-ESI-MS= liquid chromatography-electrospray ionization-mass spectrometry, u_c=uncertainty of experimentally determined value, LOQ=the limit of quantification, LLQ=lower limit of quantification

2. Leukotrienes are classified into two classes: LTB$_4$ and cysteinyl leukotrienes (Cys-LTs, i.e. LTC4, LTD4 and LTE$_4$) (75, 82). Leukotrienes have been measured in EBC by EIA (76, 78, 83-87), gas chromatography/mass spectrometry (GC/MS) (88), and liquid chromatography/mass spectrometry (LC/MS) (89).

EBC leukotrienes of healthy subjects: In the majority of studies, normal subjects present LTB$_4$ levels in the range of 0-150 pg/ml. Some investigators, however, report extremely low levels of EBC LTB$_4$, despite the use of the same EIA kit (21, 84, 85, 90). LTB$_4$ was detectable in the majority of healthy non-smokers with the exception of two studies, one using a LC/MS method with a lower limit of detection of 100 pg/ml that is above the usual levels of LTB$_4$ measured in EBC (91), and another using a silicone-coated glass condenser (92). In the latter, salivary contamination was proposed as a plausible source of LTB$_4$ in EBC, therefore questioning the use of EBC for monitoring LTB$_4$ levels in exhaled air (92). However, another study showed a significant correlation between EBC and induced sputum levels of LTB4 in a population of smokers, suggesting a more significant role of EBC LTB$_4$ in smokers (86).

Cys-LTs levels in normal subjects are often near or even below the lower limits of detection of the EIA used (59). The upper limits of Cys-LTs values in normal subjects in two studies reach 50 pg/ml (76, 87), yet the majority of the measurements are below 25 pg/ml (76, 87, 93). A single study reported significantly higher concentrations of Cys-LTs (94), however these have to be further validated. One study has measured separately LTC$_4$, LTD$_4$, and LTE$_4$ and another assessed only LTE$_4$ (78); however, given their low concentrations in EBC and the fact that LTC$_4$ and LTD$_4$ are rapidly converted to LTE$_4$, only the measurement of LTE$_4$ may be of interest in EBC.

3. Isoprostanes are formed by free-radical lipid peroxidation of arachidonic acid, representing in vivo biomarkers of oxidative stress (95). The most studied isoprostane is 8-epi-PGF$_{2a}$, also known as 8-isoprostane (96). The method of choice for 8-isoprostane measurements in EBC is EIA, but GC/MS has also been used in two studies on intubated subjects (97, 98). A recent study has used a combination of immunoseparation and liquid chromatography-electrospray ionization-mass spectrometry (LC-ESI-MS/MS) operating in multiple reaction monitoring mode (99).

EBC 8-isoprostane of healthy subjects: Major studies including healthy non-smokers are summarized in Table 4 and 8-isoprostane was detectable in the majority of normal subjects. The highest

TABLE 4

LEVELS OF 8-ISOPROSTANE MEASURED IN HEALTHY NON-SMOKERS (NOTE: WHERE HEALTHY EX-SMOKERS WERE USED A COMMENT IS ADDED)

8-isoprostane (8-iso-PGF2α) Study	Normal Values	Subjects (n)	Methodology (collection device, measurement)	Comments
Antczak et al. (83)	§17.5±2.4 pg/ml	15	Not reported, EIA	LOD: 4 pg/ml
Antczak et al(76)	§21.9±4.5 pg/ml	16	Custom built, EIA	LOD: 5 pg/ml
Battaglia et al.(100)	$3.6 (2.9-7.6) pg/ml	15	Ecoscreen, ELISA	LOD: 5 pg/ml
Biernacki et al. (90)	*6.2±0.4 pg/ml	12	Ecoscreen, EIA	LOD: 4 pg/ml
Brindicci et al.(62)	§11.5±0.9 pg/ml	10	Ecoscreen, EIA	
Borrill et al.(103)	?8.9±4.0 pg/ml	10	EcoScreen, EIA	LOD: 5 pg/ml
Carpagnano etl al.(102)	*4.7±1.8 pg/ml	15	Ecoscreen, EIA	LOD: 4 pg/ml
Carpagnano et al.(101)	*6.1±1.3 pg/ml	23	Ecoscreen, EIA	LOD: 4 pg/ml
Chow et al.(20)	†0.07(0.04-0.13)	26	Ecoscreen, EIA	LOD: 5pg/ml, 46% ex smokers
Corradi et al.(21)	$4.30 (0.0-9.61) pg/ml	8	Ecoscreen, CELISA	Groups according to genotypes
	8.23 (3.4-11.6) pg/ml	14		
Cruz et al(65)	$18-29years: 4.00(4.00-12.94) 30-39years: 6.41(4.00-14.34) 40-49years: 7.85(4.00-13.27) 50-59years: 9.11(4.00-12.33) 60-80years: 9.90(6.76-16.71)	55	Ecoscreen, competitive EIA	Assay sensitivity: 4 pg/ml. Age groups studied, 75 subjects studied but levels undetectable in 20 subjects
Dentener et al.(114)	$ 6.4 (3.5-13.5)	11	Ecoscreen, EIA	2 smokers

continued

TABLE 4

LEVELS OF 8-ISOPROSTANE MEASURED IN HEALTHY NON-SMOKERS (NOTE: WHERE HEALTHY EX-SMOKERS WERE USED A COMMENT IS ADDED) *(continued)*

8-isoprostane (8-iso-PGF2α) Study	Normal Values	Subjects (n)	Methodology (collection device, measurement)	Comments
Heinicke et al.(115)	*trained, sea level 2.77±0.65 pg/ml Sedentary, sea level 2.95±0.95 pg/ml	15	Custom built, EIA	LOD: 1pg/ml. Studied trained and sedentary subjects at sea level and altitude
Ko et al.(116)	¥6.0 (4.2-9.7) pg/ml	18	Ecoscreen, EIA	LOD: 4 pg/ml
Kostikas et al.(30)	*20±7 pg/ml	10	Glass condenser, EIA	LOD: 4 pg/ml
Lehtonen et al.(107)	§11.9±2.8pg/ml	15	Ecoscreen, EIA	LOD: 1.95pg/ml, quit smoking at least 5 years ago
Li et al. (117)	*12.6±2.2pg/ml	22	Ecoscreen, EIA	LOD: 4pg/ml, BMI 23.3±2.0
Makinen et al.(108)	§9.9±0.9pg/ml	14	Ecoscreen, EIA	
Makris et al.(118)	§5.6±0.7pg/ml	12	Custom built, EIA	LOD: 4pg/ml, 5 ex-smokers
Mazur et al.(119)	Exact values not reported, resultes presented in a figure	14	Ecoscreen, EIA	LOD: 5pg/ml
Montuschi et al.(120)	§10.8± 0.8 pg/ml	10	Ecoscreen, EIA	LOD: 4 pg/ml
Montuschi et al.(121)	§15.8±1.6 pg/ml	10	Glass condenser, EIA	LOD: 4 pg/ml

continued

TABLE 4

LEVELS OF 8-ISOPROSTANE MEASURED IN HEALTHY NON-SMOKERS (NOTE: WHERE HEALTHY EX-SMOKERS WERE USED A COMMENT IS ADDED) *(continued)*

8-isoprostane (8-iso-PGF2α) Study	Normal Values	Subjects (n)	Methodology (collection device, measurement)	Comments
Montuschi et al.(122)	§16.9±0.7 pg/ml 15.8±0.3 pg/ml	9	Glass condenser, EIA	LOD: 4 pg/ml, 2 study groups
Montuschi et al.(123)	€15.2 (1.7) pg/ml	10	Glass condenser, EIA	LOD: 4 pg/ml
Pelclova et al.(109)	‡43±10pg/ml	25	Ecoscreen, LC-ESI-MS	LOD: 1 pg/ml, 8 smokers
Petrosyan et al.(36)	* 5.5±1.9 pg/ml non obese 4.0±0.2 pg/ml obese	10 9	Ecoscreen, EIA	LOD: 4pg/ml
Psathakis et al.(124)	†20.75 (16.06-25.44) pg/ml	12	Custom built, EIA	LOD: 1pg/ml, com- pared different condensers, 13% of measurements were missing
Rosias et al.(125)	#silicone 2.0(1.3-3.5) Glass 2.9(1.4-3.7) Optimised glass 3.6(2.2-4.9) Ecoscreen 2.5(1.6-3.4)	30	Silicone, glass, Ecoscreen, optimized glass condenser, EIA	
Samitas et al.(113)	§16.4±1.6pg/ml	19	Ecoscreen, EIA	LOD: 5pg/ml
Tufvesson et al.(93)	§1.5±0.2 pg/ml	12	Ecoscreen, EIA	LOD: 5 pg/ml
Zhao et al.(126)	¥3.5(2.6-7.9)pg/ml	20	Ecoscreen, EIA	LOD: 4pg/ml

Symbols: *Mean ± SD, †Mean (95% CI), §Mean ± SEM, ▯Mean ± SEM (95% CI), ¥Median (25th, 75th percentile), $Median (range), £range, ‡ mean±uc, ∞ Geometric mean (SD)

Abbreviations: LOD=lower limit of detection, EIA=enzyme immunoassay, RIA=radioimmunoassay, LC-MS= liquid chromatography/mass spectrometry, GC-MS=gas chromatography/mass spectrometry, LC-ESI-MS= liquid chromatography-electrospray ionization-mass spectrometry, u_c=uncertainty of experimentally determined value values in healthy subjects may reach 50 pg/ml, but the majority of measurements are below 30 pg/ml. However, there are major differences between studies, with some investigators reporting normal values of EBC 8-isoprostane lower than 10 pg/ml (90, 100-102).

D. pH

EBC pH most likely reflects airway acidification at all levels of the respiratory tract (127, 128). Despite some methodological issues that remain to be elucidated, such as the effect of CO_2 on EBC pH (2), pH is considered to be the most validated measurement performed in EBC samples today (129). In most studies deaeration with an intert gas (usually argon) has been used to enhance the stability of pH measurements (30, 72), although some investigators have measured pH directly after sample collection (127, 130-134). Most investigators have used a pH-meter (30, 72), although scarcely blood gas analyzers have been used (135, 136). Measurement of EBC pH after deaeration remains the current "gold-standard", as it has been extensively validated and it has been found to represent a simple, robust and reproducible biomarker (129). However, two studies comparing EBC pH measurements with two commercially available collecting devices (Ecoscreen and RTube) have provided contradictory results (94, 137), suggesting that a single collecting device should be used in longitudinal studies. Finally, Kullmann et al. suggested that the determination of pH at a standard EBC CO_2 level provided more reproducible pH values (136), but further studies are needed in that direction.

EBC pH of healthy subjects: The largest study on dearated EBC pH included 404 healthy subjects (with more than 200 adults) and provided a median value of 8.0 and a mean value of 7.85, with a maximal value of 8.4 and with 6.4% of the subjects presenting pH ≤7.3(138). Based on that study and on previous ones, the lower limit of normal dearated EBC pH values that may separate healthy inviduals from patients with pronounced airway inflammation (such as COPD, bronchiectasis or unstable asthma) is approximately 7.4 (30, 138).

E. Additional biomarkers

Several other biomarkers have been assessed in EBC of healthy subjects, including CRP (39, 149), adenosine (81, 150, 151), aldehydes (152-155), glutathione (156), glucose (157), ammonia (64, 66, 81, 127, 135, 158-160), urea (161), acetone (160), ethanol (160), methanol (160), thiobarbituric acid reactive substances (TBARs) (9, 17, 21, 34, 35, 38), proteins (20, 66, 68, 112, 162-167), albumin (39), histamine (87), elements and ions (66, 168), interferon-γ (167) and several cytokines, such as interleukins and tumor necrosis factor-alpha (TNF-α) (68, 69, 114, 125, 141, 162, 169, 170). However, we believe that the pursuit of normal values for those biomarkers is not yet feasible and further studies focusing on standardization of measurements are needed in that direction.

Effects of Demographic Characteristics on EBC Biomakers in Healthy Subjects

- **Smoking:** Differences in biomarkers in EBC between smokers and non-smokers are summarized in Table 6. In general, smokers have elevated EBC levels of H_2O_2 (9, 13, 14, 18, 25) and 8-isoprostane (120) compared to non-smokers, and 8 isoprostane levels tended to distinguish healthy non smokers from healthy smokers (119). Moreover smoking history (pack/years) of healthy smokers correlated with EBC 8 isoprostane levels (62). Additionally, some investigators report increased levels of certain NO-derived compounds (50, 56, 68) in healthy smokers, but those findings are not consistent with other studies (51).
- **Alcoholism:** pH, hydrogen peroxide, reduced and oxidized EBC glutathione were measured in otherwise healthy subjects with and without a history of alcohol abuse (most of them were also smokers). When compared to control values the redox potential of the chronic alcohol abusers was shifted to a more oxidized state (171).
- **Obesity:** EBC IL-6 (172) levels were found to be elevated in obese subjects compared to normal-weight ones. Results are contradictory concerning 8-isoprostane levels, with one study (172) finding no difference and an other reporting higher levels in obese controls than in non-obese controls (36). Also in the study of Komakula et al. no significant association was found between BMI of normal subjects and the levels of 8-isoprostane (173). Although one study reported that EBC H_2O_2 levels were not correlated with body mass index (9) another found that H_2O_2 in obese controls was higher than in non-obese controls (36). A reduction of exhaled pH

TABLE 5

LEVELS OF EBC pH MEASURED IN HEALTHY NON-SMOKERS (NOTE: WHERE HEALTHY EX-SMOKERS WERE USED A COMMENT IS ADDED)

pH Study	Normal values	Subjects (n)	Methodology (collection device, measurement)	Comments
Accordino et al.(139)	*Winter 7.88±0.08 Autumn 7.89±0.14 Summer 7.84±0.10	10	Custom built, pH-meter	Argon deaeration
Bloemen et al.(134)	¥ 6.17 (5.96- 6.31)	20	Rtube, pH-meter	Without deaeration
Bloemen et al.(134)	¥ 6.17 (5.96-6.31)	21	Rtube, pH-meter	Without deaeration
Borrill et al.(140)	†7.61(7.52-7.70)	12	Ecoscreen, pH-meter	Argon gas deaeration
Borrill et al.(103)	$7.39 (7.29-7.75)	10	Ecoscreen, pH-meter	Argon gas deaeration
Carpagnano et al.(141)	§7.9±0.1	7	Ecoscreen, pH-meter	Argon gas deaeration
Carpagnano et al.(142)	*7.85±0.14	15	Ecoscreen, pH-meter	Argon gas deaeration
Carpagnano et al.(143)	*7.99±0.03	10	Ecoscreen, pH-meter	Argon gas deaeration
Corradi et al.(21)	$7.91 (7.70-8.08)	8	Ecoscreen, pH -meter	Argon gas deaeration.
	8.01 (7.80-8.11)	14		Groups according to genotypes.
Cruz et al(65)	$18-29years: 8.12(7.23-8.84) 30-39years: 8.21(6.74-8.64) 40-49years: 8.20(7.75-8.68) 50-59years: 8.25(7.94-8.60) 60-80years: 7.74(5.52-8.23)	75	Ecoscreen, pH-meter	Helion deaeration, age groups studied

continued

TABLE 5

LEVELS OF EBC pH MEASURED IN HEALTHY NON-SMOKERS (NOTE: WHERE HEALTHY EX-SMOKERS WERE USED A COMMENT IS ADDED) *(continued)*

pH Study	Normal values	Subjects (n)	Methodology (collection device, measurement)	Comments
Czebe et al.(112)	*Ecoscreen: 6.45±0.20 RTube: 6.19±0.23 Anacon: 6.10±0.26	12	Ecoscreen, Rtube, Anacon. CO_2 standardisation method	
Czebe et al.(144)	*6.44±0.16	19	Ecoscreen, CO_2 standardisation method	
Do et al.(145)	*7.6±0.2	5	Rtube, pH-meter	Argon gas deaeration
Effros et al.(127)	§7.24±0.24 (6.11-8.34)	10	Custom built	Without deaeration
Gessner et al.(135)	*7.46±0.48	12	Ecoscreen, blood gas analyzer	Without deaeration
Hauswirth et al. (70)	¥before deaeration 6.17 (5.50-6.78) After deaeration 8.09 (7.41-8.23)	270	Rtube, dry ice-samples thawed and pH measured with pH-meter	African Americans. 24 smokers
Hunt et al.(72)	€7.65±0.20	19	Custom built, pH-meter	Argon gas deaeration
Kostikas et al.(30)	†7.57 (7.51-7.64)	10	Glass condenser, pH-meter	Argon gas deaeration
Kullmann et al.(146)	*6.36±0.03 6.30±0.03	12	Ecoscreen, Blood gas analyzer, CO_2 standardization method	2 consecutive baseline measurements
Niimi et al.(147)	*8.26±0.20	16	Ecoscreen, pH-meter	Argon gas deaeration
Ojoo et al.(130)	$6.08 (5.58-6.64)	15	Custom built, pH-meter	Without deaeration
Paget-Brown et al.(138)	¥8.0 (7.8-8.1)	404	Rtube, pH-meter	Argon gas deaeration

continued

TABLE 5

Levels of EBC pH Measured in Healthy Non-Smokers (Note: Where healthy Ex-Smokers Were Used a Comment is Added) *(continued)*

pH Study	Normal values	Subjects (n)	Methodology (collection device, measurement)	Comments
Petrosyan et al.(36)	* 7.77±0.05 non obese 7.79±0.09 obese	10 9	Ecoscreen, pH -meter	Argon gas deaeration
Prieto et al.(145)	√ Ecoscreen -deaerated: 8.17 (8.08-8.26) -non deaerated: 6.99 (6.85-7.13) Rtube: -deaerated: 8.05 (7.92-8.17) -non deaerated: 6.67 (6.53-6.81)	6	Ecoscreen, Rtube, pH -meter	Before and after gas deaeration. Samples analyzed immediately and after freezing for 8 weeks.
Riediker et al.(148)	*8.20±0.13	15	R Tube, pH-meter	Nitrogen deaeration. Studied the acute effect of exercise.
Rolla et al.(64)	¥6.60 (6.42-6.76)	12	R Tube, pH-meter	Argon gas deaeration
Soyer et al.(94)	¥7.55 (6.88-7.90) 7.54 (7.09-7.93)	30	Ecoscreen, pH-meter Rtube, pH-meter	Argon gas deaeration
Tate et al.(131)	*6.15±0.16	12	Custom built, pH-meter	Without deaeration
Ueno et al.(39)	* before deaeration 6.16±0.07 After deaeration 7.69 ±0.1	58	Ecoscreen, pH-meter	Before and after deaeration
Valenzuela et al.(40)	*7.69±0.24	37	Custom built, pH-meter	Argon gas deaeration
Vaughan et al.(129)	*7.70±0.49	76	Rtube, pH-meter	Argon gas deaeration
Zhao et al.(126)	¥7.70(7.62-7.74)	20	Ecoscreen, pH-meter	Nitrogen gas deaeration

Symbols: *Mean ±SD, †Mean (95% CI), §Mean ±SEM, €Mean (SEM), ¥Median (25th, 75th percentile), $Median (range), £range, √ mean (95% CI) was observed in obese subjects compared to healthy volunteers (143), whereas in the study of Petrosyan et al. pH did not differ among non-obese and obese control subjects (36). Finally, no differences in the levels of LTB4 and nitrates were detected between obese and non-obese controls (36).

• **Gender:** Controversial data exist on the impact of gender on EBC H_2O_2 levels. Nowak et al. report that female never smokers exhale more H_2O_2 compared to male volunteers (9), whereas Szkudlarek et al. report no such difference (38). EBC pH values (65, 134, 138, 174), nitrite (65), nitrate (65) and 8-isoprostane (65) did not differ between males and females.

COMPARISON OF THE LEVELS OF SOME EBC BIOMARKERS IN HEALTHY SMOKERS VS. NON-SMOKERS

Biomarker	Study	Levels in smokers compared to non-smokers
H_2O_2	(14) (25) (9) (18) (13)	↑
	(26, 39, 175)	↔
NO_2^-/NO_3^-	(51, 63)	↔
Nitrate (NO_3^-)	(50)	↑
Nitrite (NO_2^-)	(68, 70)	↑
	(51) (39, 56)	↔
Nitrotyrosine	(51) (176)	↔
PGE2	(77)	↔
LTB4	(85, 88)	↑
	(111)	↔
LTD4	(88)	↑
LTE4	(88)	↑
8-isoprostane	(103, 120)	↑
	(111, 119, 177)	↔
pH	(39, 103, 111, 134, 174, 177)	↔
Aldehydes	(152)	↑ malondialdehyde, acrolein, n-hexanal
	(153)	↑ malondialdehyde, hexanal, heptanal ↔ nonanal
Glutathione	(156)	↑
Total protein	(68)	↑

Symbols: ↑ increased, ↔ no change.

- **Age:** Two studies demonstrated that H_2O_2 levels of healthy controls correlate with age (9, 33). As far as pH is concerned, although some studies show that pH does not differ with age (134, 138, 174), Cruz et al. (65) showed that pH after deaeration was lower in the 60- to 80-age group. In the same study 8-isoprostane levels showed a relationship with age, with the youngest groups having lower levels (65). Contrary to the above mentioned markers, TBARs(9), ammonia (133), nitrite (65) and nitrate (65) do not differ with age.
- **Height:** No correlation was found with pH levels (134).

Conclusions

Efforts to interpret the results of clinical trials and to determine reference values of EBC markers are extremely difficult tasks, due to the absence of many large clinical studies focusing on healthy subjects and the lack of standardization of the currently used methodologies. The diversity of sample collection devices, many of which are custom made, differences in collection techniques, sample storage and analysis, as well as issues related to the stability and reproducibility of mediators' measurements represent only a few of the confounding factors in EBC collection. From the mediators studied in this chapter, deaerated EBC pH represents the only biomarker with established normal values. There is an urgent need for proper standardization of EBC collection and evaluation of biomarkers in studies involving large numbers of normal subjects in order to establish normal values of mediators, with H_2O_2, 8-isoprostane and LTB4 representing the most promising biomarkers today. Such studies, followed by longitudinal studies and clinical trials using EBC biomarkers, may lead to the introduction of EBC in clinical practice.

References

1. Horvath I, Hunt J, Barnes PJ, Alving K, Antczak A, Baraldi E, et al. Exhaled breath condensate: methodological recommendations and unresolved questions. Eur Respir J. 2005 Sep; 26(3):523-48.

2. Silkoff PE, Erzurum SC, Lundberg JO, George SC, Marczin N, Hunt JF, et al. ATS workshop proceedings: exhaled nitric oxide and nitric oxide oxidative metabolism in exhaled breath condensate. Proc Am Thorac Soc. 2006 Apr; 3(2):131-45.

3. de Laurentiis G, Paris D, Melck D,

Maniscalco M, Marsico S, Corso G, et al. Metabonomic analysis of exhaled breath condensate in adults by nuclear magnetic resonance spectroscopy. Eur Respir J. 2008 Nov;32(5):1175-83.

4. Jobsis Q, Raatgeep HC, Schellekens SL, Hop WC, Hermans PW, de Jongste JC. Hydrogen peroxide in exhaled air of healthy children: reference values. Eur Respir J. 1998 Aug;12(2): 483-5.

5. Gallati H, Pracht I. [Horseradish peroxidase: kinetic studies and optimization of peroxidase activity determination using the substrates H2O2 and 3,3',5,5'-tetramethylbenzidine]. J Clin Chem Clin Biochem. 1985 Aug;23(8): 453-60.

6. Dekhuijzen PN, Aben KK, Dekker I, Aarts LP, Wielders PL, van Herwaarden CL, et al. Increased exhalation of hydrogen peroxide in patients with stable and unstable chronic obstructive pulmonary disease. Am J Respir Crit Care Med. 1996 Sep;154(3 Pt 1): 813-6.

7. Hyslop PA, Sklar LA. A quantitative fluorimetric assay for the determination of oxidant production by polymorphonuclear leukocytes: its use in the simultaneous fluorimetric assay of cellular activation processes. Anal Biochem. 1984 Aug 15;141(1):280-6.

8. Ruch W, Cooper PH, Baggiolini M. Assay of H2O2 production by macrophages and neutrophils with homovanillic acid and horse-radish peroxidase. J Immunol Methods. 1983 Oct 28;63(3):347-57.

9. Nowak D, Kalucka S, Bialasiewicz P, Krol M. Exhalation of H2O2 and thiobarbituric acid reactive substances (TBARs) by healthy subjects. Free

Radic Biol Med. 2001 Jan 15;30(2): 178-86.

10. Svensson S, Olin AC, Larstad M, Ljungkvist G, Toren K. Determination of hydrogen peroxide in exhaled breath condensate by flow injection analysis with fluorescence detection. J Chromatogr B Analyt Technol Biomed Life Sci. 2004 Oct 5;809(2):199-203.

11. van Beurden WJ, van den Bosch MJ, Janssen WC, Smeenk FW, Dekhuijzen PN, Harff GA. Fluorimetric analysis of hydrogen peroxide with automated measurement. Clin Lab. 2003;49(11-12):637-43.

12. Kietzmann D, Kahl R, Muller M, Burchardi H, Kettler D. Hydrogen peroxide in expired breath condensate of patients with acute respiratory failure and with ARDS. Intensive Care Med. 1993;19(2):78-81.

13. Zappacosta B, Persichilli S, Mormile F, Minucci A, Russo A, Giardina B, et al. A fast chemiluminescent method for H(2)O(2) measurement in exhaled breath condensate. Clin Chim Acta. 2001 Aug 20;310(2):187-91.

14. Gerritsen WB, Zanen P, Bauwens AA, van den Bosch JM, Haas FJ. Validation of a new method to measure hydrogen peroxide in exhaled breath condensate. Respir Med. 2005 Sep;99(9):1132-7.

15. Razola SS, Ruiz BL, Diez NM, Mark HB, Jr., Kauffmann JM. Hydrogen peroxide sensitive amperometric biosensor based on horseradish peroxidase entrapped in a polypyrrole electrode. Biosens Bioelectron. 2002 Dec;17(11-12):921-8.

16. Thanachasai S, Rokutanzono S, Yoshida S, Watanabe T. Novel hydrogen peroxide sensors based on perox-

idase-carrying poly[pyrrole-co-[4-(3-pyrrolyl)butanesulfonate]] copolymer films. Anal Sci. 2002 Jul;18(7):773-7.

17. Antczak A, Nowak D, Shariati B, Krol M, Piasecka G, Kurmanowska Z. Increased hydrogen peroxide and thiobarbituric acid-reactive products in expired breath condensate of asthmatic patients. Eur Respir J. 1997 Jun; 10(6):1235-41.

18. Nowak D, Antczak A, Krol M, Pietras T, Shariati B, Bialasiewicz P, et al. Increased content of hydrogen peroxide in the expired breath of cigarette smokers. Eur Respir J. 1996 Apr; 9(4):652-7.

19. Antczak A, Kurmanowska Z, Kasielski M, Nowak D. Inhaled glucocorticosteroids decrease hydrogen peroxide level in expired air condensate in asthmatic patients. Respir Med. 2000 May;94(5):416-21.

20. Chow S, Campbell C, Sandrini A, Thomas PS, Johnson AR, Yates DH. Exhaled breath condensate biomarkers in asbestos-related lung disorders. Respir Med. 2009 Aug;103(8):1091-7.

21. Corradi M, Alinovi R, Goldoni M, Vettori M, Folesani G, Mozzoni P, et al. Biomarkers of oxidative stress after controlled human exposure to ozone. Toxicol Lett. 2002 Aug 5;134(1-3): 219-25.

22. Emelyanov A, Fedoseev G, Abulimity A, Rudinski K, Fedoulov A, Karabanov A, et al. Elevated concentrations of exhaled hydrogen peroxide in asthmatic patients. Chest. 2001 Oct;120(4):1136-9.

23. Fireman E, Shtark M, Priel IE, Shiner R, Mor R, Kivity S, et al. Hydrogen peroxide in exhaled breath condensate (EBC) vs eosinophil count in induced sputum (IS) in parenchymal vs airways lung diseases. Inflammation. 2007 Apr;30(1-2):44-51.

24. Ganas K, Loukides S, Papatheodorou G, Panagou P, Kalogeropoulos N. Total nitrite/nitrate in expired breath condensate of patients with asthma. Respir Med. 2001 Aug;95(8):649-54.

25. Gerritsen WB, Asin J, Zanen P, van den Bosch JM, Haas FJ. Markers of inflammation and oxidative stress in exacerbated chronic obstructive pulmonary disease patients. Respir Med. 2005 Jan;99(1):84-90.

26. Guatura SB, Martinez JA, Santos Bueno PC, Santos ML. Increased exhalation of hydrogen peroxide in healthy subjects following cigarette consumption. Sao Paulo Med J. 2000 Jul 6;118(4):93-8.

27. Ho LP, Faccenda J, Innes JA, Greening AP. Expired hydrogen peroxide in breath condensate of cystic fibrosis patients. Eur Respir J. 1999 Jan; 13(1):103-6.

28. Horvath I, Donnelly LE, Kiss A, Kharitonov SA, Lim S, Chung KF, et al. Combined use of exhaled hydrogen peroxide and nitric oxide in monitoring asthma. Am J Respir Crit Care Med. 1998 Oct;158(4):1042-6.

29. Kwiatkowska S, Szkudlarek U, Luczynska M, Nowak D, Zieba M. Elevated exhalation of hydrogen peroxide and circulating IL-18 in patients with pulmonary tuberculosis. Respir Med. 2007 Mar;101(3):574-80.

30. Kostikas K, Papatheodorou G, Ganas K, Psathakis K, Panagou P, Loukides S. pH in expired breath condensate of patients with inflammatory airway diseases. Am J Respir Crit Care Med. 2002 May 15;165(10):1364-70.

31. Loukides S, Horvath I, Wodehouse T, Cole PJ, Barnes PJ. Elevated levels of expired breath hydrogen peroxide in bronchiectasis. Am J Respir Crit Care Med. 1998 Sep;158(3):991-4.

32. Loukides S, Bouros D, Papatheodorou G, Panagou P, Siafakas NM. The relationships among hydrogen peroxide in expired breath condensate, airway inflammation, and asthma severity. Chest. 2002 Feb;121(2):338-46.

33. Luczynska M, Szkudlarek U, Dziankowska-Bartkowiak B, Waszczykowska E, Kasielski M, Sysa-Jedrzejowska A, et al. Elevated exhalation of hydrogen peroxide in patients with systemic sclerosis. Eur J Clin Invest. 2003 Mar;33(3):274-9.

34. Majewska E, Kasielski M, Luczynski R, Bartosz G, Bialasiewicz P, Nowak D. Elevated exhalation of hydrogen peroxide and thiobarbituric acid reactive substances in patients with community acquired pneumonia. Respir Med. 2004 Jul;98(7):669-76.

35. Nowak D, Kasielski M, Antczak A, Pietras T, Bialasiewicz P. Increased content of thiobarbituric acid-reactive substances and hydrogen peroxide in the expired breath condensate of patients with stable chronic obstructive pulmonary disease: no significant effect of cigarette smoking. Respir Med. 1999 Jun;93(6):389-96.

36. Petrosyan M, Perraki E, Simoes D, Koutsourelakis I, Vagiakis E, Roussos C, et al. Exhaled breath markers in patients with obstructive sleep apnoea. Sleep Breath. 2008 Aug;12(3):207-15.

37. Rysz J, Kasielski M, Apanasiewicz J, Krol M, Woznicki A, Luciak M, et al. Increased hydrogen peroxide in the exhaled breath of uraemic patients unaffected by haemodialysis. Nephrol Dial Transplant. 2004 Jan;19(1):158-63.

38. Szkudlarek U, Maria L, Kasielski M, Kaucka S, Nowak D. Exhaled hydrogen peroxide correlates with the release of reactive oxygen species by blood phagocytes in healthy subjects. Respir Med. 2003 Jun;97(6):718-25.

39. Ueno T, Kataoka M, Hirano A, Iio K, Tanimoto Y, Kanehiro A, et al. Inflammatory markers in exhaled breath condensate from patients with asthma. Respirology. 2008 Sep;13(5): 654-63.

40. Valenzuela OF, Encina MP. Design and evaluation of a device for collecting exhaled breath condensate. J Bras Pneumol. 2009 Jan;35(1):69-72.

41. Kharitonov SA, Barnes PJ. Clinical aspects of exhaled nitric oxide. Eur Respir J. 2000 Oct;16(4):781-92.

42. Ricciardolo FL, Di Stefano A, Sabatini F, Folkerts G. Reactive nitrogen species in the respiratory tract. Eur J Pharmacol. 2006 Mar 8;533(1-3): 240-52.

43. Eiserich JP, Patel RP, O'Donnell VB. Pathophysiology of nitric oxide and related species: free radical reactions and modification of biomolecules. Mol Aspects Med. 1998 Aug-Oct;19(4-5):221-357.

44. Osoata GO, Hanazawa T, Brindicci C, Ito M, Barnes PJ, Kharitonov S, et al. Peroxynitrite elevation in exhaled breath condensate of COPD and its inhibition by fudosteine. Chest. 2009 Jun;135(6):1513-20.

45. Marzinzig M, Nussler AK, Stadler J, Marzinzig E, Barthlen W, Nussler NC, et al. Improved methods to measure end products of nitric oxide in biological flu-

ids: nitrite, nitrate, and S-nitrosothiols. Nitric Oxide. 1997 Apr;1(2):177-89.

46. Green LC, Wagner DA, Glogowski J, Skipper PL, Wishnok JS, Tannenbaum SR. Analysis of nitrate, nitrite, and [15N]nitrate in biological fluids. Anal Biochem. 1982 Oct;126(1):131-8.

47. Misko TP, Schilling RJ, Salvemini D, Moore WM, Currie MG. A fluorometric assay for the measurement of nitrite in biological samples. Anal Biochem. 1993 Oct;214(1):11-6.

48. Nguyen TA, Woo-Park J, Hess M, Goins M, Urban P, Vaughan J, et al. Assaying all of the nitrogen oxides in breath modifies the interpretation of exhaled nitric oxide. Vascul Pharmacol. 2005 Dec;43(6):379-84.

49. Dweik RA, Laskowski D, Abu-Soud HM, Kaneko F, Hutte R, Stuehr DJ, et al. Nitric oxide synthesis in the lung. Regulation by oxygen through a kinetic mechanism. J Clin Invest. 1998 Feb 1;101(3):660-6.

50. Corradi M, Pesci A, Casana R, Alinovi R, Goldoni M, Vettori MV, et al. Nitrate in exhaled breath condensate of patients with different airway diseases. Nitric Oxide. 2003 Feb;8(1):26-30.

51. Balint B, Donnelly LE, Hanazawa T, Kharitonov SA, Barnes PJ. Increased nitric oxide metabolites in exhaled breath condensate after exposure to tobacco smoke. Thorax. 2001 Jun; 56(6):456-61.

52. Apyari VV, Dmitrienko SG, Ostrovskaya VM, Anaev EK, Zolotov YA. Use of polyurethane foam and 3-hydroxy-7,8-benzo-1,2,3,4-tetrahydroquinoline for determination of nitrite by diffuse reflectance spectroscopy and colorimetry. Anal Bioanal Chem. 2008 Jul;391(5):1977-82.

53. Franklin P, Moeller A, Hall GL, Horak F, Jr., Patterson H, Stick SM. Variability of nitric oxide metabolites in exhaled breath condensate. Respir Med. 2006 Jan;100(1):123-9.

54. Eu JP, Liu L, Zeng M, Stamler JS. An apoptotic model for nitrosative stress. Biochemistry. 2000 Feb 8;39(5): 1040-7.

55. Rahman I, Biswas SK, Kode A. Oxidant and antioxidant balance in the airways and airway diseases. Eur J Pharmacol. 2006 Mar 8;533(1-3): 222-39.

56. Corradi M, Montuschi P, Donnelly LE, Pesci A, Kharitonov SA, Barnes PJ. Increased nitrosothiols in exhaled breath condensate in inflammatory airway diseases. Am J Respir Crit Care Med. 2001 Mar;163(4):854-8.

57. Reiter CD, Teng RJ, Beckman JS. Superoxide reacts with nitric oxide to nitrate tyrosine at physiological pH via peroxynitrite. J Biol Chem. 2000 Oct 20;275(42):32460-6.

58. Balint B, Kharitonov SA, Hanazawa T, Donnelly LE, Shah PL, Hodson ME, et al. Increased nitrotyrosine in exhaled breath condensate in cystic fibrosis. Eur Respir J. 2001 Jun;17(6):1201-7.

59. Hanazawa T, Kharitonov SA, Barnes PJ. Increased nitrotyrosine in exhaled breath condensate of patients with asthma. Am J Respir Crit Care Med. 2000 Oct;162(4 Pt 1):1273-6.

60. Celio S, Troxler H, Durka SS, Chladek J, Wildhaber JH, Sennhauser FH, et al. Free 3-nitrotyrosine in exhaled breath condensates of children fails as a marker for oxidative stress in stable cystic fibrosis and asthma. Nitric Oxide. 2006 Jul 11.

61. Larstad M, Soderling AS, Caidahl K, Olin

AC. Selective quantification of free 3-nitrotyrosine in exhaled breath condensate in asthma using gas chromatography/tandem mass spectrometry. Nitric Oxide. 2005 Sep;13(2):134-44.

62. Brindicci C, Ito K, Torre O, Barnes PJ, Kharitonov SA. Effects of aminoguanidine, an inhibitor of inducible nitric oxide synthase, on nitric oxide production and its metabolites in healthy control subjects, healthy smokers, and COPD patients. Chest. 2009 Feb;135(2):353-67.

63. Liu J, Sandrini A, Thurston MC, Yates DH, Thomas PS. Nitric oxide and exhaled breath nitrite/nitrates in chronic obstructive pulmonary disease patients. Respiration. 2007;74(6): 617-23.

64. Rolla G, Bruno M, Bommarito L, Heffler E, Ferrero N, Petrarulo M, et al. Breath analysis in patients with end-stage renal disease: effect of haemodialysis. Eur J Clin Invest. 2008 Oct;38(10):728-33.

65. Cruz MJ, Sanchez-Vidaurre S, Romero PV, Morell F, Munoz X. Impact of age on pH, 8-isoprostane, and nitrogen oxides in exhaled breath condensate. Chest. 2009 Feb;135(2):462-7.

66. Effros RM, Hoagland KW, Bosbous M, Castillo D, Foss B, Dunning M, et al. Dilution of respiratory solutes in exhaled condensates. Am J Respir Crit Care Med. 2002 Mar 1;165(5): 663-9.

67. Hunt J, Byrns RE, Ignarro LJ, Gaston B. Condensed expirate nitrite as a home marker for acute asthma. Lancet. 1995 Nov 4;346(8984):1235-6.

68. Garey KW, Neuhauser MM, Robbins RA, Danziger LH, Rubinstein I. Markers of inflammation in exhaled breath condensate of young healthy smokers. Chest. 2004 Jan;125(1):22-6.

69. Gessner C, Hammerschmidt S, Kuhn H, Hoheisel G, Gillissen A, Sack U, et al. Breath condensate nitrite correlates with hyperinflation in chronic obstructive pulmonary disease. Respir Med. 2007 Nov;101(11):2271-8.

70. Hauswirth DW, Sundy JS, Mervin-Blake S, Fernandez CA, Patch KB, Alexander KM, et al. Normative values for exhaled breath condensate pH and its relationship to exhaled nitric oxide in healthy African Americans. J Allergy Clin Immunol. 2008 Jul;122(1):101-6.

71. Ho LP, Innes JA, Greening AP. Nitrite levels in breath condensate of patients with cystic fibrosis is elevated in contrast to exhaled nitric oxide. Thorax. 1998 Aug;53(8):680-4.

72. Hunt JF, Fang K, Malik R, Snyder A, Malhotra N, Platts-Mills TA, et al. Endogenous airway acidification. Implications for asthma pathophysiology. Am J Respir Crit Care Med. 2000 Mar; 161(3 Pt 1):694-9.

73. Leslie CC. Regulation of the specific release of arachidonic acid by cytosolic phospholipase A2. Prostaglandins Leukot Essent Fatty Acids. 2004 Apr;70(4):373-6.

74. Smith WL. The eicosanoids and their biochemical mechanisms of action. Biochem J. 1989 Apr 15;259(2):315-24.

75. Funk CD. Prostaglandins and leukotrienes: advances in eicosanoid biology. Science. 2001 Nov 30;294 (5548):1871-5.

76. Antczak A, Montuschi P, Kharitonov S, Gorski P, Barnes PJ. Increased exhaled cysteinyl-leukotrienes and 8-isoprostane in aspirin-induced asth-

ma. Am J Respir Crit Care Med. 2002 Aug 1;166(3):301-6.

77. Kostikas K, Papatheodorou G, Psathakis K, Panagou P, Loukides S. Prostaglandin E2 in the expired breath condensate of patients with asthma. Eur Respir J. 2003 Nov;22(5):743-7.

78. Montuschi P, Barnes PJ. Exhaled leukotrienes and prostaglandins in asthma. J Allergy Clin Immunol. 2002 Apr;109(4):615-20.

79. Montuschi P, Ragazzoni E, Valente S, Corbo G, Mondino C, Ciappi G, et al. Validation of 8-isoprostane and prostaglandin E(2) measurements in exhaled breath condensate. Inflamm Res. 2003 Dec;52(12):502-7.

80. Huszar E, Szabo Z, Jakab A, Barta I, Herjavecz I, Horvath I. Comparative measurement of thromboxane A2 metabolites in exhaled breath condensate by different immunoassays. Inflamm Res. 2005 Aug;54(8):350-5.

81. Vass G, Huszar E, Barat E, Valyon M, Kiss D, Penzes I, et al. Comparison of nasal and oral inhalation during exhaled breath condensate collection. Am J Respir Crit Care Med. 2003 Mar 15;167(6):850-5.

82. Claesson HE, Odlander B, Jakobsson PJ. Leukotriene B4 in the immune system. Int J Immunopharmacol. 1992 Apr;14(3):441-9.

83. Antczak A, Kharitonov SA, Montuschi P, Gorski P, Barnes PJ. Inflammatory response to sputum induction measured by exhaled markers. Respiration. 2005 Nov-Dec;72(6):594-9.

84. Carpagnano GE, Barnes PJ, Geddes DM, Hodson ME, Kharitonov SA. Increased leukotriene B4 and interleukin-6 in exhaled breath condensate in cystic fibrosis. Am J Respir Crit Care Med. 2003 Apr 15;167(8):1109-12.

85. Carpagnano GE, Kharitonov SA, Foschino-Barbaro MP, Resta O, Gramiccioni E, Barnes PJ. Increased inflammatory markers in the exhaled breath condensate of cigarette smokers. Eur Respir J. 2003 Apr;21(4):589-93.

86. Kostikas K, Gaga M, Papatheodorou G, Karamanis T, Orphanidou D, Loukides S. Leukotriene B4 in exhaled breath condensate and sputum supernatant in patients with COPD and asthma. Chest. 2005 May;127(5):1553-9.

87. Bucchioni E, Csoma Z, Allegra L, Chung KF, Barnes PJ, Kharitonov SA. Adenosine 5'-monophosphate increases levels of leukotrienes in breath condensate in asthma. Respir Med. 2004 Jul;98(7):651-5.

88. Cap P, Chladek J, Pehal F, Maly M, Petru V, Barnes PJ, et al. Gas chromatography/mass spectrometry analysis of exhaled leukotrienes in asthmatic patients. Thorax. 2004 Jun;59(6):465-70.

89. Montuschi P, Martello S, Felli M, Mondino C, Barnes PJ, Chiarotti M. Liquid chromatography/mass spectrometry analysis of exhaled leukotriene B4 in asthmatic children. Respir Res. 2005;6:119.

90. Biernacki WA, Kharitonov SA, Barnes PJ. Increased leukotriene B4 and 8-isoprostane in exhaled breath condensate of patients with exacerbations of COPD. Thorax. 2003 Apr;58(4):294-8.

91. Montuschi P, Martello S, Felli M, Mondino C, Chiarotti M. Ion trap liquid chromatography/tandem mass spectrometry analysis of leukotriene B4 in exhaled breath condensate. Rapid Commun Mass Spectrom. 2004;18(22):2723-9.

92. Gaber F, Acevedo F, Delin I, Sundblad BM, Palmberg L, Larsson K, et al. Saliva is one likely source of leukotriene B4 in exhaled breath condensate. Eur Respir J. 2006 Dec;28(6): 1229-35.

93. Tufvesson E, Bjermer L. Methodological improvements for measuring eicosanoids and cytokines in exhaled breath condensate. Respir Med. 2006 Jan;100(1):34-8.

94. Soyer OU, Dizdar EA, Keskin O, Lilly C, Kalayci O. Comparison of two methods for exhaled breath condensate collection. Allergy. 2006 Aug; 61(8):1016-8.

95. Janssen LJ. Isoprostanes: an overview and putative roles in pulmonary pathophysiology. Am J Physiol Lung Cell Mol Physiol. 2001 Jun; 280(6):L1067-82.

96. Milne GL, Musiek ES, Morrow JD. F2-isoprostanes as markers of oxidative stress in vivo: an overview. Biomarkers. 2005 Nov;10 Suppl 1:S10-23.

97. Carpenter CT, Price PV, Christman BW. Exhaled breath condensate isoprostanes are elevated in patients with acute lung injury or ARDS. Chest. 1998 Dec;114(6):1653-9.

98. Moloney ED, Mumby SE, Gajdocsi R, Cranshaw JH, Kharitonov SA, Quinlan GJ, et al. Exhaled breath condensate detects markers of pulmonary inflammation after cardiothoracic surgery. Am J Respir Crit Care Med. 2004 Jan 1;169(1):64-9.

99. Syslova K, Kacer P, Kuzma M, Klusackova P, Fenclova Z, Lebedova J, et al. Determination of 8-isoprostaglandin F(2alpha) in exhaled breath condensate using combination of immunoseparation and LC-ESI-MS/MS. J Chromatogr B Analyt Technol Biomed Life Sci. 2008 May 1;867 (1):8-14.

100. Battaglia S, den Hertog H, Timmers MC, Lazeroms SP, Vignola AM, Rabe KF, et al. Small airways function and molecular markers in exhaled air in mild asthma. Thorax. 2005 Aug;60(8):639-44.

101. Carpagnano GE, Kharitonov SA, Foschino-Barbaro MP, Resta O, Gramiccioni E, Barnes PJ. Supplementary oxygen in healthy subjects and those with COPD increases oxidative stress and airway inflammation. Thorax. 2004 Dec;59(12):1016-9.

102. Carpagnano GE, Resta O, Foschino-Barbaro MP, Spanevello A, Stefano A, Di Gioia G, et al. Exhaled Interleukine-6 and 8-isoprostane in chronic obstructive pulmonary disease: effect of carbocysteine lysine salt monohydrate (SCMC-Lys). Eur J Pharmacol. 2004 Nov 28;505(1-3): 169-75.

103. Borrill ZL, Roy K, Vessey RS, Woodcock AA, Singh D. Non-invasive biomarkers and pulmonary function in smokers. Int J Chron Obstruct Pulmon Dis. 2008;3(1):171-83.

104. Corhay JL, Henket M, Nguyen D, Duysinx B, Sele J, Louis R. Leukotriene B4 Contributes to Exhaled Breath Condensate and Sputum Neutrophil Chemotaxis in COPD. Chest. 2009 May 8.

105. Hoffmeyer F, Harth V, Merget R, Goldscheid N, Hainze E, Degens P, et al. Exhaled breath condensate analysis: evaluation of a methodological setting for epidemiological field studies. J Physiol Pharmacol. 2007 Nov;58 Suppl 5(Pt 1):289-98.

106. Ko FW, Leung TF, Wong GW, Ngai J, To KW, Ng S, et al. Measurement of tumor necrosis factor-alpha, leukotriene B4, and interleukin 8 in the exhaled breath condensate in patients with acute exacerbations of chronic obstructive pulmonary disease. Int J Chron Obstruct Pulmon Dis. 2009;4(1):79-86.

107. Lehtonen H, Oksa P, Lehtimaki L, Sepponen A, Nieminen R, Kankaanranta H, et al. Increased alveolar nitric oxide concentration and high levels of leukotriene B(4) and 8-isoprostane in exhaled breath condensate in patients with asbestosis. Thorax. 2007 Jul;62(7):602-7.

108. Makinen T, Lehtimaki L, Kinnunen H, Nieminen R, Kankaanranta H, Moilanen E. Bronchial diffusing capacity of nitric oxide is increased in patients with allergic rhinitis. Int Arch Allergy Immunol. 2009;148(2):154-60.

109. Pelclova D, Fenclova Z, Kacer P, Navratil T, Kuzma M, Lebedova JK, et al. 8-isoprostane and leukotrienes in exhaled breath condensate in Czech subjects with silicosis. Ind Health. 2007 Dec;45(6):766-74.

110. Piotrowski WJ, Antczak A, Marczak J, Nawrocka A, Kurmanowska Z, Gorski P. Eicosanoids in exhaled breath condensate and BAL fluid of patients with sarcoidosis. Chest. 2007 Aug;132(2):589-96.

111. Tanou K, Koutsokera A, Kiropoulos TS, Maniati M, Papaioannou AI, Georga K, et al. Inflammatory and oxidative stress biomarkers in allergic rhinitis: the effect of smoking. Clin Exp Allergy. 2009 Mar;39(3):345-53.

112. Czebe K, Barta I, Antus B, Valyon M, Horvath I, Kullmann T. Influence of condensing equipment and temperature on exhaled breath condensate pH, total protein and leukotriene concentrations. Respir Med. 2008 May;102(5):720-5.

113. Samitas K, Chorianopoulos D, Vittorakis S, Zervas E, Economidou E, Papatheodorou G, et al. Exhaled cysteinyl-leukotrienes and 8-isoprostane in patients with asthma and their relation to clinical severity. Respir Med. 2009 May;103(5):750-6.

114. Dentener MA, Creutzberg EC, Pennings HJ, Rijkers GT, Mercken E, Wouters EF. Effect of infliximab on local and systemic inflammation in chronic obstructive pulmonary disease: a pilot study. Respiration. 2008;76(3):275-82.

115. Heinicke I, Boehler A, Rechsteiner T, Bogdanova A, Jelkmann W, Hofer M, et al. Moderate altitude but not additional endurance training increases markers of oxidative stress in exhaled breath condensate. Eur J Appl Physiol. 2009 Jul;106(4):599-604.

116. Ko FW, Lau CY, Leung TF, Wong GW, Lam CW, Hui DS. Exhaled breath condensate levels of 8-isoprostane, growth related oncogene alpha and monocyte chemoattractant protein-1 in patients with chronic obstructive pulmonary disease. Respir Med. 2006 Apr;100(4):630-8.

117. Li Y, Chongsuvivatwong V, Geater A, Liu A. Are biomarker levels a good follow-up tool for evaluating obstructive sleep apnea syndrome treatments? Respiration. 2008;76(3):317-23.

118. Makris D, Paraskakis E, Korakas P, Karagiannakis E, Sourvinos G, Siafakas NM, et al. Exhaled breath con-

densate 8-isoprostane, clinical parameters, radiological indices and airway inflammation in COPD. Respiration. 2008;75(2):138-44.

119. Mazur W, Stark H, Sovijarvi A, Myllarniemi M, Kinnula VL. Comparison of 8-Isoprostane and Interleukin-8 in Induced Sputum and Exhaled Breath Condensate from Asymptomatic and Symptomatic Smokers. Respiration. 2009 Mar 2.

120. Montuschi P, Collins JV, Ciabattoni G, Lazzeri N, Corradi M, Kharitonov SA, et al. Exhaled 8-isoprostane as an in vivo biomarker of lung oxidative stress in patients with COPD and healthy smokers. Am J Respir Crit Care Med. 2000 Sep;162(3 Pt 1): 1175-7.

121. Montuschi P, Corradi M, Ciabattoni G, Nightingale J, Kharitonov SA, Barnes PJ. Increased 8-isoprostane, a marker of oxidative stress, in exhaled condensate of asthma patients. Am J Respir Crit Care Med. 1999 Jul;160(1):216-20.

122. Montuschi P, Nightingale JA, Kharitonov SA, Barnes PJ. Ozone-induced increase in exhaled 8-isoprostane in healthy subjects is resistant to inhaled budesonide. Free Radic Biol Med. 2002 Nov 15;33(10):1403-8.

123. Montuschi P, Kharitonov SA, Ciabattoni G, Corradi M, van Rensen L, Geddes DM, et al. Exhaled 8-isoprostane as a new non-invasive biomarker of oxidative stress in cystic fibrosis. Thorax. 2000 Mar; 55(3):205-9.

124. Psathakis K, Papatheodorou G, Plataki M, Panagou P, Loukides S, Siafakas NM, et al. 8-Isoprostane, a marker of oxidative stress, is increased in the expired breath condensate of patients with pulmonary sarcoidosis. Chest. 2004 Mar; 125(3):1005-11.

125. Rosias PP, Robroeks CM, Kester A, den Hartog GJ, Wodzig WK, Rijkers GT, et al. Biomarker reproducibility in exhaled breath condensate collected with different condensers. Eur Respir J. 2008 May;31(5):934-42.

126. Zhao JJ, Shimizu Y, Dobashi K, Kawata T, Ono A, Yanagitani N, et al. The relationship between oxidative stress and acid stress in adult patients with mild asthma. J Investig Allergol Clin Immunol. 2008;18(1): 41-5.

127. Effros RM, Casaburi R, Su J, Dunning M, Torday J, Biller J, et al. The effects of volatile salivary acids and bases on exhaled breath condensate pH. Am J Respir Crit Care Med. 2006 Feb 15;173(4):386-92.

128. Hunt J. Exhaled breath condensate pH: reflecting acidification of the airway at all levels. Am J Respir Crit Care Med. 2006 Feb 15;173(4):366-7.

129. Vaughan J, Ngamtrakulpanit L, Pajewski TN, Turner R, Nguyen TA, Smith A, et al. Exhaled breath condensate pH is a robust and reproducible assay of airway acidity. Eur Respir J. 2003 Dec;22(6):889-94.

130. Ojoo JC, Mulrennan SA, Kastelik JA, Morice AH, Redington AE. Exhaled breath condensate pH and exhaled nitric oxide in allergic asthma and in cystic fibrosis. Thorax. 2005 Jan; 60(1):22-6.

131. Tate S, MacGregor G, Davis M, Innes JA, Greening AP. Airways in cystic fibrosis are acidified: detection by

exhaled breath condensate. Thorax. 2002 Nov;57(11):926-9.

132. Noble DD, McCafferty JB, Greening AP, Innes JA. Respiratory heat and moisture loss is associated with eosinophilic inflammation in asthma. Eur Respir J. 2006 Nov 29.

133. Brooks SM, Haight RR, Gordon RL. Age does not affect airway pH and ammonia as determined by exhaled breath measurements. Lung. 2006 Jul-Aug;184(4):195-200.

134. Bloemen K, Lissens G, Desager K, Schoeters G. Determinants of variability of protein content, volume and pH of exhaled breath condensate. Respir Med. 2007 Jun;101(6):1331-7.

135. Gessner C, Hammerschmidt S, Kuhn H, Seyfarth HJ, Sack U, Engelmann L, et al. Exhaled breath condensate acidification in acute lung injury. Respir Med. 2003 Nov;97(11):1188-94.

136. Kullmann T, Barta I, Lazar Z, Szili B, Barat E, Valyon M, et al. Exhaled breath condensate pH standardised for CO2 partial pressure. Eur Respir J. 2007 Mar;29(3):496-501.

137. Prieto L, Ferrer A, Palop J, Domenech J, Llusar R, Rojas R. Differences in exhaled breath condensate pH measurements between samples obtained with two commercial devices. Respir Med. 2007 Aug;101(8):1715-20.

138. Paget-Brown AO, Ngamtrakulpanit L, Smith A, Bunyan D, Hom S, Nguyen A, et al. Normative data for pH of exhaled breath condensate. Chest. 2006 Feb;129(2):426-30.

139. Accordino R, Visentin A, Bordin A, Ferrazzoni S, Marian E, Rizzato F, et al. Long-term repeatability of exhaled breath condensate pH in asthma. Respir Med. 2008 Mar;102(3):377-81.

140. Borrill Z, Starkey C, Vestbo J, Singh D. Reproducibility of exhaled breath condensate pH in chronic obstructive pulmonary disease. Eur Respir J. 2005 Feb;25(2):269-74.

141. Carpagnano GE, Foschino Barbaro MP, Cagnazzo M, Di Gioia G, Giliberti T, Di Matteo C, et al. Use of exhaled breath condensate in the study of airway inflammation after hypertonic saline solution challenge. Chest. 2005 Nov;128(5):3159-66.

142. Carpagnano GE, Foschino Barbaro MP, Resta O, Gramiccioni E, Valerio NV, Bracciale P, et al. Exhaled markers in the monitoring of airways inflammation and its response to steroid's treatment in mild persistent asthma. Eur J Pharmacol. 2005 Sep 5;519(1-2):175-81.

143. Carpagnano GE, Spanevello A, Sabato R, Depalo A, Turchiarelli V, Foschino Barbaro MP. Exhaled pH, exhaled nitric oxide, and induced sputum cellularity in obese patients with obstructive sleep apnea syndrome. Transl Res. 2008 Jan; 151(1):45-50.

144. Czebe K, Kullmann T, Csiszer E, Barat E, Horvath I, Antus B. Variability of exhaled breath condensate pH in lung transplant recipients. Respiration. 2008;75(3):322-7.

145. Do R, Bartlett KH, Chu W, Dimich-Ward H, Kennedy SM. Within- and between-person variability of exhaled breath condensate pH and NH4+ in never and current smokers. Respir Med. 2008 Mar;102(3):457-63.

146. Kullmann T, Barta I, Antus B, Horvath I. Drinking influences exhaled breath

condensate acidity. Lung. 2008 Jul-Aug;186(4):263-8.

147. Niimi A, Nguyen LT, Usmani O, Mann B, Chung KF. Reduced pH and chloride levels in exhaled breath condensate of patients with chronic cough. Thorax. 2004 Jul;59(7):608-12.

148. Riediker M, Danuser B. Exhaled breath condensate pH is increased after moderate exercise. J Aerosol Med. 2007 Spring;20(1):13-8.

149. Zietkowski Z, Tomasiak-Lozowska MM, Skiepko R, Mroczko B, Szmitkowski M, Bodzenta-Lukaszyk A. High-sensitivity C-reactive protein in the exhaled breath condensate and serum in stable and unstable asthma. Respir Med. 2009 Mar;103(3): 379-85.

150. Csoma Z, Huszar E, Vizi E, Vass G, Szabo Z, Herjavecz I, et al. Adenosine level in exhaled breath increases during exercise-induced bronchoconstriction. Eur Respir J. 2005 May;25(5):873-8.

151. Huszar E, Vass G, Vizi E, Csoma Z, Barat E, Molnar Vilagos G, et al. Adenosine in exhaled breath condensate in healthy volunteers and in patients with asthma. Eur Respir J. 2002 Dec;20(6):1393-8.

152. Andreoli R, Manini P, Corradi M, Mutti A, Niessen WM. Determination of patterns of biologically relevant aldehydes in exhaled breath condensate of healthy subjects by liquid chromatography/atmospheric chemical ionization tandem mass spectrometry. Rapid Commun Mass Spectrom. 2003;17(7):637-45.

153. Corradi M, Rubinstein I, Andreoli R, Manini P, Caglieri A, Poli D, et al. Aldehydes in exhaled breath conden-sate of patients with chronic obstructive pulmonary disease. Am J Respir Crit Care Med. 2003 May 15;167(10):1380-6.

154. Corradi M, Pignatti P, Manini P, Andreoli R, Goldoni M, Poppa M, et al. Comparison between exhaled and sputum oxidative stress biomarkers in chronic airway inflammation. Eur Respir J. 2004 Dec;24(6):1011-7.

155. Barregard L, Sallsten G, Andersson L, Almstrand AC, Gustafson P, Andersson M, et al. Experimental exposure to wood smoke: effects on airway inflammation and oxidative stress. Occup Environ Med. 2008 May;65(5):319-24.

156. Nuttall SL, Routledge HC, Manney S. Circulating and exhaled markers of nitric oxide and antioxidant activity after smoking. Circulation. 2002 Nov 12;106(20):e145-6; discussion e-6.

157. Baker EH, Clark N, Brennan AL, Fisher DA, Gyi KM, Hodson ME, et al. Hyperglycemia and cystic fibrosis alter respiratory fluid glucose concentrations estimated by breath condensate analysis. J Appl Physiol. 2007 May;102(5):1969-75.

158. Effros RM, Biller J, Foss B, Hoagland K, Dunning MB, Castillo D, et al. A simple method for estimating respiratory solute dilution in exhaled breath condensates. Am J Respir Crit Care Med. 2003 Dec 15;168(12): 1500-5.

159. Svensson S, Isacsson AC, Ljungkvist G, Toren K, Olin AC. Optimization and validation of an ion chromatographic method for the simultaneous determination of sodium, ammonium and potassium in exhaled breath condensate. J Chromatogr B Analyt

Technol Biomed Life Sci. 2005 Jan 5;814(1):173-7.

160. Cap P, Dryahina K, Pehal F, Spanel P. Selected ion flow tube mass spectrometry of exhaled breath condensate headspace. Rapid Commun Mass Spectrom. 2008 Sep;22(18):2844-50.

161. Folesani G, Corradi M, Goldoni M, Manini P, Acampa O, Andreoli R, et al. Urea in exhaled breath condensate of uraemics and patients with chronic airway diseases. Acta Biomed. 2008;79 Suppl 1:79-86.

162. Gessner C, Scheibe R, Wotzel M, Hammerschmidt S, Kuhn H, Engelmann L, et al. Exhaled breath condensate cytokine patterns in chronic obstructive pulmonary disease. Respir Med. 2005 Oct;99(10):1229-40.

163. Kurova VS, Anaev EC, Kononikhin AS, Fedorchenko KY, Popov IA, Kalupov TL, et al. Proteomics of exhaled breath: methodological nuances and pitfalls. Clin Chem Lab Med. 2009;47(6):706-12.

164. Hoffmann HJ, Tabaksblat LM, Enghild JJ, Dahl R. Human skin keratins are the major proteins in exhaled breath condensate. Eur Respir J. 2008 Feb;31(2):380-4.

165. Fumagalli M, Dolcini L, Sala A, Stolk J, Fregonese L, Ferrari F, et al. Proteomic analysis of exhaled breath condensate from single patients with pulmonary emphysema associated to alpha1-antitrypsin deficiency. J Proteomics. 2008 Jul 21;71(2):211-21.

166. Scheideler L, Manke HG, Schwulera U, Inacker O, Hammerle H. Detection of nonvolatile macromolecules in breath. A possible diagnostic tool? Am Rev Respir Dis. 1993 Sep;148(3):778-84.

167. Edme JL, Tellart AS, Launay D, Neviere R, Grutzmacher C, Boulenguez C, et al. Cytokine concentrations in exhaled breath condensates in systemic sclerosis. Inflamm Res. 2008 Apr;57(4):151-6.

168. Griese M, Noss J, Schramel P. Elemental and ion composition of exhaled air condensate in cystic fibrosis. J Cyst Fibros. 2003 Sep;2(3):136-42.

169. Rozy A, Czerniawska J, Stepniewska A, Wozbinska B, Goljan A, Puscinska E, et al. Inflammatory markers in the exhaled breath condensate of patients with pulmonary sacroidosis. J Physiol Pharmacol. 2006 Sep;57 Suppl 4:335-40.

170. Schumann C, Triantafilou K, Krueger S, Hombach V, Triantafilou M, Becher G, et al. Detection of erythropoietin in exhaled breath condensate of non-hypoxic subjects using a multiplex bead array. Mediators Inflamm. 2006;2006(5):18061.

171. Yeh MY, Burnham EL, Moss M, Brown LA. Non-invasive evaluation of pulmonary glutathione in the exhaled breath condensate of otherwise healthy alcoholics. Respir Med. 2008 Feb;102(2):248-55.

172. Carpagnano GE, Kharitonov SA, Resta O, Foschino-Barbaro MP, Gramiccioni E, Barnes PJ. Increased 8-isoprostane and interleukin-6 in breath condensate of obstructive sleep apnea patients. Chest. 2002 Oct;122(4):1162-7.

173. Komakula S, Khatri S, Mermis J, Savill S, Haque S, Rojas M, et al. Body mass index is associated with reduced exhaled nitric oxide and higher exhaled 8-isoprostanes in asthmatics. Respir Res. 2007;8:32.

174. Varnai VM, Ljubicic A, Prester L, Macan J. Exhaled breath condensate pH in adult Croatian population without respiratory disorders: how healthy a population should be to provide normative data? Arh Hig Rada Toksikol. 2009 Mar;60(1):87-97.

175. Corradi M, Goldoni M, Caglieri A, Folesani G, Poli D, Corti M, et al. Collecting exhaled breath condensate (EBC) with two condensers in series: a promising technique for studying the mechanisms of EBC formation, and the volatility of selected bio-markers. J Aerosol Med Pulm Drug Deliv. 2008 Mar;21(1):35-44.

176. Goen T, Muller-Lux A, Dewes P, Musiol A, Kraus T. Sensitive and accurate analyses of free 3-nitrotyrosine in exhaled breath condensate by LC-MS/MS. J Chromatogr B Analyt Technol Biomed Life Sci. 2005 Nov 5;826(1-2):261-6.

177. Antonopoulou S, Loukides S, Papatheodorou G, Roussos C, Alchanatis M. Airway inflammation in obstructive sleep apnea: is leptin the missing link? Respir Med. 2008 Oct;102(10):1399-405.

Exhaled Breath Condensate in Asthma: Application in Clinical Practice

John Hunt

*T*he medical profession throughout the globe has been shifting toward servitude to a distorted incarnation of "evidence-based medicine". Evidence plays unequivocally valuable roles in many aspects of medical care. It helps to overcome the blind persistence in a physician's ways predicated on one prior anecdote. It helps increase the chances of successful interventions. If used correctly, it can help in health policy decisions. However, evidence based medicine is also a powerful tool of manipulation and control. In the case of "asthma" the growing influence of a tyrannical evidence-controlled mentality can be particularly troublesome. If the evidence relies on a false understanding of "asthma" at the core, then all that elutes from the evidence is unreliable. That is the case in asthma today. From the point of view of most evidence-based papers and guidelines, patients with asthma

Correspondence

Dr. John Hunt

Pediatric Pulmonology, Allergy & Immunology Department, University of Virginia, Charlottesville, VA 22908
email jfh2m@virginia.edu

are generally lumped under one umbrella. This is a major disservice that can be obviated by improved efforts at delineating underlying diagnoses in patients with asthma. Exhaled breath condensate assays play a role in this most important process of returning to a mentality in which we are optimizing care of the individual patient, instead of the group as a whole.

Each individual patient is unique. Just because they happen to have recurrent episodes of reversible airflow obstruction ("asthma") does not turn them into clones of the subjects enrolled in large clinical trials of others with "asthma". Exhaled breath condensate assays, as used in the research literature, have already helped physicians realize the heterogeneity of "asthma". Some patients have high oxidative burdens (best demonstrated in EBC) (1). Some patients do not. Some patients have greater expression of the leukotriene mediators, as found in EBC (2). Others do not. Many patients with acute exacerbations of asthma even have pronounced airway acidification, non-invasively identified in EBC (3). These assays in EBC have allowed a window to be opened on underlying abnormalities that were previously difficult to see. These research findings have participated in a process of opening up the eyes and brains of physicians, and they can continue to do so.

Thus, clinical use #1 of EBC is to provide little bits of evidence that can help physicians feel empowered to fight for their patients, confident that their patients are individuals, different than all other patients with asthma, and may well not be optimally treated by inflexible obedience to guidelines. This concept provides reinvigoration to the concept of personalized medicine, which is a critical component of the provision of health care, and to which exhaled breath assays can further contribute (see next). Helping to reassert the uniqueness of the individual patient may be the most important contribution of EBC assays.

Phenotyping asthma patients

As noted, asthma is not a disease, but a symptom. There are multiple causes and multiple confounders. The diagnostic process for asthma starts, not stops, with the identification of asthma. What comes next in the diagnostic process? A search for causation. History, physical and objective physiologic parameters such as spirometry can provide highly useful information, but provide no objective information about inflammation or chemistry or infection or genetically-programmed responses.

The quest for a non-invasive inflammometer has been a Holy Grail of lung disease researchers. It remains absolutely elusive. This results in part because "inflammation" is itself a highly heterogeneous term. Instead of an inflammometer, perhaps we should be seeking more specific information. And EBC can help with that.

In the clinical setting, keeping in mind all the barriers to getting a diagnostic test available, it is safe to say that the time is approaching when EBC will be clearly useful.

Exhaled breath condensate pH

One example that is of particular interest to the current author is the EBC pH assay. The author has a conflict-of-interest to disclose in this regard for the author invented the EBC pH test. It is perhaps better to call these disclosures a "synergy-of-interest" which is a phrase both less accusatory and more confirming. EBC pH is a non-invasive assessment of the presence of acidity in the airway. EBC pH correlates with certain markers of inflammation in asthma (4, 5). It is useful at distinguishing group mean differences (3, 5). EBC pH benefits from extensive normative databases (6-9). It has undergone the most complete validation testing of the EBC biomarkers so far studied (10-12) (with hydrogen peroxide coming in a close second). EBC pH also benefits from there needing to be only minimal standardization issues to address. EBC pH doesn't require special sample storage or transport conditions (13).

Notably, EBC pH reflects lower airway pH in a carefully performed cow lung model (10). It does not appear to be a perfect reflection of lower airway pH as measured invasively, for several reasons. First, EBC pH contains volatile acids and bases that emanate from throughout the communicating respiratory tract. In contrast, invasive pH measurements are generally proximal and limited in locations. So an area of airway acidification may be missed by a wired probe in the lung, but identified by EBC. In contrast, a small area of acidification in an airway may be identified by a fortuitously located wired probe, but be lost in the noise of the rest of the airway which may contribute to EBC volatiles substantially, resulting in a pH that is normal.

Second, EBC pH can certainly be affected by acids arising more proximally in the respiratory tract (14). For example, gastro-pharyngeal acid reflux has been found to lower EBC pH markedly, although transiently, even when the patient doesn't recognize that they are refluxing (15, 16). This acidification may or may not encroach upon the lower airway.

Third, EBC pH can be readily performed in the clinical setting without expensive equipment (15, 16).

But, what does one do if one finds a patient who has a low EBC pH? Does this mean he has a need for more inhaled steroids? Not necessarily at all. What it means is that, at the time the sample was collected, the patient's airway pH was low. It does not delineate where in the airway tree the acidification is present. It could be alveolar, or it could be hypopharyngeal, or anywhere in between. Is the physician going to want to neutralize the acidity with inhaled basic buffer? Perhaps someday. This makes the most sense, for it focuses directly on a core airway problem. But there are no currently approved medications for the purpose of neutralizing airway acidity. So why would a physician want to perform an EBC pH test for clinical purposes?

The answer, for the time being, is to identify gastro-pharyngeal acid reflux and its potential for aspiration into the lower airway. Indeed, this is not just a small issue. Currently, leading respiratory physicians throughout the globe are nearly unanimous in our recognition of the lack of a rational modality to identify if a patient has esophageal reflux disease contributing to a cough or other respiratory symptoms. Expenditures for proton-pump inhibitors in the setting of respiratory disease are in the billions of US dollars.

This issue of reflux-induced respiratory disease presents a classic example of where both anecdote-based medicine and evidence-based medicine lead to poor medical care. Many physicians are convinced of the utility of proton pump inhibitor medications for the treatment and miraculous improvement in some patients with asthma or cough. The literature meanwhile does not strongly support that such drugs improve the average patient with generic asthma (17), although it does support use in exercise-triggered asthma (18). Additionally a recent article supports a complete lack of efficacy in poorly controlled asthma of this class of acid blockade medication (19). The danger here is obvious. *Clearly* some patients have acid reflux contributing to their disease. All respiratory physicians have convincingly seen this. But the major evidence now seems to support not treating asthma patients with proton pump inhibitors. Beware. The data actually support the contention that we should not treat *ALL* asthma patients with acid blockade. But that does not mean we cannot treat selected patients in our practices, and indeed the literature again supports such practice (17). How about if it is a patient who has a low EBC pH whenever they cough? That is a pretty convincing data set that acid is relevant. There are two primary sources of acid: the lungs, and the stomach. We can't treat the lung source yet. So it makes sense to try to treat the stomach source. It would be foolish to ignore such patient-based data, simply because proton pump inhibitors did not show efficacy in asthma in a group of other people who did not have the same characteristics as the patient in clinic right now. Likewise, treating all patients who have asthma with acid blockade makes little sense, for most will not benefit from it, and may even be harmed (20). The answer for what a doctor should do with any individual patient who has chronic cough, asthma, and possibly reflux is supplied by neither the evidence base nor anecdotes. But EBC may supply precisely that needed answer.

EBC pH cannot be perfect. There are non-gastric causes of airway acidification that may confound an individual's EBC pH data (21). Fortunately, low EBC pH is overwhelmingly most common in the setting of acute exacerbations of asthma, not in stable asthma, and such exacerbations can be recognized clinically. Nonetheless, even an asymptomatic cold can profoundly and rapidly acidify EBC (22). As noted previously, no one test will give a comprehensive answer.

In regard to phenotyping asthma, EBC pH is just one potential marker. It identifies asthma patients with acidic airways (an important phenotype), and clinically helps because many of those patients have reflux and aspiration contributing to the acidity, and gastric acid can be blocked with available pharmacotherapeutics. In the future, EBC pH may be useful for titrating airway alkalinization therapy for acute asthma exacerbations.

Markers of oxidative stress and strain in exhaled breath condensate

Other compounds in EBC can likely be used as clinical tests in the relatively near future. For example, there are numerous anti-oxidant therapies on the market currently. Although these drugs and nutritional supplements have not been found to be terribly useful in the treatment of generic "asthma", they have not been extensively tested in the setting of patients with "asthma" who also have evidence of abnormal oxidative processes (which may well not be common to all patients who have "asthma". EBC hydrogen peroxide (H_2O_2) is another of the more thoroughly technically-validated markers (13, 23). It is often considered a marker of oxidative stress. Actually, H_2O_2 is not a marker of oxidative stress so much as a marker of potential stress. It is the precursor of the prototypical oxidant, the hydroxyl radical ($OH^\bullet$). If the native antioxidant systems are well-balanced with production of oxidants, then there is no major stress/no tissue injury. However measurement of H_2O_2 may well tell of a tendency toward stress.

H_2O_2 can be measured in EBC with relative ease with devices, such as the ECoCheck (Jaeger, Germany), but only because of the efforts and expenses industry has undertaken to bring automated equipment to the hospitals. There are numerous additional methods of measuring H_2O_2 in the typical research laboratory setting that could be taken to the clinic with effort.

Measurement of oxidative *strain* can also be undertaken, most notably by using levels of 8-isoprostane (2) and aldehydes in EBC. These compounds are the result of the effect of unbalanced oxidants on lipids. The lipids are effectively burned by these oxidants. This destruction is strain, the response to the oxidative stress. These compounds may be of particular interest, because they s-peak to the net balance of oxidative overflow and the ability of the organism to defend against the oxidant stress. Evidence of strain is evidence that oxidation is injurious.

Systems have been developed that rapidly analyze EBC aldehydes at the bedside (www.fredthedevice.com). 8-isoprostane remains a laboratory-based test.

Why should a doctor care about measuring oxidative stress and strain? Because these are rightfully thought to be central pathologic mechanisms of many respiratory diseases. And because the evidence base has failed to provide sufficient support for the use of any of the multiple available anti-oxidant regimens. This is because of a failure of evidence based techniques, not of biology. The evidence fails to prequalify subjects to study by determining if they have a pathology that includes oxidative stress and strain (24), instead lumping everyone together into syndromes such as "asthma" and not surprisingly obtaining at most marginally useful data.

Leukotrienes in EBC

Finally, another EBC marker may be approaching clinical utility, although has hurdles to move through yet. EBC leukotrienes are reported to be assayable in EBC (25, 26) and there are numerous papers examining the assays as well as their use in studying respiratory diseases. The most experienced groups with these assays provide the most consistent data. These EBC assays are of particular interest because they hold some promise for predicting which individual patients might benefit from leukotriene modifiers. Again, the point here is that while leukotriene modifiers may appear to be less effective than inhaled steroids for the treatment of asthma if one looks at the broad evidence, the reality is that in any one specific patient, leukotriene modification may be overwhelmingly more effective than inhaled steroid. But one needs to identify that patient. Measurement of their leukotriene levels (their leukotriene stress) seems likely to provide utility (27).

Many diverse additional molecules have been identified in EBC that may become of clinical value in the future. Additionally, metabolomics in EBC is an intriguing concept that may become useful for phenotyping (28). But none of these others have the clinical data, regulatory, and industry support necessary to serve as a clinically applicable test just yet.

Conclusion

One cannot think of any test in medicine without considering the overall environment. This is certainly true of exhaled breath condensate. EBC pH is already in clinical use, but as yet only for the purpose of identifying airway acidity when reflux-induced respiratory symptoms is on the differential diagnosis list. In the future, EBC pH may be useful in titrating inhaled pH modulatory medications. EBC H_2O_2 and aldehydes measurements are available now with rapid assay devices, and these may be appropriate tests, not perhaps for diagnosis, but for individualization of patient care for those physicians and patients who are interested in neutraceuticals and redox balance. This interest should increase over time, if the data emerge that guiding anti-oxidant therapy based on relevant measures of stress is more effective than simply dosing up with anti-oxidants at arbitrary doses. Leukotriene measurement does not yet have sufficient industry support to make it clinically available. Each EBC test considered for clinical applicability needs to satisfy many factors that are not commonly considered by the academic researcher.

Most importantly, the test needs to be useful for individual patient management, readily available, and supported by the health care financial systems.

References

1. Zhao JJ, Shimizu Y, Dobashi K, Kawata T, Ono A, Yanagitani N, et al. The relationship between oxidative stress and acid stress in adult patients with mild asthma. J Investig Allergol Clin Immunol. 2008;18(1):41-5.

2. Samitas K, Chorianopoulos D, Vittorakis S, Zervas E, Economidou E, Papatheodorou G, et al. Exhaled cysteinyl-leukotrienes and 8-isoprostane in patients with asthma and their relation to clinical severity. Respir Med. 2009 May;103(5):750-6.

3. Hunt JF, Fang K, Malik R, Snyder A, Malhotra N, Platts-Mills TA, et al. Endogenous airway acidification. Implications for asthma pathophysiology. Am J Respir Crit Care Med. 2000 Mar;161(3 Pt 1):694-9.

4. Kostikas K, Koutsokera A, Papiris S, Gourgoulianis KI, Loukides S. Exhaled breath condensate in patients with asthma: implications for application in clinical practice. Clin Exp Allergy. 2008 Apr;38(4):557-65.

5. Kostikas K, Papatheodorou G, Ganas K, Psathakis K, Panagou P, Loukides S. pH in expired breath condensate of patients with inflammatory airway diseases. Am J Respir Crit Care Med. 2002 May 15;165(10):1364-70.

6. Varnai VM, Ljubicic A, Prester L, Macan J. Exhaled breath condensate pH in adult Croatian population without respiratory disorders: how healthy a population should be to provide normative data? Arh Hig Rada Toksikol. 2009 Mar;60(1):87-97.

7. Paget-Brown AO, Ngamtrakulpanit L, Smith A, Bunyan D, Hom S, Nguyen A, et al. Normative data for pH of exhaled breath condensate. Chest. 2006 Feb;129(2):426-30.

8. Hauswirth DW, Sundy JS, Mervin-Blake S, Fernandez CA, Patch KB, Alexander KM, et al. Normative values for exhaled breath condensate pH and its relationship to exhaled nitric oxide in healthy African Americans. J Allergy Clin Immunol. 2008 Jul;122(1):101-6.

9. Nicolaou NC, Lowe LA, Murray CS, Woodcock A, Simpson A, Custovic A. Exhaled breath condensate pH and childhood asthma: unselected birth cohort study. Am J Respir Crit Care Med. 2006 Aug 1;174(3):254-9.

10. Bunyan D, Smith A, Davidson W, Yu Y, Urban P, Naccara L, et al. Correlation of exhaled breath condensate pH with invasively measured airway pH in the cow. Eur Respir J. 2005;26:2407.

11. Vaughan J, Ngamtrakulpanit L, Pajewski TN, Turner R, Nguyen TA, Smith A, et al. Exhaled breath condensate pH is a robust and repro-

ducible assay of airway acidity. Eur Respir J. 2003 Dec;22(6):889-94.

12. Wells K, Vaughan J, Pajewski TN, Hom S, Ngamtrakulpanit L, Smith A, et al. Exhaled breath condensate pH assays are not influenced by oral ammonia. Thorax. 2005 Jan;60(1):27-31.

13. Horvath I, Hunt J, Barnes PJ, Alving K, Antczak A, Baraldi E, et al. Exhaled breath condensate: methodological recommendations and unresolved questions. Eur Respir J. 2005 Sep;26(3):523-48.

14. Ricciardolo FL, Gaston B, Hunt J. Acid stress in the pathology of asthma. J Allergy Clin Immunol. 2004 Apr;113(4):610-9.

15. Hunt J, Yu Y, Burns J, Gaston B, Ngamtrakulpanit L, Bunyan D, et al. Identification of acid reflux cough using serial assays of exhaled breath condensate pH. Cough. 2006;2:3.

16. Walsh B. Non-invasive diagnosis of acid reflux cough. Respir Ther. 2005; 1:69-71.

17. Sopo SM, Radzik D, Calvani M. Does treatment with proton pump inhibitors for gastroesophageal reflux disease (GERD) improve asthma symptoms in children with asthma and GERD? A systematic review. J Investig Allergol Clin Immunol. 2009;19(1):1-5.

18. Peterson KA, Samuelson WM, Ryujin DT, Young DC, Thomas KL, Hilden K, et al. The role of gastroesophageal reflux in exercise-triggered asthma: a randomized controlled trial. Dig Dis Sci. 2009 Mar;54(3):564-71.

19. Mastronarde JG, Anthonisen NR, Castro M, Holbrook JT, Leone FT, Teague WG, et al. Efficacy of esomeprazole for treatment of poorly controlled asthma. N Engl J Med. 2009 Apr 9; 360(15):1487-99.

20. Insogna KL. The effect of proton pump-inhibiting drugs on mineral metabolism. Am J Gastroenterol. 2009 Mar;104(2 Suppl):S2-4.

21. Walsh BK, Mackey DJ, Pajewski T, Yu Y, Gaston BM, Hunt JF. Exhaled-breath condensate pH can be safely and continuously monitored in mechanically ventilated patients. Respir Care. 2006 Oct;51(10):1125-31.

22. Ngamtrakulpanit L, Vaughan J, Nguyen A, Urban P, Hom S, Smith A. Exhaled breath condensate acidification during rhinovirus cold. Am J Respir Crit Care Med. 2003;167: A446.

23. Fireman E, Shtark M, Priel IE, Shiner R, Mor R, Kivity S, et al. Hydrogen peroxide in exhaled breath condensate (EBC) vs eosinophil count in induced sputum (IS) in parenchymal vs airways lung diseases. Inflammation. 2007 Apr;30(1-2):44-51.

24. Hoshino Y, Mishima M. Redox-based therapeutics for lung diseases. Antioxid Redox Signal. 2008 Apr;10(4): 701-4.

25. Montuschi P, Barnes PJ. Exhaled leukotrienes and prostaglandins in asthma. J Allergy Clin Immunol. 2002 Apr;109(4):615-20.

26. Baraldi E, Carraro S, Alinovi R, Pesci A, Ghiro L, Bodini A, et al. Cysteinyl leukotrienes and 8-isoprostane in exhaled breath condensate of children with asthma exacerbations. Thorax. 2003 Jun;58(6):505-9.

27. Montuschi P, Mondino C, Koch P, Barnes PJ, Ciabattoni G. Effects of a

leukotriene receptor antagonist on exhaled leukotriene E4 and prostanoids in children with asthma. J Allergy Clin Immunol. 2006Aug; 118(2): 347-53.

28. Carraro S, Rezzi S, Reniero F, Heberger K, Giordano G, Zanconato S, et al. Metabolomics applied to exhaled breath condensate in childhood asthma. Am J Respir Crit Care Med. 2007 May 15;175(10):986-90.

Exhaled Breath Condensate in COPD: Application in Clinical Practice

Paolo Montuschi

 xhaled breath consists of a gaseous phase that contains volatile biomolecules (e.g., nitric oxide, carbon monoxide and volatile organic compounds) and a liquid phase, known as exhaled breath condensate (EBC), that is mainly formed by water vapour, but also contains aerosol particles in which non-volatile biomolecules have been detected (1-3). As it is completely non-invasive, EBC might also be suitable for longitudinal studies, and for monitoring the efficacy of pharmacotherapy in patients with COPD. Different profiles of biomarkers might reflect different aspects of lung inflammation or oxidative stress, that is an important component of inflammation. Identification of selective profiles of biomarkers in lung diseases might be of value for differential diagnosis in respiratory medicine. However, the possible application of EBC analysis in the clinical setting requires the elucidation of several methodological aspects, including the standardization of this

Correspondence

Prof. Paolo Montuschi

Department of Pharmacology, Faculty of Medicine, Catholic University of the Sacred Heart, Largo F. Vito 1, 00168 Rome, Italy
e-mail: pmontuschi@rm.unicatt.it

technique and validation of the analytical methods commonly used to measure biomolecules in EBC. This article summarizes the results of the EBC analysis in patients with COPD, discusses some methodological aspects, presents advantages and limitations of this technique, and proposes directions for future research.

Analysis of EBC in Patients with COPD and Healthy Smokers

Several biomolecules including leukotrienes, prostaglandins, iso-prostanes, hydrogen peroxide, nitric oxide-derived products, hydrogen ions, and adenosine triphoshpate have been measured in healthy subjects. Some inflammatory mediators are elevated in patients with chronic obstructive pulmonary disease (COPD) (4).

Eicosanoids

In most studies, LT and prostanoid concentrations in EBC have been measured by commercially available immunoassays that are generally not validated. The limitations of this approach and the need for a robust analytical methodology for a specific and quantitative assessment of eicosanoid concentrations in EBC have been discussed (5-7). The presence of LTB_4 (8, 9), 8-isoprostane (10, 11), and PGE_2 (10) in EBC has been definitively demonstrated by mass spectrometry. Radioimmunoassays for 8-isoprostane ($15\text{-}F_{2t}$-isoprostane) and PGE_2 have been qualitatively validated by using high performance liquid chromatography (12).

Leukotrienes

Leukotriene (LT) B_4 concentrations in EBC are elevated in steroid-naive and steroid-treated patients with stable COPD (13, 14) compared with healthy smokers. In patients with COPD (13), the profile of LTs in EBC is different from that in patients with asthma (15). LTE_4 is elevated in patients with asthma (15), but not in patients with COPD (13). Exhaled LTB_4 is elevated in both patients with asthma and COPD, but this increase is more pronounced in patients with COPD (13). In patients with exacerbations of COPD, LTB_4 concentrations in EBC are decreased 2 weeks after treatment with antibiotics and this effect persists after 2 months (16).

Prostanoids

Compared with healthy non-smokers, PGE_2 concentrations in EBC are increased in steroid-naive and steroid-treated patients with stable COPD (13). There is a correlation between exhaled PGE_2 and LTB_4 concentrations in both COPD groups of patients (13). These data might indicate higher production of PGE_2, an endogenous biomolecule that may have anti-inflammatory effects in the airways, in conditions of increased lung inflammation. Non-selective cyclo-oxygenase (COX) inhibition by oral ibuprofen (400 mg q.i.d. for 2 days) reduces PGE_2 concentrations in EBC in patients with COPD (17). This effect might be relevant to the modulation of airway inflammation. Selective COX-2 inhibition by oral rofecoxib (25 mg once a day for 5 days) has no effect on PGE_2 and LTB_4 concentrations in EBC in patients with stable COPD (17). Taken together, these findings indicate that PGE_2 in EBC in patients with COPD is mainly derived from COX-1 activity (17). The pathophysiological implications of selective and non-selective inhibition of COX for lung inflammation in patients with COPD have to be clarified.

Isoprostanes

Isoprostanes are prostaglandin-like compounds that are produced in vivo independently of COX enzymes, principally by peroxidation of arachidonic acid due to free radicals (18). Isoprostanes are considered among the best markers of oxidative stress (19, 20). 8-Isoprostane, a compound that belongs to the F_2 class of isoprostanes, is measurable in EBC in healthy non-smokers (10, 21, 22), and its concentrations in EBC are elevated in healthy smokers and, to a lesser extent, in current and ex-smokers with stable COPD (21). Similar EBC 8-isoprostane concentrations in current and ex-smokers with COPD might indicate that oxidative stress due to chronic smoking reaches a point at which smoking cessation has little, if any, effect (21). Increased 8-isoprostane concentrations in EBC in healthy smokers and patients with stable COPD has been confirmed by other authors (23-27) . 8-Isoprostane concentrations in E-BC may reflect the degree of emphysema assessed by high resolution computed tomography (25). In patients with exacerbations of COPD, 8-isoprostane concentrations in EBC are higher than in healthy subjects (16, 27) and decreased after antibiotic treatment (16). One study reported that 8-isoprostane concentrations in EBC are at least 10-fold lower than those in sputum supernatants (27). Inhalation of aminoguanidine, a relatively selective inhibitor of inducible nitric oxide-synthase (iNOS), has no effect on 8-isoprostane concentrations in EBC in patients with COPD, healthy smokers and healthy non-smokers (28).

Hydrogen peroxide

Hydrogen peroxide in EBC has been measured by spectrophotometry (29-31), fluorimetric assays (32-35), and chemiluminescence (36, 37). A wide variability in the mean hydrogen peroxide concentrations in EBC in healthy, nonsmoking adults, has been reported (0.01 nM - 0.45 µM) (29, 38). Even under strictly controlled conditions, there is a high degree of day-to-day variability that highlights the fact that standardization of the experimental technique is required (32).

In healthy non-smokers and subjects with mild asthma, one study reported that hydrogen peroxide concentrations in EBC depend on the expiratory flow rate (32). Compared with healthy non-smokers, exhaled hydrogen peroxide concentrations are increased in healthy smokers and this increase is more pronounced in patients with stable COPD (30, 39, 40). In these patients, hydrogen peroxide concentrations in EBC do not seem to be dependent on smoking (40). Exhaled hydrogen peroxide in EBC is further elevated in patients with COPD exacerbations (30, 41). EBC hydrogen peroxide concentrations increase immediately after maximal exercise in patients with stable COPD (42).

The effect of inhaled glucocorticoids on exhaled hydrogen peroxide concentrations in patients with COPD is not established (43, 44). One study showed that beclomethasone at a dose of 500 µg twice daily for 2 weeks had no effect on hydrogen peroxide concentrations in EBC in non-smoking patients with stable COPD (43). By contrast, another study reported that HFA-beclomethasone dipropionate at a dose of 400 µg twice daily for 4 weeks and fluticasone dipropionate at a dose of 375 µg twice daily for 4 weeks reduced hydrogen peroxide concentrations in EBC in patients with stable to moderate COPD (44). In patients with COPD who required hospital admission because of exacerbations due to lower respiratory tract infections, exhaled hydrogen peroxide concentrations were not reduced during treatment with intravenous dexamethasone, inhaled salbutamol/ipratropium and antibiotics as needed

(45). By contrast, other studies reported reduced hydrogen peroxide concentrations in EBC after intravenous glucocorticoid treatment in patients with exacerbation of COPD (41, 46). In patients with stable COPD, treatment with oral N-acetyl-cysteine, which can have antioxidant effects, at a daily dose of 600 mg for 12 months reduced hydrogen peroxide concentrations in EBC starting from 9 months (47), whereas a similar study showed a much earlier effect starting from 15 days (48). Despite some evidence of reduced oxidant stress, a multicenter trial has shown that N-acetyl-cysteine is ineffective at prevention of deterioration in lung function and prevention of exacerbations in patients with COPD (49). Hydrogen peroxide concentrations in EBC in patients with COPD are transiently increased 30 min after inhalation of N-acetyl-cysteine given by nebulization (50). The clinical relevance of these findings is not currently known. More controlled studies to establish the effects of pharmacological therapy on hydrogen peroxide concentrations in EBC in patients with COPD are required. As with other biomolecules, a reliable methodology for EBC analysis is essential for planning and interpreting the results of interventional studies.

NO-derived products

Patients with COPD have higher S-nitrosothiols concentrations in E-BC than healthy non-smokers (51). Whether elevated S-nitrosothiols merely reflects NO production or whether they are functionally involved in the pathophysioly of COPD has to be clarified. Concentrations of peroxynitrite, measured using oxidation of 2',7'-dichlorofluorescin in EBC collected at high pH, are increased in patients with moderately to severe COPD compared with those in healthy smokers and non-smokers and are negatively correlated with FEV_1 (52). Nitrite and nitrates are end-products of NO metabolism. Nitrite has been measured in the EBC from healthy non-smokers and was found increased in patients with COPD (51). Another study reported similar nitrite/nitrates concentrations in EBC in patients with COPD and healthy subjects (53). In patients with COPD nitrite concentrations in EBC correlate with hyperinflation (54). Smoking induces an acute increase in nitrate, but not nitrite, concentrations in EBC in healthy smokers (55). In a double-blind, placebo-controlled study, inhibition of iNOS with inhalation of aminoguanidine given by nebulization resulted in a significant, but not complete, inhibition of peroxynitrite production as reflected by its concentrations in EBC in patients with COPD and healthy smokers 60 minutes after inhalation (28). Inhalation of aminoguanidine has no effect on peroxynitrite concentrations in EBC in healthy non-smokers (28). Aminoguanidine reduces nitrite/nitrate concentrations in EBC in patients with COPD at 60 minutes and 120 minutes after inhalation, whereas in healthy smokers and healthy non-smokers reduction in nitrite/nitrate concentrations in EBC following aminoguanidine inhalation is observed only at 60 minutes (28). iNOS inhibition with aminoguanidine has no effect on nitrotyrosine concentrations in EBC in patients with COPD, healthy smokers and healthy non-smokers (28). Taken together, these data indicate that both constitutive and inducible NOS isoforms might contribute to the elevated pulmonary peroxynitrite and nitrite/nitrate production in patients with COPD (28).

pH

EBC pH is a robust and reproducible assay of airway acidity (56, 57). Mean EBC pH values are lower in patients with COPD compared with patients with asthma and healthy subjects (23). In patients with COPD, pH values in EBC are correlated with sputum neutrophilia and hydrogen peroxide concentrations in EBC (23). In this study, pH values in EBC in patients with COPD were similar irrespective of treatment with inhaled glucocorticosteroids (23). However, controlled studies to establish the effects of glucocorticoids on EBC pH values in patients with COPD are warranted. pH values in EBC are negatively correlated with gastro-oesophageal reflux disease symptoms in patients with COPD and healthy controls (58).

Aldehydes

Measurement of malondialdehyde (MDA), a product of lipid peroxidation, in biological fluids is a widely used test for oxidative stress, but its reliability for assessing oxidative stress in vivo is questionable (59). MDA and other aldheydes (hexanal, heptanal, and nonanal) have been measured in EBC using liquid chromatography-tandem mass sapectrometry (60). MDA, hexanal, and heptanal concentrations in EBC are increased in patients with COPD as compared with non-smoking subjects, whereas only MDA is elevated in patients with COPD compared with healthy smokers (60).

Adenosine triphosphate

Adenosine triphosphate (ATP) was detected in EBC in healthy non-smokers, healthy smokers and patients with exacerbation of COPD. There was no difference in ATP concentrations in the three study groups (61).

Other markers

A wide inter-individual variability (from undetectable to 1.4 mg) in the amount of total proteins in EBC (62) has been reported even in healthy subjects. Although amylase concentrations can be detected by very sensitive analytical techniques, amylase concentrations in EBC are generally undetectable or very low, indicating little, if any, salivary contamination of EBC (63, 64). Compared with healthy non-smokers, healthy smokers and patients with stable COPD, interleukin (IL)-1, IL-6, IL-8, IL-10, IL-12p70, and tumor necrosis factor (TNF) concentrations in EBC measured by a multiplex bead array test combined with flow cytometry have been found increased in patients with exacerbation of COPD(65). Compared with healthy non-smokers, IL-1 and IL-12 concentrations in EBC were increased in patients with COPD (65). Healthy smokers had increased concentrations of all cytokines in EBC compared to healthy non-smokers and, with the exception of IL-1 , to patients with stable COPD (65). One study reported elevated macrophage migration inhibitory factor, IL-12, regulated on activation normal T cell expressed and secreted (RANTES), and soluble intracellular adhesion molecule-1 in EBC in patients with moderate to severe COPD with no effect after treatment with infliximab, an anti-TNF- antibody (66). In all published studies, cytokines in EBC were measured by immunoassays that are very sensitive and work well in buffer, but their behavior in EBC has not been established. Concentrations of cytokines measured in EBC are very low and close to the lower limit of quantification of the immunoassays used. At these concentrations, the analytical variability is very high. This makes it difficult the interpretation of results. The presence of cytokines in E-BC has not been definitively demonstrated and an accurate quantification of their concentrations in EBC has not yet been provided. This relevant issue needs to be formally addressed by a specific and robust analytical methodology.

Metabolomics, the study of molecules generated by metabolic

pathways, has been applied to the analysis of EBC (67). Metabolomic analysis of EBC by nuclear magnetic resonance spectroscopy discriminates between patients with COPD, laringectomised patients and healthy subjects (67). When samples were collected using a commercially available condenser, saliva spectra were highly different from corresponding EBC samples (67). These data exclude significant salivary contamination.

Advantages and Limitations

Measurements of biomolecules in EBC may provide insights into the pathophysiology of COPD. Measurement of surrogate markers of pulmonary inflammation in EBC might be useful for identifying subgroups of healthy chronic smokers who are more susceptible to COPD, phenotyping of COPD, assessing the effect of anti-inflammatory therapy in patients with COPD, identifying those patients who are most likely to benefit from pharmacological therapy, and testing new drugs for COPD. The identification of selective profiles of inflammatory markers in patients with COPD might be useful for a more accurate selection of patients with COPD in clinical trials.

At present, the lack of standardization of EBC analysis is the principal limitation of this technique. This can account for most of the variability of the results reported in different studies and makes it difficult between-laboratory comparison of data. Other current limitations of EBC analysis are: the size of the published studies that is generally relatively small; the fact that this technique is unable to provide any information on the inflammatory cells involved in the pathophysiology of COPD; the fact EBC reflects lung rather than systemic inflammation has to be demonstrated; the origin (airways vs alveolar region) and cellular sources of biomolecules in E-BC that have to be identified.

Methodological Issues and Future Research

Methodological aspects of EBC analysis have been discussed in details (5, 68) and in another chapter of this book. These include flow- and time-dependence of biomolecules in EBC; the effects of temperature, humidity, and collecting system materials on measurements; possible nasal, saliva and sputum contamination; be-

INFLAMMATORY BIOMARKERS IN EXHALED BREATH CONDENSATE IN PATIENTS WITH COPD

Biomarker	Method	Values	References
Leukotrienes			
LTB$_4$	EIA	*100.6 (73.5-145.0) pg/ml	[13]
	EIA	§8.5 ± 0.8 pg/ml	[16]
	EIA	§§86.7 ± 19 pg/ml	[14]
LTE$_4$	EIA	*23.3 (9.1-31.3) pg/ml	[13]
Prostanoids			
PGE$_2$	EIA	*98.0 (57.0-128.4) pg/ml	[13]
PGE$_2$	RIA	#93.5 (84.0-105.5) pg/ml	[17]
PGF$_{2a}$	EIA	*15.0 (10.9-19.0) pg/ml	[13]
PGD$_{2a}$-MOX	EIA	*11.2 (8.7-15.0) pg/ml	[13]
Isoprostanes			
8-Isoprostane	EIA	§45 ± 3.6 pg/ml	[21]
	RIA	#47.9 (40.5-51.9) pg/ml	[17]
	EIA	¶47 (95% CI, 41-53) pg/ml	[24]
	EIA	§43.7 ± 2.8 pg/ml	[28]
	EIA	§6.0 ± 0.7 pg/ml	[16]
	EIA	§18.1 ± 2.0 pg/ml	[25]
	EIA	#14.2 [9.5-26.4]	[26]
Hydrogen peroxide	spectrophotometry	§0.205 ± 0.054 mM	[30]
	spectrophotometry	*2.6 (1.9-3.5) mM	[44]
	spectrofluorimetry	§0.48 ± 0.67 mM	[41]
	fluorimetry	§0.22 ± 0.03 mM	[36]
	spectrophotometry	§0.50 ± 0.11 mM	[39]
NO-derived products			
S-Nitrosothiols	spectrophotometry	§0.24 ± 0.04 µM	[51]
Peroxynitrite^△	fluorimetry	§§7.9 ± 3.0 nM	[52]
Peroxynitrite^△	fluorimetry	§295.1 ± 52.7 nM	[28]
Nitrite	spectrophotometry	§2.62 ± 0.52 µM	[51]
Nitrite/nitrates	fluorimetry	§37.8 ± 3.4 mM	[28]
Nitrite/nitrates	fluorimetry	*10.2 (2.0-93.8) µM	[53]
Nitrotyrosine	EIA	§24.6 ± 2.2 ng/ml	[28]
Hydrogen ions	pH meter	7.16 (7.09-7.23)	[23]
Aldehydes			
MDA	GC/MS/MS	§57.2 ± 2.4 nmol/l	[60]
hexanal	GC/MS/MS	§63.5 ± 4.4 nmol/l	[60]
heptanal	GC/MS/MS	§26.6 ± 3.9 nmol/l	[60]

continued

INFLAMMATORY BIOMARKERS IN EXHALED BREATH CONDENSATE IN PATIENTS WITH COPD *(con.)*

Biomarker	Method	Values	References
ATP	bioluminescence	§141 ± 44 pM	[61]
Cytokines			
IL-1b	multiplex fluorescent bead immunoassay	**not available	[65]
IL-6	multiplex fluorescent bead immunoassay	**not available	[65]
	EIA	§8.0 ± 0.1 pg/ml	[71]
IL-8	multiplex fluorescent bead immunoassay	**not available	[65]
IL-10	multiplex fluorescent bead immunoassay	**not available	[65]
IL-12p70	multiplex fluorescent bead immunoassay	**not available	[65]
	multiplex bead immunoassay	*3.75 (3.15-5.02) pg/ml	[66]
sICAM-1	multiplex bead immunoassay	*22.8 (16.6-35.6) pg/ml	[66]
MIF	multiplex bead immunoassay	§37.2 ± 8.9 (pg/ml)	[66]
RANTES	multiplex bead immunoassay	§22.5 ± 1.7 pg/ml	[66]
TNF a	multiplex fluorescent bead immunoassay	**not available	[65]

Values are expressed as §mean ± SEM, §§mean ± SD, *median with the minimum to maximum range, mean with 95% confidence intervals for the differences, #median with interquartile range, or. ^^Peroxynitrite was measured using oxidation of 2',7'-dichlorofluorescin in EBC collected at high pH. **Data are presented as figures, numerical data are not available.

For some biomarkers, there is a high variability in the concentrations reported in different studies. This can be partially explained by the lack of standardization of the exhaled breath condensate method and different analytical techniques.

Abbreviations: ATP, adenosine triphospahte; sICAM-1, soluble intracellular adhesion molecule-1; IL, interleukin; LT, leukotriene; MDA, malondialdehyde; MIF, macrophage migration inhibitory factor; MOX, methoxime, a stable PGD_2 metabolite; NO, nitric oxide; PG, prostaglandin; regulated on activation normal T cell expressed and secreted, RANTES; tumor necrosis factor a, TNF a.

tween-day, diurnal, and analytical variability of measurements; comparison of different condenser devices; storage issues; whether sample pre-treatment is required; characterization of the physico-chemical properties of different biomolecules in EBC; whether use of reference indicators to estimate biomolecule concentrations in the airway lining fluid and to normalize for variations in non-volatile biomolecules in EBC due to variations in aerosol particle dilution by water vapor is required. To achieve this, measurement of conductivity of EBC has been proposed (69).

Standardization of procedures for sample collection and storage and validation of the analytical techniques for measuring different biomolecules in EBC are currently the priorities in this research area (70). A robust analytical methodology is essential for the development of EBC analysis. Future research in this field should aim at developing: reference analytical techniques (e.g., mass spectrometry) to provide definitive evidence for the presence of biomolecules in EBC and an accurate quantitative assessment of their concentrations; development of sensitive, specific, and reproducible immunoassays or validation of those already available to be used routinely.

Controlled studies are required to establish the utility of EBC analysis as a tool for assessing the response to pharmacological therapy in patients with COPD. Future research in this area should also include: identification of reference values for different inflammatory biomarkers in healthy subjects and quantitative assessment of their concentrations in patients with stable COPD of different severity and in patients with COPD exacerbations; studies on the reproducibility of measurements to address between-day, diurnal, and analytical variability; large longitudinal studies in patients with COPD; studies aiming at clarifying the relationships of EBC markers with symptoms, lung function, and other indices and/or methods for quantifying lung inflammation in patients with COPD. As the behaviour of biomolecules in EBC may be different, standardized procedures need to be implemented for each individual biomolecule.

Whether, and when, analysis of EBC will have clinical applications is difficult to predict. In any case, this technique should be part of an integrated approach that consists of clinical assessment, lung function testing, and possibly sputum induction. Due to the relative lack of noninvasive methods for assessing and monitoring airway inflammation and therapeutic intervention in patients with COPD, further research in this area is warranted.

Acknowledgements

Supported by Catholic University of the Sacred Heart, Fondi di Ateneo 2007-2010.

References

1. Montuschi P. Indirect monitoring of lung inflammation. Nat Rev Drug Discov. 2002 Mar;1(3):238-42.
2. Montuschi P, (editor). New perspectives in monitoring lung inflammation: analysis of exhaled breath condensate. Florida: Boca Raton: CRC Press; 2005.
3. Horvath I, Hunt J, Barnes PJ, Alving K, Antczak A, Baraldi E, et al. Exhaled breath condensate: methodological recommendations and unresolved questions. Eur Respir J. 2005 Sep;26 (3):523-48.
4. Montuschi P. Exhaled breath condensate analysis in patients with COPD. Clin Chim Acta. 2005 Jun; 356(1-2):22-34.
5. Montuschi P. Analysis of exhaled breath condensate: methodological issues. New perspectives in monitoring lung inflammation: analysis of exhaled breath condensate: Boca Raton: CRC Press; 2005. p. 11-30.
6. Montuschi P. Isoprostane, prostanoids, and leukotrienes in exhaled breath condensate. New perspectives in monitoring lung inflammation: analysis of exhaled breath condensate Boca Raton: CRC Press; 2005. p. 53-66.
7. Montuschi P. LC/MS/MS analysis of leukotriene B4 and other eicosanoids in exhaled breath condensate for assessing lung inflammation. J Chromatogr B Analyt Technol Biomed Life Sci. 2009 May 1;877(13):1272-80.
8. Montuschi P, Martello S, Felli M, Mondino C, Chiarotti M. Ion trap liquid chromatography/tandem mass spectrometry analysis of leukotriene B4 in exhaled breath condensate. Rapid Commun Mass Spectrom. 2004;18(22):2723-9.
9. Montuschi P, Martello S, Felli M, Mondino C, Barnes PJ, Chiarotti M. Liquid chromatography/mass spectrometry analysis of exhaled leukotriene B4 in asthmatic children. Respir Res. 2005;6:119.
10. Carpenter CT, Price PV, Christman BW. Exhaled breath condensate isoprostanes are elevated in patients with acute lung injury or ARDS. Chest. 1998 Dec;114(6):1653-9.
11. Syslova K, Kacer P, Kuzma M, Klusackova P, Fenclova Z, Lebedova J, et al. Determination of 8-iso-prostaglandin F(2alpha) in exhaled breath condensate using combination of immunoseparation and LC-ESI-MS/MS. J Chromatogr B Analyt Technol Biomed Life Sci. 2008 May 1;867(1): 8-14.
12. Montuschi P, Ragazzoni E, Valente S, Corbo G, Mondino C, Ciappi G, et al. Validation of 8-isoprostane and prostaglandin E(2) measurements in exhaled breath condensate. Inflamm Res. 2003 Dec;52(12):502-7.

13. Montuschi P, Kharitonov SA, Ciabattoni G, Barnes PJ. Exhaled leukotrienes and prostaglandins in COPD. Thorax. 2003 Jul;58(7):585-8.

14. Kostikas K, Gaga M, Papatheodorou G, Karamanis T, Orphanidou D, Loukides S. Leukotriene B4 in exhaled breath condensate and sputum supernatant in patients with COPD and asthma. Chest. 2005 May; 127(5):1553-9.

15. Montuschi P, Barnes PJ. Exhaled leukotrienes and prostaglandins in asthma. J Allergy Clin Immunol. 2002 Apr;109(4):615-20.

16. Biernacki WA, Kharitonov SA, Barnes PJ. Increased leukotriene B4 and 8-isoprostane in exhaled breath condensate of patients with exacerbations of COPD. Thorax. 2003 Apr; 58(4):294-8.

17. Montuschi P, Macagno F, Parente P, Valente S, Lauriola L, Ciappi G, et al. Effects of cyclo-oxygenase inhibition on exhaled eicosanoids in patients with COPD. Thorax. 2005 Oct;60 (10):827-33.

18. Morrow JD, Hill KE, Burk RF, Nammour TM, Badr KF, Roberts LJ, 2nd. A series of prostaglandin F2-like compounds are produced in vivo in humans by a non-cyclooxygenase, free radical-catalyzed mechanism. Proc Natl Acad Sci U S A. 1990 Dec; 87(23):9383-7.

19. Montuschi P, Barnes PJ, Roberts LJ, 2nd. Isoprostanes: markers and mediators of oxidative stress. FASEB J. 2004 Dec;18(15):1791-800.

20. Montuschi P, Barnes P, Roberts LJ, 2nd. Insights into oxidative stress: the isoprostanes. Curr Med Chem. 2007;14(6):703-17.

21. Montuschi P, Collins JV, Ciabattoni G, Lazzeri N, Corradi M, Kharitonov SA, et al. Exhaled 8-isoprostane as an in vivo biomarker of lung oxidative stress in patients with COPD and healthy smokers. Am J Respir Crit Care Med. 2000 Sep;162(3 Pt 1): 1175-7.

22. Montuschi P, Corradi M, Ciabattoni G, Nightingale J, Kharitonov SA, Barnes PJ. Increased 8-isoprostane, a marker of oxidative stress, in exhaled condensate of asthma patients. Am J Respir Crit Care Med. 1999 Jul;160 (1):216-20.

23. Kostikas K, Papatheodorou G, Ganas K, Psathakis K, Panagou P, Loukides S. pH in expired breath condensate of patients with inflammatory airway diseases. Am J Respir Crit Care Med. 2002 May 15;165(10):1364-70.

24. Kostikas K, Papatheodorou G, Psathakis K, Panagou P, Loukides S. Oxidative stress in expired breath condensate of patients with COPD. Chest. 2003 Oct;124(4):1373-80.

25. Makris D, Paraskakis E, Korakas P, Karagiannakis E, Sourvinos G, Siafakas NM, et al. Exhaled breath condensate 8-isoprostane, clinical parameters, radiological indices and airway inflammation in COPD. Respiration. 2008;75(2):138-44.

26. Ko FW, Lau CY, Leung TF, Wong GW, Lam CW, Hui DS. Exhaled breath condensate levels of 8-isoprostane, growth related oncogene alpha and monocyte chemoattractant protein-1 in patients with chronic obstructive pulmonary disease. Respir Med. 2006 Apr;100(4):630-8.

27. Mazur W, Stark H, Sovijarvi A, Myllarniemi M, Kinnula VL. Comparison

of 8-isoprostane and interleukin-8 in induced sputum and exhaled breath condensate from asymptomatic and symptomatic smokers. Respiration. 2009;78(2):209-16.

28. Brindicci C, Ito K, Torre O, Barnes PJ, Kharitonov SA. Effects of aminoguanidine, an inhibitor of inducible nitric oxide synthase, on nitric oxide production and its metabolites in healthy control subjects, healthy smokers, and COPD patients. Chest. 2009 Feb;135(2):353-67.

29. Nowak D, Kalucka S, Bialasiewicz P, Krol M. Exhalation of H2O2 and thiobarbituric acid reactive substances (TBARs) by healthy subjects. Free Radic Biol Med. 2001 Jan 15;30(2): 178-86.

30. Dekhuijzen PN, Aben KK, Dekker I, Aarts LP, Wielders PL, van Herwaarden CL, et al. Increased exhalation of hydrogen peroxide in patients with stable and unstable chronic obstructive pulmonary disease. Am J Respir Crit Care Med. 1996 Sep;154(3 Pt 1):813-6.

31. Horvath I, Donnelly LE, Kiss A, Kharitonov SA, Lim S, Chung KF, et al. Combined use of exhaled hydrogen peroxide and nitric oxide in monitoring asthma. Am J Respir Crit Care Med. 1998 Oct;158(4):1042-6.

32. Schleiss MB, Holz O, Behnke M, Richter K, Magnussen H, Jorres RA. The concentration of hydrogen peroxide in exhaled air depends on expiratory flow rate. Eur Respir J. 2000 Dec;16(6):1115-8.

33. Ho LP, Faccenda J, Innes JA, Greening AP. Expired hydrogen peroxide in breath condensate of cystic fibrosis patients. Eur Respir J. 1999 Jan;13(1): 103-6.

34. Jobsis Q, Raatgeep HC, Hermans PW, de Jongste JC. Hydrogen peroxide in exhaled air is increased in stable asthmatic children. Eur Respir J. 1997 Mar;10(3):519-21.

35. van Beurden WJ, van den Bosch MJ, Janssen WC, Smeenk FW, Dekhuijzen PN, Harff GA. Fluorimetric analysis of hydrogen peroxide with automated measurement. Clin Lab. 2003;49(11-12):637-43.

36. van Beurden WJ, Harff GA, Dekhuijzen PN, van den Bosch MJ, Creemers JP, Smeenk FW. An efficient and reproducible method for measuring hydrogen peroxide in exhaled breath condensate. Respir Med. 2002 Mar;96(3):197-203.

37. Zappacosta B, Persichilli S, Mormile F, Minucci A, Russo A, Giardina B, et al. A fast chemiluminescent method for H(2)O(2) measurement in exhaled breath condensate. Clin Chim Acta. 2001 Aug 20;310(2):187-91.

38. Antczak A, Nowak D, Shariati B, Krol M, Piasecka G, Kurmanowska Z. Increased hydrogen peroxide and thiobarbituric acid-reactive products in expired breath condensate of asthmatic patients. Eur Respir J. 1997 Jun;10(6):1235-41.

39. De Benedetto F, Aceto A, Dragani B, Spacone A, Formisano S, Cocco R, et al. Validation of a new technique to assess exhaled hydrogen peroxide: results from normals and COPD patients. Monaldi Arch Chest Dis. 2000 Jun;55(3):185-8.

40. Nowak D, Kasielski M, Antczak A, Pietras T, Bialasiewicz P. Increased content of thiobarbituric acid-reactive substances and hydrogen peroxide in the expired breath condensate of

patients with stable chronic obstructive pulmonary disease: no significant effect of cigarette smoking. Respir Med. 1999 Jun;93(6):389-96.

41. Oudijk EJ, Gerritsen WB, Nijhuis EH, Kanters D, Maesen BL, Lammers JW, et al. Expression of priming-associated cellular markers on neutrophils during an exacerbation of COPD. Respir Med. 2006 Oct;100(10): 1791-9.

42. Mercken EM, Hageman GJ, Schols AM, Akkermans MA, Bast A, Wouters EF. Rehabilitation decreases exercise-induced oxidative stress in chronic obstructive pulmonary disease. Am J Respir Crit Care Med. 2005 Oct 15;172(8):994-1001.

43. Ferreira IM, Hazari MS, Gutierrez C, Zamel N, Chapman KR. Exhaled nitric oxide and hydrogen peroxide in patients with chronic obstructive pulmonary disease: effects of inhaled beclomethasone. Am J Respir Crit Care Med. 2001 Sep 15;164(6): 1012-5.

44. van Beurden WJ, Harff GA, Dekhuijzen PN, van der Poel-Smet SM, Smeenk FW. Effects of inhaled corticosteroids with different lung deposition on exhaled hydrogen peroxide in stable COPD patients. Respiration. 2003 May-Jun;70(3):242-8.

45. van Beurden WJ, Smeenk FW, Harff GA, Dekhuijzen PN. Markers of inflammation and oxidative stress during lower respiratory tract infections in COPD patients. Monaldi Arch Chest Dis. 2003 Oct-Dec;59(4):273-80.

46. Gerritsen WB, Asin J, Zanen P, van den Bosch JM, Haas FJ. Markers of inflammation and oxidative stress in exacerbated chronic obstructive pulmonary disease patients. Respir Med. 2005 Jan;99(1):84-90.

47. Kasielski M, Nowak D. Long-term administration of N-acetylcysteine decreases hydrogen peroxide exhalation in subjects with chronic obstructive pulmonary disease. Respir Med. 2001 Jun;95(6):448-56.

48. De Benedetto F, Aceto A, Dragani B, Spacone A, Formisano S, Pela R, et al. Long-term oral n-acetylcysteine reduces exhaled hydrogen peroxide in stable COPD. Pulm Pharmacol Ther. 2005;18(1):41-7.

49. Decramer M, Rutten-van Molken M, Dekhuijzen PN, Troosters T, van Herwaarden C, Pellegrino R, et al. Effects of N-acetylcysteine on outcomes in chronic obstructive pulmonary disease (Bronchitis Randomized on NAC Cost-Utility Study, BRONCUS): a randomised placebo-controlled trial. Lancet. 2005 Apr 30-May 6;365 (9470):1552-60.

50. Rysz J, Stolarek RA, Luczynski R, Sarniak A, Wlodarczyk A, Kasielski M, et al. Increased hydrogen peroxide concentration in the exhaled breath condensate of stable COPD patients after nebulized N-acetylcysteine. Pulm Pharmacol Ther. 2007;20(3):281-9.

51. Corradi M, Montuschi P, Donnelly LE, Pesci A, Kharitonov SA, Barnes PJ. Increased nitrosothiols in exhaled breath condensate in inflammatory airway diseases. Am J Respir Crit Care Med. 2001 Mar;163(4):854-8.

52. Osoata GO, Hanazawa T, Brindicci C, Ito M, Barnes PJ, Kharitonov S, et al. Peroxynitrite elevation in exhaled breath condensate of COPD and its

inhibition by fudosteine. Chest. 2009 Jun;135(6):1513-20.

53. Liu J, Sandrini A, Thurston MC, Yates DH, Thomas PS. Nitric oxide and exhaled breath nitrite/nitrates in chronic obstructive pulmonary disease patients. Respiration. 2007;74 (6):617-23.

54. Gessner C, Hammerschmidt S, Kuhn H, Hoheisel G, Gillissen A, Sack U, et al. Breath condensate nitrite correlates with hyperinflation in chronic obstructive pulmonary disease. Respir Med. 2007 Nov;101(11): 2271-8.

55. Balint B, Donnelly LE, Hanazawa T, Kharitonov SA, Barnes PJ. Increased nitric oxide metabolites in exhaled breath condensate after exposure to tobacco smoke. Thorax. 2001 Jun; 56(6):456-61.

56. Vaughan J, Ngamtrakulpanit L, Pajewski TN, Turner R, Nguyen TA, Smith A, et al. Exhaled breath condensate pH is a robust and reproducible assay of airway acidity. Eur Respir J. 2003 Dec;22(6):889-94.

57. Hunt J. Exhaled breath condensate: an evolving tool for noninvasive evaluation of lung disease. J Allergy Clin Immunol. 2002 Jul;110(1):28-34.

58. Terada K, Muro S, Sato S, Ohara T, Haruna A, Marumo S, et al. Impact of gastro-oesophageal reflux disease symptoms on COPD exacerbation. Thorax. 2008 Nov;63(11):951-5.

59. Halliwell B. Lipid peroxidation, antioxidants and cardiovascular disease: how should we move forward? Cardiovasc Res. 2000 Aug 18;47 (3):410-8.

60. Corradi M, Rubinstein I, Andreoli R, Manini P, Caglieri A, Poli D, et al. Aldehydes in exhaled breath condensate of patients with chronic obstructive pulmonary disease. Am J Respir Crit Care Med. 2003 May 15;167 (10):1380-6.

61. Lazar Z, Huszar E, Kullmann T, Barta I, Antus B, Bikov A, et al. Adenosine triphosphate in exhaled breath condensate of healthy subjects and patients with chronic obstructive pulmonary disease. Inflamm Res. 2008 Aug;57(8):367-73.

62. Scheideler L, Manke HG, Schwulera U, Inacker O, Hammerle H. Detection of nonvolatile macromolecules in breath. A possible diagnostic tool? Am Rev Respir Dis. 1993 Sep;148 (3):778-84.

63. Effros RM, Hoagland KW, Bosbous M, Castillo D, Foss B, Dunning M, et al. Dilution of respiratory solutes in exhaled condensates. Am J Respir Crit Care Med. 2002 Mar 1;165(5): 663-9.

64. Hoffmann HJ, Tabaksblat LM, Enghild JJ, Dahl R. Human skin keratins are the major proteins in exhaled breath condensate. Eur Respir J. 2008 Feb;31(2):380-4.

65. Gessner C, Scheibe R, Wotzel M, Hammerschmidt S, Kuhn H, Engelmann L, et al. Exhaled breath condensate cytokine patterns in chronic obstructive pulmonary disease. Respir Med. 2005 Oct;99(10):1229-40.

66. Dentener MA, Creutzberg EC, Pennings HJ, Rijkers GT, Mercken E, Wouters EF. Effect of infliximab on local and systemic inflammation in chronic obstructive pulmonary dis-

ease: a pilot study. Respiration. 2008;76(3):275-82.

67. de Laurentiis G, Paris D, Melck D, Maniscalco M, Marsico S, Corso G, et al. Metabonomic analysis of exhaled breath condensate in adults by nuclear magnetic resonance spectroscopy. Eur Respir J. 2008 Nov; 32(5):1175-83.

68. Montuschi P, Barnes PJ. Analysis of exhaled breath condensate for monitoring airway inflammation. Trends Pharmacol Sci. 2002 May;23(5): 232-7.

69. Effros RM, Biller J, Foss B, Hoagland K, Dunning MB, Castillo D, et al. A simple method for estimating respiratory solute dilution in exhaled breath condensates. Am J Respir Crit Care Med. 2003 Dec 15;168(12): 1500-5.

70. Montuschi P. Analysis of exhaled breath condensate in respiratory medicine: methodological aspects and potential clinical applications. Ther Adv Respir Dis. 2007 Oct;1(1): 5-23.

71. Bucchioni E, Kharitonov SA, Allegra L, Barnes PJ. High levels of interleukin-6 in the exhaled breath condensate of patients with COPD. Respir Med. 2003 Dec;97(12):1299-302.

Exhaled Biomarkers in Asthma in Children

Emmanouil Paraskakis • *Athanasios Chatzimichael* • *Andrew Bush*

Measurement of airway inflammation is a hot topic in respiratory medicine. There are important general principles. The first is that the investigator needs to specify carefully the question being asked. A difference between groups of patients (acute exacerbation of asthma vs. stable asthma, or asthma vs. normal) may be statistically significant, and give a valuable indication about mechanisms of disease, but the overlap is usually too great for the measurement to be a clinically useful tool. The difference between mechanistically useful and the much more demanding clinical utility is often confused. Secondly, there is no such thing as a perfect "inflammometer". There is a lot of controversy about "inflammometry", but none about the use of spirometry in the clinic; this is because we appreciate that spirometry is only part of the picture, not the whole, whereas there seems to be a relentless quest for a biomarker which will replace all other aspects of clinical manage-

Correspondence

Dr. Emmanouil Paraskakis
Assistant Professor of Pediatrics, Respiratory Unit, Pediatric Department, University of Thrace, Alexandroupolis, Greece
e-mail: eparaska@med.duth.gr

ment! The third principle is to consider what aspects of inflammation are of interest, because this will determine the best tool to use. So for example, if mechanisms of recruitment of inflammatory cells from the bone marrow are of interest, then a blood sample may be required; if airway inflammatory events, then induced sputum may be the best tool. One size does not fit all.

It is also important to note that monitoring airway inflammation is not necessary or appropriate for everyone. Mild asthmatics can be managed satisfactorily without these sophisticated measurements, and indeed in one study, adding in monitoring of sputum eosinophils made no difference to outcome (1). Another group have suggested (2) it is in specific groups of patients with discordance between inflammation and symptoms (either many symptoms and little inflammation, for example obesity, or severe inflammation and little in the way of symptoms, an exacerbation prone phenotype) that inflammometry may be most useful. Inflammatory monitoring is not useful in many cases, including those in whom basic asthma care has not been optimised (3, 4).

Asthma is a complex chronic disease mainly characterized by airway inflammation (5-10). Treatment aims at reducing or eliminating airway inflammation, but this is not measured in clinical practice; we are like cardiologists treating hypertension without actually measuring the blood pressure. Recent studies have shown that monitoring asthma using conventional methods such as peak flow or lung function testing is suboptimal since in asthmatic children airway inflammation may persist despite apparent clinical stability and normal spirometry (7). The invasive techniques which are considered as gold standard such as bronchoscopic biopsy and bronchoalveolar lavage (BAL) often are not justified in paediatrics because of the need of anaesthesia, the risk of the procedure and patient's discomfort (6). Moreover these invasive procedures could not be performed serially. Therefore there has been growing interest in non-invasive methods (7, 11-15).

A number of inflammatory volatile and non volatile biomarkers that could increase our understanding on the pathophysiology of asthma and augment the effectiveness of our anti-inflammatory treatment can non-invasively be measured in exhaled breath(11-16). Inflammatory biomarkers of asthma in children such as exhaled nitric oxide, carbon monoxide, ethane, pentane and a number of volatile and non volatile biomarkers in exhaled breath condensate will be discussed.

Exhaled Nitric Oxide

Nitric Oxide (NO) is a relatively unstable diatomic free radical gas produced in vivo when L-arginine is oxidized to L-citrulline (11, 12, 17-19). Nitric oxide synthesis is catalyzed by NO synthases (NOS) of which three isoforms have been identified, the neuronal nitric oxide synthase (nNOS), the endothelial nitric oxide synthase (eNOS), and the inducible one (iNOS) (11, 12, 17-19). The constitutive nitric oxide synthases (i.e. nNOS and eNOS) are activated by rises in the intracellular calcium and can be stimulated by mediators such as histamine, leucotrienes, bradykinine, acetylocholine and platelet activating factor (11, 12, 17-19). Endothelial NOS is found in endothelial cells of pulmonary blood vessels, bronchial epithelium, type II alveolar epithelial cells, nasal mucosa and the membrane of ciliary microtubules (13, 17, 18). Neuronal NOS are located in nerves in the human airways(17-19). The inducible nitric oxide synthase iNOS has been detected in macrophages, airway smooth muscle cells, fibroblasts, respiratory epithelial cells, endothelial cells, mast cells and neutrophils (17, 18, 20). The upregulation of the iNOS by inflammatory cytokines seems to be the main source of increased production of NO by epithelial cells and alveolar macrophages in asthma. After synthesis the gas diffuses into the airway lumen leading to increased levels of NO in exhaled breath (17, 19).

NO is usually measured by chemiluminescence assay, based on detection of photons when NO reacts with ozone. According to an American Thoracic Society (ATS)/European Respiratory Society (ERS) task force recommendation, FeNO (Fractional exhaled Nitric Oxide) should be measured using an expiratory flow of 50 mL/s^2. Available methods to measure FeNO are the online method using the single breath technique which can be performed by children older than five years old and the offline method, analysing exhaled gas first collected in a reservoir which is able to assess FeNO in children younger than five years old (17, 19). A recent study has helped to establish the range of normal values of FeNO which is between 15 and 25 ppb in children aged of 4 to 17 years old (21).

A substantial number of studies have shown that mean FeNO is significantly higher in steroid-naive asthmatic children than controls(17, 22, 23). FeNO in atopic asthmatic children correlates with eosinophil counts in induced sputum and BAL, eosinophil infiltration of the airway wall (7, 17, 19), serum total IgE, specific IgE to house dust mite and with a number of positive skin prick tests (24-29).

Several studies have confirmed that FeNO levels in atopic subjects are elevated, even in the absence of respiratory tract symptoms. FeNO levels of atopic asthmatics are higher than those of non-atopic asthmatics and atopy appears to be at least a co-factor of FeNO (17, 24, 26, 30, 31).

The exhaled NO signal can be partitioned into airway and alveolar components by measuring exhaled NO at multiple flows and applying mathematical models (23, 32). The airway NO flux and alveolar NO concentration can be elevated in children with asthma and have been correlated with markers of airway inflammation in several studies (23, 32). The alveolar NO concentration is significantly elevated in children with asthma when compared to normal children and atopic non-asthmatic children, which is different from FeNO (atopic asthmatics and atopic non-asthmatics both elevated) (23). The airway NO flux was found to be elevated in both the asthmatic and atopic group when compared to normal subjects (23). Alveolar NO concentration was higher in the subgroup of children whose asthma was poorly controlled, suggesting that alveolar NO may be indicative of asthma control (23). Moreover partitioning of the exhaled NO signal revealed that airway NO flux correlated with bronchial wall thickening estimated using HRCT and reticular basement membrane thickening assessed by endobronchial biopsy (33).

In steroid-naive asthmatic children, treatment with low dose of ICS (fluticasone) have been showed to reduce FeNO (11-13, 17, 20, 34, 35). FeNO in adult subjects with mild asthma indicated the onset and cessation of anti-inflammatory action of inhaled steroids [budesonide] in a dose-dependent manner (13, 20). A more rapid increase of FeNO was seen after stopping treatment with budesonide 400 mcg/day compared with 100 mcg/day (13, 20). Studies have shown that FeNO gradually decreases during the first week of regular treatment with ICS to reach a nadir at approximately the 4th week of treatment (36).

The leukotriene receptor antagonist montelukast also reduces FENO but to a lesser extent than low dose ICS (37-41). Studies on the effect of short acting β2-agonists are still controversial (42-44). A number of studies have found that short acting β2-agonists increase FeNO levels, possibly by their effect on airway calibre and ventilated airway surface, but not all could confirm this finding (17, 42-44). Similar findings are reported for the effects of long acting β2-agonists (LABA) on FENO (45-47).

Most studies demonstrated no correlations between FeNO and pulmonary function tests such as forced expiratory volume in 1 s (FEV$_1$), peak expiratory flow (PEF) although a few showed weak correlations (17, 23, 48, 49). Likewise some studies showed a correlation between symptoms (recent symptoms, symptom frequency, symptom scores, symptom control or rescue b2-agonist use) whereas others did not (11, 25, 49, 50).

Several studies have examined the diagnostic utility of FeNO measurements in young children with conflicting results (33, 51-53). An increasing number of studies have shown acceptable sensitivity, increasing with the age of the children, and high specificity while other studies found FeNO to perform poorly in distinguishing asthma and non-asthma in individual subjects (51, 53).

A limited number of studies have shown that children with elevated FeNO values were more likely to respond to fluticasone than to montelukast implicating that FeNO levels may predict steroid responsiveness (17, 22).

FeNO may be able to predict deterioration in asthma in children, since it is suggested that FeNO rose prior to an exacerbation or following steroid withdrawal in currently asymptomatic young patients(17, 54).

In paediatric and adult studies of allergic asthmatic subjects using ICS, treatment decisions or dose titration based on FeNO showed a significant reduction in the severity of AHR, reduction in exacerbations requiring oral prednisone in children and ICS dose requirements in adults (54-57). Although adult and paediatric studies differed in study design and population and showed varying outcomes all of them have shown that benefits may be reached when incorporating FeNO measurements in treatment decisions (54, 57).

However, further research is needed to evaluate if the assessment of FeNO levels is useful for titration of ICS dose in atopic asthmatic children. Future studies using individual cut-offs, based on a patient's baseline values - as a "personal best" FeNO in the same way we used to do with PEFR or frequent monitoring of FeNO at home may augment the usefulness of FENO measurements in treatment decisions.

In conclusion FeNO provides the clinician with valuable, additional information regarding underlying airway inflammation (6, 58), even allowing the use of specific mathematical models to estimate proximal and distal inflammation.

The use of FeNO is complementary to lung function testing, and only part of the clinical picture. In atopic asthmatic children its use seems to increase the diagnostic accuracy, enables us to administer ICS more effectively and distinguishes patients who will benefit from ICS from those who will not. Moreover FeNO seems to be efficient in predicting exacerbations and successful steroid reduction or withdrawal. In children under five years old, where the diagnosis of asthma is extremely challenging, FeNO assessment may help at the diagnosis and allow for better targeting and monitoring of anti-inflammatory treatment, but more data are needed.

Sputum Induction

Sputum induction is a relatively non invasive technique allowing the assessment of lung inflammatory profile in asthmatic children (57, 59-61). Studies from adults have shown that the cellular composition of sputum induction correlates rather well with bronchial wash or bronchoalveolar lavage but not with bronchial biopsies (62).

Induced sputum is usually attained by inhalation of hypertonic normal saline for 10-20 minutes. The child is asked to produce sputum at 2-5 minutes intervals and close monitoring for FEV_1 (forced expiratory volume in one second) and PEF (peak expiratory flow) changes is undertaken (59).

A number of studies have shown the safety of the procedure in children with stable, acute and severe asthma aged 5-14 years old (59, 63, 64). The success rate of sputum induction in children is reported to be 68-100% (59). The usual side effect reported are cough, bronchoconstriction, vomiting or anxiety. The side effects are mild, easily reversed and rarely the procedure needs to be discontinued (in 3% of the children). However it should be mentioned that in most of the studies pretreatment with β2 agonist is effective in bronchospasm avoidance. With β2 agonist pretreatment a fall in lung function of 10% of base line reported only in 6% of the children (63).

Sputum eosinophils represent the cardinal marker of airway inflammation in asthmatic children (61). The values of eosinophils count in normal/healthy children have been reported to have an upper limit of 2.5% of sputum cells (65). Children with stable asthma exhibit increased eosinophils and may exhibit increased bronchial epithelial cell number of in their sputum (65, 66). Children with asymptomatic airway hyperresponsiveness show normal cell count (67). Young patients with acute asthma showed to have increased number of eosinophils, mast cells and eosinophilic cationic protein in their induced sputum (68). Some children exhibit accompanying sputum neutrophilia with increased levels of interleukin-8 (68).

Corticosteroid therapy seems to lower the percentage of sputum eosinophils (68-70). Sputum eosinophils decrease correlates well with asthma control (57, 60, 71). Moreover recent studies have shown that sputum eosinophils seem to be a useful marker in steroid step down therapy, since dose reduction was successful in all treated children with no eosinophils in their induced sputum (57). The number of eosinophils was shown to be a significant predictor of medication reduction failure (57). Additionally sputum eosinophils were associated with higher bronchodilator reversibility, fractional exhaled nitric oxide (FeNO) levels, sputum eosinophilic cationic protein, greater asthma severity, more prednisone courses and lower FEV_1/FVC ratio (72). Additionally, the use of sputum induction, as it has been shown in a number of adult studies, is helpful to identify the non-eosinophilic or neutrophilic asthma which may require different therapeutic approach (71, 73).

Sputum induction could additionally provide research information if new techniques are used, such as flow cytometry (62), DNA extraction for genetic studies (74) or PCR for IL-8 of the induced sputum (75).

Despite the safety, tolerability and the useful information provided by sputum induction the method is not widely used probably because of some limitations of the method, such as the requirement of substantial amount of time to perform and process the sample average time needed three hours) and the need of experienced technical support to process, stain and interpret the samples (72).

In summary, sputum induction is a safe well tolerated method which in experienced hands is able to provide useful information on the inflammatory profile of different asthmatic phenotypes and help the clinician retain asthma control, predict exacerbation and reduce steroid treatment more safely.

Exhaled Carbon Monoxide (eCO)

Exhaled CO represents a marker of oxidative stress of the airways

(20). The data from children are still limited. Children with severe asthma may have increased levels of eCO, despite steroid treatment. At the moment there are insufficient data to recommend eCO for clinical purposes.

Exhaled Ethane/Pentane

Exhaled ethane and pentane are markers of lipid hyperoxidation. Exhaled ethane is elevated in adult asthmatics, reduced in steroid-treated patients, and correlate with FeNO and airway obstruction. The data from children are too limited for clinical use.

Exhaled Breath Condensate (EBC)

Exhaled breath condensate (EBC) is a new method that may serve as a tool to study airway inflammation and oxidative stress through the detection of non-volatile substances in the exhaled air. Exhaled breath contains water vapor and micro-droplets (which are generated by shear forces and derived especially during turbulent air flow) and appears to reflect the airway lining fluid that covers the respiratory track surface (16). The non-volatile compounds are mainly the molecules that likely derive from droplets of airway fluid. Changes in condensate markers may mirror local abnormalities of airway extracellular lining fluid, so exhaled breath analysis may be used to quantify lung inflammation.

EBC has been reported to be successfully collected in children, with 100% completion of the procedure, without any significant fall in FEV_1 after the procedure neither in asthmatic nor in healthy children, and generally no significant adverse effects reported so far (52, 76). Frequently repeated measurements can be applied with no harmful effects on children as young as 4 years old even during disease exacerbation (76, 77). Moreover, with some modifications (like sedation and the use of facemask) reasonable amounts can be safely collected from younger children, infants and newborns (52, 78-80).

The mean volume of EBC collected from children has been reported to be 1.5 ml (range 0.5-3 ml). The EBC volume is correlated with age length, weight and minute ventilation (Vm) in infants, and probable with disease of the subjects (52, 76, 80, 81).

Non Volatile compounds derived from EBC

Many inflammatory mediators can be measured in EBC, of molecular weight 40-70kDa (81).

Eicosanoid family

F2-isoprostanes: (F2-IPs)

Isoprostanes (IPs) are products of non-enzymatic peroxidation of arachidonic acid by oxygen species (ROS) and may serve as a marker of oxidative stress. 8-isoprostane (8-IP) may induce s-mooth-muscle contraction *in vitro* in asthma and contribute to lung injury.

The levels of 8-IP in EBC are increased in steroid-naive and steroid-treated stable or unstable asthmatic children, and in children during asthma exacerbation but not in atopic children without asth-ma (77, 82, 83). Moreover increased 8-IP concentrations in EBC were found in children with exercise induced bronchoconstriction (EIB) suggesting a role for oxidative stress in bronchial hyperreactiv-ity (32). No difference was reported in exhaled 8-isoprostane levels between atopic children without asthma and healthy children (84). These results may indicate that atopy does not seem to be predis-posing factor for IP elevation although exhaled 8-IP has been showed to reduce after allergen avoidance in asthmatic children (35). Although asthmatic children using inhaled steroids have a trend towards a lower 8-IP levels than those of steroid-naive group, most studies have shown that low or high dose inhaled or even oral corticosteroids do not affect the levels 8-IP in asthmatic children (82, 85, 86). Similarly treatment with oral montelukast had no effect on exhaled 8-IP of atopic children with or without asthma (84).

As emphasized by the majority of authors, there is possibly residual inflammation and oxidative stress in children with asthma despite corticosteroid treatment, implicating the need for antioxi-dant treatment for the disease in the future (16, 87, 88). Clinical tri-als with antioxidants in childhood asthma are awaited, and these drugs could be monitored by the levels of 8-IP in EBC.

Cys -Leukotrienes (LT C4/ D4/ E4):

Leukotrienes LTC4, LTD4 and LTE4 are the cysteinyl-leukotrienes (Cys-LTs) and can be quantified in EBC in children (89). Cys-LTs are generated from arachidonic acid by the 5-lipoxygenase pathway and are released mainly by mast cells and macrophages in the airways. They are also produced by eosinophils recruited to the conducting airways when asthmatic inflammation is active (during early and late-phase allergic reactions). Leukotrienes in turn, cause further eosinophil migration into the airways. Ccys-LTs can induce smooth-muscle contraction, microvascular leakage, and mucus hyper-secretion (16).

LTD4 and LTE4 are detectable in EBC of normal children and children with airway disease in the majority of studies (90, 91). LTC4 is frequently undetectable or close to detection limit (92, 93). EBC concentrations of cys-LTs in children with stable asthma (both steroid-naive and ICS-treated) have been found to be significantly higher than in normal children (94). Specifically, Cys-LT levels have been found elevated in mild to moderate persistent asthma but not in children with mild intermittent asthma compared with normal control subjects (95). In children with an asthma exacerbation, Cys-LTs have been found to be elevated compared with healthy children, or with stable asthmatic children (77, 83). Exhaled LTE4 levels are increased in both steroid-naive and steroid-treated atopic asthmatic children but not in atopic nonasthmatic children compared with control subjects (84, 96). There is no difference in exhaled LTE4 values between atopic children without asthma and healthy children (84).

ICS treatment does not seem to affect the LTD4 and LTC4 concentrations in EBC of children with stable asthma (83, 89). On the contrary LTE4 values are reduced significantly after treatment with inhaled low dose fluticasone (96). There was a significant relationship found between EBC cysLTs levels and reticular basement membrane thickness, estimated with endobronchial biopsy (97); indicating that Cys-LTs may play a role in the pathophysiology of remodeling. Additionally, EBC Cys-LT values are elevated in asthmatic children with exercise induced bronchocontriction (EIB) and correlate with the decrease in FEV_1 after exercise (98).

In atopic children with asthma (but not atopic children without asthma), oral montelukast significantly reduced exhaled LTE4 and dependent on initial baseline values, indicating that children with higher baseline LTE4 levels might be the most likely to have a significant reduction in exhaled LTE4 from leukotriene receptor antagonists (LTRAs) (84, 99). In clinical practice, not all patients treated with cys-LT antagonists show a clinical improvement, therefore measurement of LTE4 might help identify children with asthma who are most likely to benefit from LTRAs (84).

LTE4 concentrations were significantly increased in nonasthmatic adults with seasonal allergic rhinitis during the pollen season in comparison with healthy controls (100).

Leukotriene B4 (LTB4)

LTB4, a potent neutrophil chemoattractant, is a weak bronchoconstrictor but it may contribute to airway narrowing by producing local neutrophil mediated oedema and mucus secretion (101, 102). Although LTB4 has not been closely linked to asthma, there is increasing evidence that neutrophils may play a role in the pathogenesis of both adult and childhood asthma (92, 101, 103, 104)

LTB4 concentrations in EBC are variably reported to be reduced or unchanged in association with ICS therapy (105-107); more work is needed to elucidate this relationship.

Prostaglandins (PG)

PGE_2 is bronchoprotective and has inhibitory effects on inflammatory cells. The impaired production of PGE_2 has been implicated in the pathophysiology of asthma. PGE_2 concentrations are similar among asthmatic and healthy children. In addition, no difference in PGE_2 levels has been noticed between steroid-naive, steroid-treated atopic asthmatic children, atopic nonasthmatic children and healthy controls (16, 84, 96). Oral montelukast does not reduce prostaglandin E_2 from baseline in steroid-naive asthmatic children (51).

Thromboxane (TX)

There are no differences in TXB2 levels between healthy children, atopic nonasthmatic children, steroid-naive atopic asthmatic children and steroid-treated atopic children with asthma (96).

Nitric Oxide Metabolites

NO metabolites, such NO_3^-, NO_2, and nitrotyrosine can be detected in the epithelial lining fluid of the normal human respiratory tract as well as in EBC.The stable oxidation end products of NO metabolism are nitrite and nitrate and 3-nitrotyrosine, and these may indicate local formation of reactive nitrogen species. NO also reacts with the anion O_2^- leading to peroxynitrite (ONOO-) formation (108, 109)

Nitrotyrosine (NT)

3-nitrotyrosine is a stable marker of protein nitration, a biological process derived from the biochemical interaction of NO with reactive oxygen species (RNS) (108, 109). The median EBC concentration of 3-NT in asthmatic children was fivefold higher than in healthy subjects with no difference between steroid-naive and unstable steroid-treated asthmatic patients indicating that ICS may not inhibit the oxidative stress (109). However this is controversial since a single-blind placebo-controlled study in asthmatic children showed that inhaled corticosteroid treatment (flunisolide) reduced nitrotyrosine levels in EBC (110).

NO_2^-/NO_3^- (nitrite, nitrate)

NO gas in aqueous solution is a free radical that reacts rapidly with reactive oxygen species to form stable oxides of nitrogen (NOx). Some NOx metabolites, such as peroxynitrite [$OONO^-$] or peroxynitrous acid, are unstable intermediates that then decompose, forming nitrite (NO_2) and nitrate (NO_3^-)(78, 79, 95, 111-115).

Children with mild or moderate asthma have been proved to have significantly elevated nitrite concentrations compared to healthy subjects (116, 117). In addition, children with asthma do not differ in nitrite levels from children with nonasthmatic, episodic cough (116). Atopy does not seem to influence nitrites in EBC, within the cough or asthmatic groups (116, 117). Nitrate levels in EBC are possibly influenced by dietary intake, and there may be a substantial contamination by nitrite derived from the oropharyngeal tract (118).

S-nitrosothiols (SNOs)

Nitrosothiols (S-NOs) are formed by interaction of NO with glutathione. They are detectable in EBC (119). Data in children are limited. Recent studies have shown that SNOs were higher in asthmatic children when compared with normal controls (119). A significant reduction in S-nitrosothiols after budesonide treatment was observed in adults with mild asthma but was not dose-dependent (20).

Lipid peroxidation products

Lipid peroxidation products are mainly the aldehydic products, namely malondialdehyde (MDA), acrolein, unsaturated aldehydes (4-hydroxyhexenal and 4-hydroxynonenal), and saturated aldehydes (hexanal, heptanal, and nonanal) which reflect oxidant induced damages (120-122). In children with asthma or acute asthma exacerbation, malondialdehyde levels are substantially higher than in con-

trol subjects and reduced after oral steroid therapy to control levels
(121).

Volatile compounds derived from EBC

Ammonia/Ammonium

Ammonia values in EBC are reportedly significantly lower in the asthmatic children than in controls, but significantly higher in ICS-treated than in steroid-naive subjects (123, 124). EBC ammonia levels before exercise were significantly greater in healthy asthmatic children. EBC ammonia does not appear to be affected by age but may be affected by EBC pH (125).

Oral formation of ammonia has been suggested, as ammonia could not be detected in subjects with tracheostomies (126) and was reduced in EBC by methods used to limit oral ammonia (127).

Hydrogen ions (pH)

Hydrogen ions are measured by microelectrode pH meter with or without deaeration with argon gas to enhance the stability of the readings (11, 12, 125, 128-130). Acidic airway pH has been shown to inhibit ciliary beating, cause bronchoconstriction, lead to coughing and increase mucous viscosity (131).

In healthy subjects, EBC pH is maintained alkaline ranging from 7.4-8.8 (129). Lower pH values were observed in the EBC of children with asthma compared to control subjects (103, 129). EBC pH (non-deaerated) from children with asthma seem to be influenced by asthma severity; it was lower in children with moderate-to-severe persistent than mild or intermittent asthma (103, 128). There is no significant difference between median pH in children with stable asthma compared with controls, but pH values are significantly higher in ICS-treated than in steroid-naive asthmatic children (16).

The pH of children with acute asthma is lower than that of patients with stable asthma, rhinitis, and controls, and patients with acute asthma normalized their pH after treatment with ICS (132). Patients with rhinitis, and eczema had also lower pH than that of controls (8, 132, 133).

Patients whose cough responds to proton pump inhibition have transient EBC acidification (decline that persisted for 10-20 min) with coughing episodes, supporting the role of airway acidification in reflux-triggered cough (134).

One study has shown that in the epidemiologic setting, EBC-pH does not differ between children with and without parentally reported symptoms suggestive of asthma (135). There are some suggestions that EBC pH may not be a reliable marker of airway acidification as the interpretation of its concentration is complicated by the dependency of NH_4^+ concentrations in the condensate and the balance of volatile salivary acids and bases in the mouth (29, 126, 136). Temperature of collection, duration of collection and storage, acute airway obstruction (after methacholine challenge), subject age, saliva pH, and profound hyperventilation and hypoventilation seem to have no effect on deaerated pH of adults subjects (125, 130).

Hydrogen peroxide (H₂O₂)

H_2O_2 is a reactive oxygen radical released from various inflammatory cells such as alveolar macrophages and leukocytes and type-II pneumocytes. H_2O_2 can be converted into hydroxyl radicals leading to peroxidative damage of airway structures and formation of volatile thiobarbituric acid-reactive substances (TBARs). Reference data for exhaled hydrogen peroxide in a large group of healthy children have been published (median H_2O_2 in the exhaled air condensate of all children was 0.13 microM, with a 2.5-97.5% range of <0.01-0.48 microM), where the observed levels were lower than those reported previously for healthy adults and were independent of age, sex and lung function (137, 138).

The median H_2O_2 level in the exhaled air condensate of the stable asthmatic children is significantly higher than in healthy controls, and tended to be lower in asthmatics using anti-inflammatory medication (137).

H_2O_2 in exhaled air condensate is elevated during a common cold, and returns to normal within 2 weeks of recovery in healthy subjects (139). Passive smoking proved not to increase H_2O_2 exhalation in healthy children (140).

However it should be mentioned that even under strictly controlled conditions, a high degree of variability persists, which may limit the usefulness of exhaled hydrogen peroxide (141).

Cytokines

An increasing number have shown that a number of interleukins and other cytokines or factors have been detected in EBC of asthmatic patients.

Interleukin-4 has been showed to be increased in asthmatic children compared to controls and the concentrations decrease after ICS treatment (142, 143). Exhaled IFN-γ has been found to be decreased in children with asthma compared to controls (142). The IL-4/IFN-γ ratio in EBC was greater in steroid-naive asthmatic children compared to control and corticosteroids appear to correct this imbalance (142). In another study, IL-4 concentrations were found increased in asthmatic children as well as subjects with increased plasma total IgE but patients with persistent asthma (receiving high-dose ICS) had higher EBC IL-4 concentrations than those on low-dose ICS (144).

EBC IL-5 is higher in children with atopic dermatitis, allergic rhinitis, and asthma in comparison with healthy controls (8). The IL-5 level is significantly higher in subjects with intermittent asthma (ICS-naive) than in moderate asthma (ICS-treated) and controls (8).

Higher concentration of IL-6 is observed in the breath condensate of adult asthmatic patients compared to controls without substantial reduction after 6-month of treatment with ICS (145). IL-8 was elevated in adult asthmatic patients (steroid-naive) compared with healthy subjects (146). IL10 levels seem to be higher in subjects with asthma compared with controls; others found EBC IL10 very close to detection limits. The levels of IL10 do not seem to be affected by corticosteroid treatment (147).

A limited number of studies have been reported that cytokines in asthma have been reported such as IL-1, IL-2, IL-13 IL-17 are found in the EBC of the asthmatics (146, 147). Growth factors such as vascular endothelial growth factor (VEGF) are detectable in a significant proportion in asthmatic children (144). Increased AA isoform of platelet-derived growth factor (PDGF-AA) is found in asthmatic children with more severe airflow limitation (144). Eotaxin (an eosinophil chemoattractact) and macrophage-derived chemokine MDC, a Th-2 specific chemokine, levels are higher in adult and child asthmatics on ICS than the steroid-naive asthmatics and controls (148, 149). Surfactant protein A (SPA) (9), thymus and activation-regulated chemokine (TARC) (149), vitronectin (150) and, and epidermal growth factor (EGF) (144), advanced glycation end-products (AGEs) (151), and hepatocyte growth factor (HGF] (104) have been studied occasionally in EBC of adult asthmatics. In addition TGF-beta, INF-gamma-inducible protein-10, RANTES, macrophage inflammatory protein 1-alpha and 1-beta were detected and found elevated in steroid-naive adults with asthma (146). TNF-alpha, were significantly upregulated in adult steroid-naive asthmatic airways compared with those of non-smoking healthy subjects (146).

Adenosine

Adenosine is a nucleotide that may be produced in allergic inflammatory conditions and may modulate persistent airway inflammation. Adenosine is able to influence leukocyte chemotaxis (152). Adenosine concentration is higher in steroid-naive adult patients with allergic asthma compared with healthy control subjects and steroid-treated patients (152). In patients with worsening symptoms of asthma adenosine concentration was elevated compared with those in a stable condition (89, 152).

Electrolytes

Limited numbers of studies have shown that, the Na+ and Cl- of the asthmatic children are significantly higher than that of healthy children (153).

Exhaled Breath Temperature

Respiratory temperature probably reflected the increased mucosal vascularity found in asthma was elevated in adult patients with asthma compared with control subjects (154). So far there are no studies measuring exhaled breath temperature asthmatic children.

New Techniques

Increasing data from recent studies indicate that new techniques such as metabolomics, genomics and proteomics all based on characterization of airway biochemical, genetic or protein fingerprints using artificial networks might in the future help to identify children with asthma or different asthmatic phenotypes with a high success rate.

Conclusions

In conclusion it is obvious that there are many methods for assessing lung inflammation with non-invasive procedures in which with combination with clinical information they can help in diagnosis, increase the knowledge for pathophysiology of asthma and eventually lead to the proper management of patients. Among them FENO, which seems to be adequately studied compared with the other biomarkers, as a marker of eosinophilic airway inflammation has the potential to serve as an indicator of the adequacy of anti-inflammatory treatment, and may help to rationalize steroid therapy in asthmatic children. Induced sputum eosinophils represent a useful marker for the evaluation of asthma control and the guidance of treatment, especially in the direction of steroid reduction, but the need for a dedicated laboratory limits its widespread use. Different markers such as 8-isoprostane, nitrate and nitrite in condensate are of an additional value to exhaled nitric oxide, and they could be useful to diagnose asthma and to indicate asthma control and severity in childhood. EBC 8-isoprostane may be helpful in monitoring oxidative stress and serve as a marker for new antioxidative treatments. Assessment of exhaled breath condensate acidification by pH in patients with coughing episodes may also help to identify patients with reflux-triggered cough.

References

1. Jayaram L, Pizzichini MM, Cook RJ, Boulet LP, Lemiere C, Pizzichini E, et al. Determining asthma treatment by monitoring sputum cell counts: effect on exacerbations. Eur Respir J. 2006 Mar;27(3):483-94.

2. Haldar P, Pavord ID, Shaw DE, Berry MA, Thomas M, Brightling CE, et al. Cluster analysis and clinical asthma phenotypes. Am J Respir Crit Care Med. 2008 Aug 1;178(3):218-24.

3. Effros RM, Biller J, Foss B, Hoagland K, Dunning MB, Castillo D, et al. A simple method for estimating respiratory solute dilution in exhaled breath condensates. Am J Respir Crit Care Med. 2003 Dec 15;168(12):1500-5.

4. Szefler SJ, Mitchell H, Sorkness CA, Gergen PJ, O'Connor GT, Morgan WJ, et al. Management of asthma based on exhaled nitric oxide in addition to guideline-based treatment for inner-city adolescents and young adults: a randomised controlled trial. Lancet. 2008 Sep 20;372(9643):1065-72.

5. Agarwal AR, Mih J, George SC. Expression of matrix proteins in an in vitro model of airway remodeling in asthma. Allergy Asthma Proc. 2003 Jan-Feb;24(1):35-42.

6. Bush A. Inflammometry and asthma: onto the next level. Pediatr Pulmonol. 2007 Jul;42(7):569-72.

7. Gibson PG, Henry RL, Thomas P. Noninvasive assessment of airway in-

flammation in children: induced sputum, exhaled nitric oxide, and breath condensate. Eur Respir J. 2000 Nov; 16(5):1008-15.

8. Profita M, La Grutta S, Carpagnano E, Riccobono L, Di Giorgi R, Bonanno A, et al. Noninvasive methods for the detection of upper and lower airway inflammation in atopic children. J Allergy Clin Immunol. 2006 Nov;118(5): 1068-74.

9. Simpson JL, Wood LG, Gibson PG. Inflammatory mediators in exhaled breath, induced sputum and saliva. Clin Exp Allergy. 2005 Sep;35(9): 1180-5.

10. Tashkin DP. The role of small airway inflammation in asthma. Allergy Asthma Proc. 2002 Jul-Aug;23(4): 233-42.

11. Kharitonov SA, Barnes PJ. Biomarkers of some pulmonary diseases in exhaled breath. Biomarkers. 2002 Jan-Feb;7(1):1-32.

12. Kharitonov SA, Barnes PJ. Exhaled biomarkers. Chest. 2006 Nov;130(5): 1541-6.

13. Kharitonov SA, Barnes PJ. Exhaled markers of pulmonary disease. Am J Respir Crit Care Med. 2001 Jun;163(7):1693-722.

14. Smith AD, Cowan JO, Brassett KP, Filsell S, McLachlan C, Monti-Sheehan G, et al. Exhaled nitric oxide: a predictor of steroid response. Am J Respir Crit Care Med. 2005 Aug 15;172(4): 453-9.

15. Strunk RC, Szefler SJ, Phillips BR, Zeiger RS, Chinchilli VM, Larsen G, et al. Relationship of exhaled nitric oxide to clinical and inflammatory markers of persistent asthma in children. J Allergy Clin Immunol. 2003 Nov;112(5): 883-92.

16. Horvath I, Hunt J, Barnes PJ, Alving K, Antczak A, Baraldi E, et al. Exhaled breath condensate: methodological recommendations and unresolved questions. Eur Respir J. 2005 Sep;26 (3):523-48.

17. Pijnenburg MW, De Jongste JC. Exhaled nitric oxide in childhood asthma: a review. Clin Exp Allergy. 2008 Feb;38(2):246-59.

18. Ricciardolo FL, Sterk PJ, Gaston B, Folkerts G. Nitric oxide in health and disease of the respiratory system. Physiol Rev. 2004 Jul;84(3):731-65.

19. ATS Workshop Proceedings: Exhaled nitric oxide and nitric oxide oxidative metabolism in exhaled breath condensate: Executive summary. Am J Respir Crit Care Med. 2006 Apr 1;173 (7):811-3.

20. Kharitonov SA, Donnelly LE, Montuschi P, Corradi M, Collins JV, Barnes PJ. Dose-dependent onset and cessation of action of inhaled budesonide on exhaled nitric oxide and symptoms in mild asthma. Thorax. 2002 Oct;57(10):889-96.

21. Buchvald F, Baraldi E, Carraro S, Gaston B, De Jongste J, Pijnenburg MW, et al. Measurements of exhaled nitric oxide in healthy subjects age 4 to 17 years. J Allergy Clin Immunol. 2005 Jun;115(6):1130-6.

22. Ojoo JC, Mulrennan SA, Kastelik JA, Morice AH, Redington AE. Exhaled breath condensate pH and exhaled nitric oxide in allergic asthma and in cystic fibrosis. Thorax. 2005 Jan;60(1):22-6.

23. Paraskakis E, Brindicci C, Fleming L, Krol R, Kharitonov SA, Wilson NM, et al. Measurement of bronchial and alveolar nitric oxide production in nor-

mal children and children with asthma. Am J Respir Crit Care Med. 2006 Aug 1;174(3):260-7.

24. Cardinale F, de Benedictis FM, Muggeo V, Giordano P, Loffredo MS, Iacoviello G, et al. Exhaled nitric oxide, total serum IgE and allergic sensitization in childhood asthma and allergic rhinitis. Pediatr Allergy Immunol. 2005 May;16(3):236-42.

25. Franklin PJ, Turner SW, Le Souef PN, Stick SM. Exhaled nitric oxide and asthma: complex interactions between atopy, airway responsiveness, and symptoms in a community population of children. Thorax. 2003 Dec;58(12): 1048-52.

26. Jouaville LF, Annesi-Maesano I, Nguyen LT, Bocage AS, Bedu M, Caillaud D. Interrelationships among asthma, atopy, rhinitis and exhaled nitric oxide in a population-based sample of children. Clin Exp Allergy. 2003 Nov; 33(11):1506-11.

27. Leung TF, Wong GW, Ko FW, Lam CW, Fok TF. Clinical and atopic parameters and airway inflammatory markers in childhood asthma: a factor analysis. Thorax. 2005 Oct;60(10): 822-6.

28. Steerenberg PA, Janssen NA, de Meer G, Fischer PH, Nierkens S, van Loveren H, et al. Relationship between exhaled NO, respiratory symptoms, lung function, bronchial hyperresponsiveness, and blood eosinophilia in school children. Thorax. 2003 Mar; 58(3):242-5.

29. Wells K, Vaughan J, Pajewski TN, Hom S, Ngamtrakulpanit L, Smith A, et al. Exhaled breath condensate pH assays are not influenced by oral ammonia. Thorax. 2005 Jan;60(1):27-31.

30. Silvestri M, Sabatini F, Spallarossa D, Fregonese L, Battistini E, Biraghi MG, et al. Exhaled nitric oxide levels in non-allergic and allergic mono- or polysensitised children with asthma. Thorax. 2001 Nov;56(11):857-62.

31. Frank TL, Adisesh A, Pickering AC, Morrison JF, Wright T, Francis H, et al. Relationship between exhaled nitric oxide and childhood asthma. Am J Respir Crit Care Med. 1998 Oct;158(4):1032-6.

32. Barreto M, Villa MP, Olita C, Martella S, Ciabattoni G, Montuschi P. 8-Isoprostane in exhaled breath condensate and exercise-induced bronchoconstriction in asthmatic children and adolescents. Chest. 2009 Jan;135(1):66-73.

33. de Blic J, Tillie-Leblond I, Emond S, Mahut B, Dang Duy TL, Scheinmann P. High-resolution computed tomography scan and airway remodeling in children with severe asthma. J Allergy Clin Immunol. 2005 Oct;116(4):750-4.

34. Beck-Ripp J, Griese M, Arenz S, Koring C, Pasqualoni B, Bufler P. Changes of exhaled nitric oxide during steroid treatment of childhood asthma. Eur Respir J. 2002 Jun;19(6): 1015-9.

35. Bodini A, Peroni D, Vicentini L, Loiacono A, Baraldi E, Ghiro L, et al. Exhaled breath condensate eicosanoids and sputum eosinophils in asthmatic children: a pilot study. Pediatr Allergy Immunol. 2004 Feb;15(1): 26-31.

36. Jatakanon A, Kharitonov S, Lim S, Barnes PJ. Effect of differing doses of inhaled budesonide on markers of airway inflammation in patients with mild

asthma. Thorax. 1999 Feb;54(2):108-14.

37. Bisgaard H, Loland L, Oj JA. NO in exhaled air of asthmatic children is reduced by the leukotriene receptor antagonist montelukast. Am J Respir Crit Care Med. 1999 Oct;160(4): 1227-31.

38. Sorkness CA, Lemanske RF, Jr., Mauger DT, Boehmer SJ, Chinchilli VM, Martinez FD, et al. Long-term comparison of 3 controller regimens for mild-moderate persistent childhood asthma: the Pediatric Asthma Controller Trial. J Allergy Clin Immunol. 2007 Jan;119(1):64-72.

39. Straub DA, Minocchieri S, Moeller A, Hamacher J, Wildhaber JH. The effect of montelukast on exhaled nitric oxide and lung function in asthmatic children 2 to 5 years old. Chest. 2005 Feb;127(2):509-14.

40. Sandrini A, Ferreira IM, Gutierrez C, Jardim JR, Zamel N, Chapman KR. Effect of montelukast on exhaled nitric oxide and nonvolatile markers of inflammation in mild asthma. Chest. 2003 Oct;124(4):1334-40.

41. Straub DA, Moeller A, Minocchieri S, Hamacher J, Sennhauser FH, Hall GL, et al. The effect of montelukast on lung function and exhaled nitric oxide in infants with early childhood asthma. Eur Respir J. 2005 Feb;25(2): 289-94.

42. Silkoff PE, Wakita S, Chatkin J, Ansarin K, Gutierrez C, Caramori M, et al. Exhaled nitric oxide after beta2-agonist inhalation and spirometry in asthma. Am J Respir Crit Care Med. 1999 Mar;159(3):940-4.

43. Kissoon N, Duckworth LJ, Blake KV, Murphy SP, Lima JJ. Effect of beta2-agonist treatment and spirometry on exhaled nitric oxide in healthy children and children with asthma. Pediatr Pulmonol. 2002 Sep;34(3):203-8.

44. Terada A, Fujisawa T, Togashi K, Miyazaki T, Katsumata H, Atsuta J, et al. Exhaled nitric oxide decreases during exercise-induced bronchoconstriction in children with asthma. Am J Respir Crit Care Med. 2001 Nov 15;164(10 Pt 1):1879-84.

45. Fuglsang G, Vikre-Jorgensen J, Agertoft L, Pedersen S. Effect of salmeterol treatment on nitric oxide level in exhaled air and dose-response to terbutaline in children with mild asthma. Pediatr Pulmonol. 1998 May; 25(5): 314-21.

46. Yates DH, Kharitonov SA, Barnes PJ. Effect of short- and long-acting inhaled beta2-agonists on exhaled nitric oxide in asthmatic patients. Eur Respir J. 1997 Jul;10(7):1483-8.

47. Overbeek SE, Mulder PG, Baelemans SM, Hoogsteden HC, Prins JB. Formoterol added to low-dose budesonide has no additional antiinflammatory effect in asthmatic patients. Chest. 2005 Sep;128(3):1121-7.

48. del Giudice MM, Brunese FP, Piacentini GL, Pedulla M, Capristo C, Decimo F, et al. Fractional exhaled nitric oxide (FENO), lung function and airway hyperresponsiveness in naive atopic asthmatic children. J Asthma. 2004 Oct;41(7):759-65.

49. Rosias PP, Dompeling E, Dentener MA, Pennings HJ, Hendriks HJ, Van Iersel MP, et al. Childhood asthma: exhaled markers of airway inflammation, asthma control score, and lung function tests. Pediatr Pulmonol. 2004 Aug;38(2):107-14.

50. Pijnenburg MW, Floor SE, Hop WC,

De Jongste JC. Daily ambulatory exhaled nitric oxide measurements in asthma. Pediatr Allergy Immunol. 2006 May;17(3):189-93.

51. Malmberg LP, Pelkonen AS, Haahtela T, Turpeinen M. Exhaled nitric oxide rather than lung function distinguishes preschool children with probable asthma. Thorax. 2003 Jun;58(6): 494-9.

52. Thomas PS, Gibson PG, Wang H, Shah S, Henry RL. The relationship of exhaled nitric oxide to airway inflammation and responsiveness in children. J Asthma. 2005 May;42(4): 291-5.

53. Narang I, Ersu R, Wilson NM, Bush A. Nitric oxide in chronic airway inflammation in children: diagnostic use and pathophysiological significance. Thorax. 2002 Jul;57(7):586-9.

54. Fritsch M, Uxa S, Horak F, Jr., Putschoegl B, Dehlink E, Szepfalusi Z, et al. Exhaled nitric oxide in the management of childhood asthma: a prospective 6-months study. Pediatr Pulmonol. 2006 Sep;41(9):855-62.

55. Pijnenburg MW, Bakker EM, Hop WC, De Jongste JC. Titrating steroids on exhaled nitric oxide in children with asthma: a randomized controlled trial. Am J Respir Crit Care Med. 2005 Oct 1;172(7):831-6.

56. Smith AD, Cowan JO, Brassett KP, Herbison GP, Taylor DR. Use of exhaled nitric oxide measurements to guide treatment in chronic asthma. N Engl J Med. 2005 May 26;352(21): 2163-73.

57. Zacharasiewicz A, Wilson N, Lex C, Erin EM, Li AM, Hansel T, et al. Clinical use of noninvasive measurements of airway inflammation in steroid reduction in children. Am J Respir Crit Care Med. 2005 May 15;171(10): 1077-82.

58. Bush A, Eber E. The value of FeNO measurement in asthma management: the motion for Yes, it's NO--or, the wrong end of the Stick! Paediatr Respir Rev. 2008 Jun;9(2):127-31.

59. Gibson PG, Grootendor DC, Henry RL, Pin I, Rytila PH, Wark P, et al. Sputum induction in children. Eur Respir J Suppl. 2002 Sep;37:44s-6s.

60. Gibson PG, Simpson JL, Hankin R, Powell H, Henry RL. Relationship between induced sputum eosinophils and the clinical pattern of childhood asthma. Thorax. 2003 Feb;58(2):116-21.

61. Gogate S, Katial R. Pediatric biomarkers in asthma: exhaled nitric oxide, sputum eosinophils and leukotriene E4. Curr Opin Allergy Clin Immunol. 2008 Apr;8(2):154-7.

62. Holz O, Kips J, Magnussen H. Update on sputum methodology. Eur Respir J. 2000 Aug;16(2):355-9.

63. Jones PD, Hankin R, Simpson J, Gibson PG, Henry RL. The tolerability, safety, and success of sputum induction and combined hypertonic saline challenge in children. Am J Respir Crit Care Med. 2001 Oct 1;164(7):1146-9.

64. Pizzichini E, Pizzichini MM, Leigh R, Djukanovic R, Sterk PJ. Safety of sputum induction. Eur Respir J Suppl. 2002 Sep;37:9s-18s.

65. Cai Y, Carty K, Henry RL, Gibson PG. Persistence of sputum eosinophilia in children with controlled asthma when compared with healthy children. Eur Respir J. 1998 Apr;11(4):848-53.

66. Piacentini GL, Vicentini L, Mazzi P, Chilosi M, Martinati L, Boner AL. Mite-antigen avoidance can reduce bron-

chial epithelial shedding in allergic asthmatic children. Clin Exp Allergy. 1998 May;28(5):561-7.

67. Pin I, Radford S, Kolendowicz R, Jennings B, Denburg JA, Hargreave FE, et al. Airway inflammation in symptomatic and asymptomatic children with methacholine hyperresponsiveness. Eur Respir J. 1993 Oct;6(9): 1249-56.

68. Norzila MZ, Fakes K, Henry RL, Simpson J, Gibson PG. Interleukin-8 secretion and neutrophil recruitment accompanies induced sputum eosinophil activation in children with acute asthma. Am J Respir Crit Care Med. 2000 Mar;161(3 Pt 1):769-74.

69. Oh JW, Lee HB, Kim CR, Yum MK, Koh YJ, Moon SJ, et al. Analysis of induced sputum to examine the effects of inhaled corticosteroid on airway inflammation in children with asthma. Ann Allergy Asthma Immunol. 1999 May;82(5):491-6.

70. Sorva R, Metso T, Turpeinen M, Juntunen-Backman K, Bjorksten F, Haahtela T. Eosinophil cationic protein in induced sputum as a marker of inflammation in asthmatic children. Pediatr Allergy Immunol. 1997 Feb;8(1): 45-50.

71. Lex C, Payne DN, Zacharasiewicz A, Li AM, Wilson NM, Hansel TT, et al. Sputum induction in children with difficult asthma: safety, feasibility, and inflammatory cell pattern. Pediatr Pulmonol. 2005 Apr;39(4):318-24.

72. Covar RA, Spahn JD, Martin RJ, Silkoff PE, Sundstrom DA, Murphy J, et al. Safety and application of induced sputum analysis in childhood asthma. J Allergy Clin Immunol. 2004 Sep;114(3):575-82.

73. Haldar P, Pavord ID. Noneosinophilic asthma: a distinct clinical and pathologic phenotype. J Allergy Clin Immunol. 2007 May;119(5):1043-52; quiz 53-4.

74. Thomou C, Paraskakis E, Neofytou E, Kalmanti M, Siafakas NM, Tzortzaki EG. Acquired somatic mutations in the microsatellite DNA, in children with bronchial asthma. Pediatr Pulmonol. 2009 Oct;44(10):1017-24.

75. Gibson PG, Wark PA, Simpson JL, Meldrum C, Meldrum S, Saltos N, et al. Induced sputum IL-8 gene expression, neutrophil influx and MMP-9 in allergic bronchopulmonary aspergillosis. Eur Respir J. 2003 Apr;21(4): 582-8.

76. Baraldi E, Ghiro L, Piovan V, Carraro S, Zacchello F, Zanconato S. Safety and success of exhaled breath condensate collection in asthma. Arch Dis Child. 2003 Apr;88(4):358-60.

77. Baraldi E, Carraro S, Alinovi R, Pesci A, Ghiro L, Bodini A, et al. Cysteinyl leukotrienes and 8-isoprostane in exhaled breath condensate of children with asthma exacerbations. Thorax. 2003 Jun;58(6):505-9.

78. Chladkova J, Krcmova I, Chladek J, Cap P, Micuda S, Hanzalkova Y. Validation of nitrite and nitrate measurements in exhaled breath condensate. Respiration. 2006;73(2):173-9.

79. Hitka P, Cerny M, Vizek M, Wilhelm J, Zoban P. Assessment of exhaled gases in ventilated preterm infants. Physiol Res. 2004;53(5):561-4.

80. Moeller A, Franklin P, Hall GL, Horak F, Jr., Wildhaber JH, Stick SM. Measuring exhaled breath condensates in infants. Pediatr Pulmonol. 2006 Feb;41(2):184-7.

81. Griese M, Noss J, von Bredow C. Protein pattern of exhaled breath condensate and saliva. Proteomics. 2002 Jun;2(6):690-6.

82. Baraldi E, Ghiro L, Piovan V, Carraro S, Ciabattoni G, Barnes PJ, et al. Increased exhaled 8-isoprostane in childhood asthma. Chest. 2003 Jul;124(1):25-31.

83. Zanconato S, Carraro S, Corradi M, Alinovi R, Pasquale MF, Piacentini G, et al. Leukotrienes and 8-isoprostane in exhaled breath condensate of children with stable and unstable asthma. J Allergy Clin Immunol. 2004 Feb;113(2):257-63.

84. Montuschi P, Mondino C, Koch P, Barnes PJ, Ciabattoni G. Effects of a leukotriene receptor antagonist on exhaled leukotriene E4 and prostanoids in children with asthma. J Allergy Clin Immunol. 2006 Aug;118(2):347-53.

85. Shahid SK, Kharitonov SA, Wilson NM, Bush A, Barnes PJ. Exhaled 8-isoprostane in childhood asthma. Respir Res. 2005;6:79.

86. Montuschi P, Nightingale JA, Kharitonov SA, Barnes PJ. Ozone-induced increase in exhaled 8-isoprostane in healthy subjects is resistant to inhaled budesonide. Free Radic Biol Med. 2002 Nov 15;33(10):1403-8.

87. Montuschi P, Corradi M, Ciabattoni G, Nightingale J, Kharitonov SA, Barnes PJ. Increased 8-isoprostane, a marker of oxidative stress, in exhaled condensate of asthma patients. Am J Respir Crit Care Med. 1999 Jul;160(1):216-20.

88. Montuschi P, Ragazzoni E, Valente S, Corbo G, Mondino C, Ciappi G, et al. Validation of 8-isoprostane and prostaglandin E(2) measurements in exhaled breath condensate. Inflamm Res. 2003 Dec;52(12):502-7.

89. Csoma Z, Huszar E, Vizi E, Vass G, Szabo Z, Herjavecz I, et al. Adenosine level in exhaled breath increases during exercise-induced bronchoconstriction. Eur Respir J. 2005 May;25(5): 873-8.

90. Montuschi P, Barnes PJ. Exhaled leukotrienes and prostaglandins in asthma. J Allergy Clin Immunol. 2002 Apr;109(4):615-20.

91. Shibata A, Katsunuma T, Tomikawa M, Tan A, Yuki K, Akashi K, et al. Increased leukotriene E4 in the exhaled breath condensate of children with mild asthma. Chest. 2006 Dec; 130(6):1718-22.

92. Cap P, Chladek J, Pehal F, Maly M, Petru V, Barnes PJ, et al. Gas chromatography/mass spectrometry analysis of exhaled leukotrienes in asthmatic patients. Thorax. 2004 Jun;59(6):465-70.

93. Cap P, Pehal F, Chladek J, Maly M. Analysis of exhaled leukotrienes in nonasthmatic adult patients with seasonal allergic rhinitis. Allergy. 2005 Feb;60(2):171-6.

94. Paredi P, Kharitonov SA, Barnes PJ. Elevation of exhaled ethane concentration in asthma. Am J Respir Crit Care Med. 2000 Oct;162(4Pt 1): 1450-4.

95. Goen T, Muller-Lux A, Dewes P, Musiol A, Kraus T. Sensitive and accurate analyses of free 3-nitrotyrosine in exhaled breath condensate by LC-MS/MS. J Chromatogr B Analyt Technol Biomed Life Sci. 2005 Nov 5;826(1-2):261-6.

96. Mondino C, Ciabattoni G, Koch P, Pistelli R, Trove A, Barnes PJ, et al. Effects of inhaled corticosteroids on exhaled leukotrienes and prostanoids in asthmatic children. J Allergy Clin Immunol. 2004 Oct;114(4):761-7.

97. Lex C, Zacharasiewicz A, Payne DN, Wilson NM, Nicholson AG, Kharitonov SA, et al. Exhaled breath condensate cysteinyl leukotrienes and airway remodeling in childhood asthma: a pilot study. Respir Res. 2006;7:63.

98. Carraro S, Corradi M, Zanconato S, Alinovi R, Pasquale MF, Zacchello F, et al. Exhaled breath condensate cysteinyl leukotrienes are increased in children with exercise-induced bronchoconstriction. J Allergy Clin Immunol. 2005 Apr;115(4):764-70.

99. Biernacki WA, Kharitonov SA, Biernacka HM, Barnes PJ. Effect of montelukast on exhaled leukotrienes and quality of life in asthmatic patients. Chest. 2005 Oct;128(4): 1958-63.

100. Failla M, Biondi G, Provvidenza Pistorio M, Gili E, Mastruzzo C, Vancheri C, et al. Intranasal steroid reduces exhaled bronchial cysteinyl leukotrienes in allergic patients. Clin Exp Allergy. 2006 Mar;36(3):325-30.

101. Csoma Z, Kharitonov SA, Balint B, Bush A, Wilson NM, Barnes PJ. Increased leukotrienes in exhaled breath condensate in childhood asthma. Am J Respir Crit Care Med. 2002 Nov 15;166(10):1345-9.

102. Kostikas K, Gaga M, Papatheodorou G, Karamanis T, Orphanidou D, Loukides S. Leukotriene B4 in exhaled breath condensate and sputum supernatant in patients with COPD and asthma. Chest. 2005 May;127 (5):1553-9.

103. Carpagnano GE, Barnes PJ, Francis J, Wilson N, Bush A, Kharitonov SA. Breath condensate pH in children with cystic fibrosis and asthma: a new noninvasive marker of airway inflammation? Chest. 2004 Jun; 125(6): 2005-10.

104. Nayeri F, Millinger E, Nilsson I, Zetterstrom, Brudin L, Forsberg P. Exhaled breath condensate and serum levels of hepatocyte growth factor in pneumonia. Respir Med. 2002 Feb;96(2):115-9.

105. Montuschi P, Martello S, Felli M, Mondino C, Barnes PJ, Chiarotti M. Liquid chromatography/mass spectrometry analysis of exhaled leukotriene B4 in asthmatic children. Respir Res. 2005;6:119.

106. Montuschi P, Martello S, Felli M, Mondino C, Chiarotti M. Ion trap liquid chromatography/tandem mass spectrometry analysis of leukotriene B4 in exhaled breath condensate. Rapid Commun Mass Spectrom. 2004;18(22):2723-9.

107. Montuschi P, Ragazzoni E, Valente S, Corbo G, Mondino C, Ciappi G, et al. Validation of leukotriene B4 measurements in exhaled breath condensate. Inflamm Res. 2003 Feb;52(2):69-73.

108. Celio S, Troxler H, Durka SS, Chladek J, Wildhaber JH, Sennhauser FH, et al. Free 3-nitrotyrosine in exhaled breath condensates of children fails as a marker for oxidative stress in stable cystic fibrosis and asthma. Nitric Oxide. 2006 Nov; 15(3):226-32.

109. Baraldi E, Giordano G, Pasquale MF, Carraro S, Mardegan A, Bonetto G, et al. 3-Nitrotyrosine, a marker of nitrosative stress, is increased in breath condensate of allergic asthmatic children. Allergy. 2006 Jan;61(1):90-6.

110. Bodini A, Peroni DG, Zardini F, Corradi M, Alinovi R, Boner AL, et al. Flunisolide decreases exhaled nitric oxide and nitrotyrosine levels in asthmatic children. Mediators Inflamm. 2006;2006(4):31919.

111. Corradi M, Pesci A, Casana R, Alinovi R, Goldoni M, Vettori MV, et al. Nitrate in exhaled breath condensate of patients with different airway diseases. Nitric Oxide. 2003 Feb;8(1): 26-30.

112. Franklin P, Moeller A, Hall GL, Horak F, Jr., Patterson H, Stick SM. Variability of nitric oxide metabolites in exhaled breath condensate. Respir Med. 2006 Jan;100(1):123-9.

113. Ganas K, Loukides S, Papatheodorou G, Panagou P, Kalogeropoulos N. Total nitrite/nitrate in expired breath condensate of patients with asthma. Respir Med. 2001 Aug;95(8): 649-54.

114. Gaston B, Drazen JM, Loscalzo J, Stamler JS. The biology of nitrogen oxides in the airways. Am J Respir Crit Care Med. 1994 Feb;149(2 Pt 1): 538-51.

115. Larstad M, Soderling AS, Caidahl K, Olin AC. Selective quantification of free 3-nitrotyrosine in exhaled breath condensate in asthma using gas chromatography/tandem mass spectrometry. Nitric Oxide. 2005 Sep;13(2):134-44.

116. Ratnawati, Morton J, Henry RL, Thomas PS. Exhaled breath condensate nitrite/nitrate and pH in relation to pediatric asthma control and exhaled nitric oxide. Pediatr Pulmonol. 2006 Oct;41(10):929-36.

117. Formanek W, Inci D, Lauener RP, Wildhaber JH, Frey U, Hall GL. Elevated nitrite in breath condensates of children with respiratory disease. Eur Respir J. 2002 Mar;19(3):487-91.

118. Marteus H, Tornberg DC, Weitzberg E, Schedin U, Alving K. Origin of nitrite and nitrate in nasal and exhaled breath condensate and relation to nitric oxide formation. Thorax. 2005 Mar;60(3):219-25.

119. Corradi M, Montuschi P, Donnelly LE, Pesci A, Kharitonov SA, Barnes PJ. Increased nitrosothiols in exhaled breath condensate in inflammatory airway diseases. Am J Respir Crit Care Med. 2001 Mar;163(4):854-8.

120. Andreoli R, Manini P, Corradi M, Mutti A, Niessen WM. Determination of patterns of biologically relevant aldehydes in exhaled breath condensate of healthy subjects by liquid chromatography/atmospheric chemical ionization tandem mass spectrometry. Rapid Commun Mass Spectrom. 2003;17(7):637-45.

121. Corradi M, Folesani G, Andreoli R, Manini P, Bodini A, Piacentini G, et al. Aldehydes and glutathione in exhaled breath condensate of children with asthma exacerbation. Am J Respir Crit Care Med. 2003 Feb 1;167(3):395-9.

122. Corradi M, Pignatti P, Manini P, Andreoli R, Goldoni M, Poppa M, et al. Comparison between exhaled and sputum oxidative stress biomarkers in chronic airway inflammation. Eur Respir J. 2004 Dec;24(6):1011-7.

123. Carraro S, Rezzi S, Reniero F, Heberger K, Giordano G, Zanconato S, et al. Metabolomics applied to exhaled breath condensate in childhood asthma. Am J Respir Crit Care Med. 2007 May 15;175(10):986-90.

124. MacGregor G, Ellis S, Andrews J, Imrie M, Innes A, Greening AP, et al. Breath condensate ammonium is lower in children with chronic asthma. Eur Respir J. 2005 Aug;26(2):271-6.

125. Brooks SM, Haight RR, Gordon RL. Age does not affect airway pH and ammonia as determined by exhaled breath measurements. Lung. 2006 Jul-Aug;184(4):195-200.

126. Effros RM, Hoagland KW, Bosbous M, Castillo D, Foss B, Dunning M, et al. Dilution of respiratory solutes in exhaled condensates. Am J Respir Crit Care Med. 2002 Mar 1;165(5):663-9.

127. Puckett JL, George SC. Partitioned exhaled nitric oxide to non-invasively assess asthma. Respir Physiol Neurobiol. 2008 Nov 30;163(1-3):166-77.

128. Leung TF, Li CY, Yung E, Liu EK, Lam CW, Wong GW. Clinical and technical factors affecting pH and other biomarkers in exhaled breath condensate. Pediatr Pulmonol. 2006 Jan;41(1):87-94.

129. Paget-Brown AO, Ngamtrakulpanit L, Smith A, Bunyan D, Hom S, Nguyen A, et al. Normative data for pH of exhaled breath condensate. Chest. 2006 Feb;129(2):426-30.

130. Vaughan J, Ngamtrakulpanit L, Pajewski TN, Turner R, Nguyen TA, Smith A, et al. Exhaled breath condensate pH is a robust and reproducible assay of airway acidity. Eur Respir J. 2003 Dec;22(6):889-94.

131. Niimi A, Nguyen LT, Usmani O, Mann B, Chung KF. Reduced pH and chloride levels in exhaled breath condensate of patients with chronic cough. Thorax. 2004 Jul;59(7):608-12.

132. Emelyanov A, Fedoseev G, Abulimity A, Rudinski K, Fedoulov A, Karabanov A, et al. Elevated concentrations of exhaled hydrogen peroxide in asthmatic patients. Chest. 2001 Oct;120(4):1136-9.

133. Brunetti L, Francavilla R, Tesse R, Fiermonte P, Fiore FP, Lore M, et al. Exhaled breath condensate cytokines and pH in pediatric asthma and atopic dermatitis. Allergy Asthma Proc. 2008 Sep-Oct;29(5):461-7.

134. Hunt J, Yu Y, Burns J, Gaston B, Ngamtrakulpanit L, Bunyan D, et al. Identification of acid reflux cough using serial assays of exhaled breath condensate pH. Cough. 2006;2:3.

135. Nicolaou NC, Lowe LA, Murray CS, Woodcock A, Simpson A, Custovic A. Exhaled breath condensate pH and childhood asthma: unselected birth cohort study. Am J Respir Crit Care Med. 2006 Aug 1;174(3):254-9.

136. Effros RM, Casaburi R, Su J, Dunning M, Torday J, Biller J, et al. The effects of volatile salivary acids and bases on exhaled breath condensate pH. Am J Respir Crit Care Med. 2006 Feb 15;173(4):386-92.

137. Jobsis Q, Raatgeep HC, Hermans PW, de Jongste JC. Hydrogen peroxide in exhaled air is increased in stable asthmatic children. Eur Respir J. 1997 Mar;10(3):519-21.

138. Jobsis Q, Raatgeep HC, Schellekens

SL, Hop WC, Hermans PW, de Jongste JC. Hydrogen peroxide in exhaled air of healthy children: reference values. Eur Respir J. 1998 Aug;12 (2):483-5.

139. Jobsis RQ, Schellekens SL, Fakkel-Kroesbergen A, Raatgeep RH, de Jongste JC. Hydrogen peroxide in breath condensate during a common cold. Mediators Inflamm. 2001 Dec; 10(6):351-4.

140. Doniec Z, Nowak D, Tomalak W, Pisiewicz K, Kurzawa R. Passive smoking does not increase hydrogen peroxide (H2O2) levels in exhaled breath condensate in 9-year-old healthy children. Pediatr Pulmonol. 2005 Jan;39(1):41-5.

141. Schleiss MB, Holz O, Behnke M, Richter K, Magnussen H, Jorres RA. The concentration of hydrogen peroxide in exhaled air depends on expiratory flow rate. Eur Respir J. 2000 Dec;16(6):1115-8.

142. Shahid SK, Kharitonov SA, Wilson NM, Bush A, Barnes PJ. Increased interleukin-4 and decreased interferon-gamma in exhaled breath condensate of children with asthma. Am J Respir Crit Care Med. 2002 May 1;165(9):1290-3.

143. Tang ML, Coleman J, Kemp AS. Interleukin-4 and interferon-gamma production in atopic and non-atopic children with asthma. Clin Exp Allergy. 1995 Jun;25(6):515-21.

144. Leung TF, Wong GW, Ko FW, Li CY, Yung E, Lam CW, et al. Analysis of growth factors and inflammatory cytokines in exhaled breath condensate from asthmatic children. Int Arch Allergy Immunol. 2005 May; 137(1):66-72.

145. Carpagnano GE, Foschino Barbaro MP, Resta O, Gramiccioni E, Valerio NV, Bracciale P, et al. Exhaled markers in the monitoring of airways inflammation and its response to steroid's treatment in mild persistent asthma. Eur J Pharmacol. 2005 Sep 5;519(1-2):175-81.

146. Matsunaga K, Yanagisawa S, Ichikawa T, Ueshima K, Akamatsu K, Hirano T, et al. Airway cytokine expression measured by means of protein array in exhaled breath condensate: correlation with physiologic properties in asthmatic patients. J Allergy Clin Immunol. 2006 Jul;118(1): 84-90.

147. Robroeks CM, Jobsis Q, Damoiseaux JG, Heijmans PH, Rosias PP, Hendriks HJ, et al. Cytokines in exhaled breath condensate of children with asthma and cystic fibrosis. Ann Allergy Asthma Immunol. 2006 Feb;96(2):349-55.

148. Ko FW, Lau CY, Leung TF, Wong GW, Lam CW, Lai CK, et al. Exhaled breath condensate levels of eotaxin and macrophage-derived chemokine in stable adult asthma patients. Clin Exp Allergy. 2006 Jan;36(1):44-51.

149. Leung TF, Wong GW, Ko FW, Lam CW, Fok TF. Increased macrophage-derived chemokine in exhaled breath condensate and plasma from children with asthma. Clin Exp Allergy. 2004 May;34(5):786-91.

150. Carpagnano GE, Kharitonov SA, Wells AU, Pantelidis P, Du Bois RM, Barnes PJ. Increased vitronectin and endothelin-1 in the breath condensate of patients with fibrosing lung disease. Respiration. 2003 Mar-Apr;70(2):154-60.

151. Gonzalez-Reche LM, Kucharczyk A, Musiol AK, Kraus T. Determination of N epsilon-(carboxymethyl)lysine in exhaled breath condensate using isotope dilution liquid chromatography/electrospray ionization tandem mass spectrometry. Rapid Commun Mass Spectrom. 2006;20(18):2747-52.

152. Huszar E, Vass G, Vizi E, Csoma Z, Barat E, Molnar Vilagos G, et al. Adenosine in exhaled breath condensate in healthy volunteers and in patients with asthma. Eur Respir J. 2002 Dec;20(6):1393-8.

153. Zacharasiewicz A, Wilson N, Lex C, Li A, Kemp M, Donovan J, et al. Repeatability of sodium and chloride in exhaled breath condensates. Pediatr Pulmonol. 2004 Mar;37(3):273-5.

154. Noble DD, McCafferty JB, Greening AP, Innes JA. Respiratory heat and moisture loss is associated with eosinophilic inflammation in asthma. Eur Respir J. 2007 Apr;29(4):676-81.

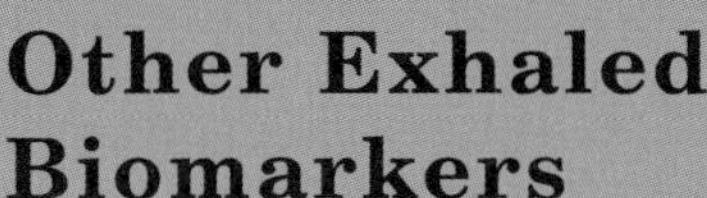

Other Exhaled Biomarkers

Paolo Paredi • Koralia Paschalaki

The Role of New Markers of Airway Inflammation

The non-invasive monitoring of airway inflammation and oxidative stress has received a lot of interest because it may provide researchers and clinicians with an objective assessment of lung disease and its underlying mechanisms.

So far, the measurement of exhaled nitric oxide (NO) and the analysis of induced sputum have offered some insight into the mechanisms of airway inflammation. However, these measurements have some limitations. For instance NO reflects the activity of the inducible NO synthase and therefore does not provide information about the other pathways of inflammation, on the other hand induced sputum provides information about the number of cells and the level of inflammatory compounds in the supernatant, however the technique is not entirely non-invasive and can induce inflam-

Correspondence

Dr. Paolo Paredi

Airway Disease Section, National Heart and Lung Institute, Imperial College School of Science, Technology and Medicine, Dovehouse Street, London SW3 6LY, UK
e-mail: p.paredi@imperial.ac.uk

mation by itself (1) and not all patients, particularly children, can provide a sample. The method for the collection of exhaled breath condensate is not standardised and the concentrations of the markers measured are close to the detection limit of the method used.

In view of these limitations, a number of additional new methods which may be complementary to the above mentioned techniques have been developed. Exhaled breath temperature and bronchial blood flow may provide information on airway inflammation and re-modelling, whereas the levels of exhaled ethane and carbon monoxide may reflect oxidative stress and lipid peroxidation. We will briefly review the methods and the results of some clinical studies investigating these new techniques.

Exhaled Breath Temperature

The histological examination of the airway wall has revealed increased vascularity and vascular engorgement in asthma (2, 3) and a reduced number of blood vessels in COPD (4). These changes contribute to airway remodelling and may play a pathogenetic role.

The bronchial circulation arises from the aorta and forms a dense peribronchial plexus of interconnecting vessels. Branches then penetrate the muscular layer to form a second complex in the submucosa. Capillary engorgement and/or leakage in this circulatory bed could directly alter airway wall thickness. Inflammatory mediators known to be released in asthma may contribute to bronchial vascular dilation. Potential candidates include histamine (5), bradykinin (5) leukotriens (6) and mediators released by autonomic sensory nerves (7). Platelet activating factor (PAF) may also increase bronchial vascular blood flow (8). There are, hence, several inflammatory mediators, each having known agonists, capable of causing bronchial vascular dilation.

A model of airway-wall thickening (9) suggests that a small increase in thickness, such as that caused by edema or vascular engorgement, may account for the increased airway resistance seen with bronchial provocation (10). In humans, it has also been hypothesised that the vascular engorgement of these vessels, and consequent thickening of the airway mucosa, leads to narrowing of the lumen of the bronchi, an increase in airway resistance, and a decrease in forced expiratory rates (11). Supporting this notion is the observation that patients with impaired left ventricular function have heightened sensitivity to methacholine (12) and that normal subjects develop similar changes in airway responsiveness upon rapid infusion of intravenous fluids (13). These studies suggest that that bronchial circulation may play a role in the pathophysiology of lung disease.

Crucially, bronchial blood flow is the main determinant of airway temperature, therefore, the measurement of the temperature of exhaled breath may be an estimate of bronchial blood flow. Because NO has vasodilating properties and plays a major role in the modulation of the pulmonary vasomotor tone (14) patients with inflammatory lung disease resulting in high levels of NO have increased airway temperature.

Method for exhaled breath temperature measurement

Exhaled breath temperature has been measured in a number of studies, some authors have investigated the rate of temperature increase (Δe^oT) during exhalation (15-17) while others have studied the mean temperature plateau value (18-20).

Exhaled breath temperature gradients (Δe^oT)

In this method Δe^oT is measured during a flow- and pressure-controlled exhalation (exhalation flow rate 5 to 6 L/min, mouth pressure 10 cm H_2O) from total lung capacity through a 2.77-mm mouthpiece (21). The temperature is measured by a fast-response (1ms) high-accuracy (0.015 ± 0.027^oC) thermometer (Picotech Ltd, Cambridge, UK) interfaced with a computer by a single-channel Picotech oscilloscope (model ADC 42, resolution 12 bits) allowing online recording of exhaled breath temperature (Figure 1).

Exhaled breath temperature tracings are analysed mathematically. The tracings have an exponential rise and the point at 63% of the total temperature increase is chosen to study the slope of the curves because it represents two time constants of the maximal ^oT change and therefore allows a better mathematical characterization of the tracings before plateau.

Δe^oT calculated between the beginning of exhalation and 63 % of the total temperature increase (a/b, where "a" is 63% of Δ^oT and "b" the time to reach "a", Figure 2) is the more reproducible parameter to characterize the curves.

Δe^oT is exhalation flow dependent. Therefore, the exhalation

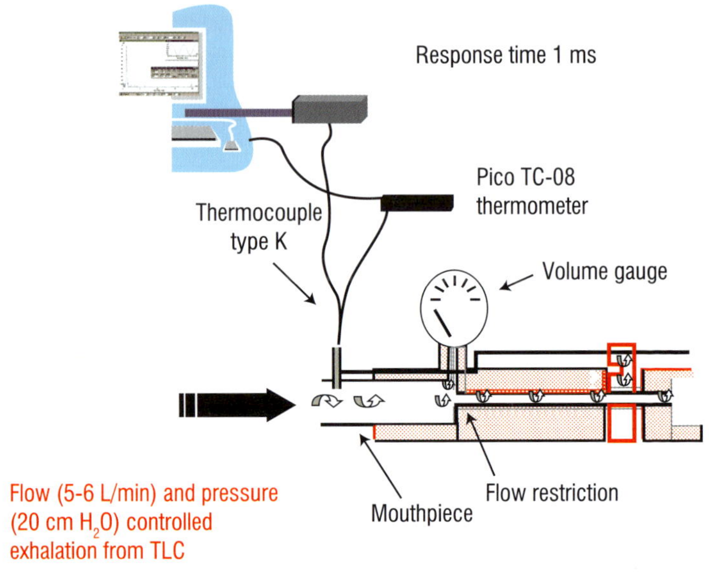

FIGURE 1

Method for the measurement of rate of temperature increase ($\Delta e^o T$).

flow rate should be standardised for example at 5-6 L/min which, in our experience, allows the measurement of exhaled air temperature even in patients with severe lung disease. The distance of the thermocouple from the edge of the mouthpiece significantly affects $\Delta e^o T$, this should also be standardised. There is a tendency for faster $\Delta e^o T$ when subjects exhale from higher baseline ambient temperatures but this is not significant for temperature changes within $\pm 3^o C$ (5.05 $\pm 0.8^o C/s$ at $28^o C$ and 4.45 $\pm 0.8^o C/s$ at $22^o C$ $p > 0.05$). The volume ventilation does not influence the $\Delta e^o T$ value.

Clinical studies

Surprisingly, contrary to asthmatic subject, patients with COPD have a lower rise of breath temperature compared to normal subjects (16). This may be due to the decreased vascularity of the bronchial vessels (22) and reduced blood supply caused by intimal proliferation and hyperplasia (23). Cudkiwicz and Armstrong performed postmortem bronchial arteriograms in 18 cases of em-

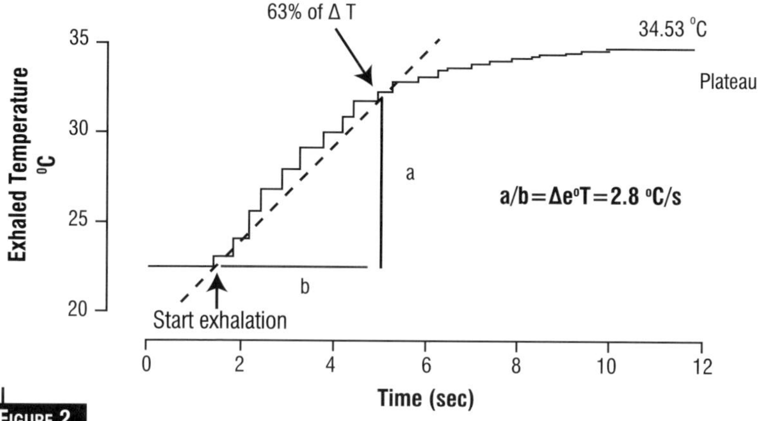

FIGURE 2

Exhaled breath temperature tracing. The a/b ratio represents the rate of temperature increase between the beginning of exhalation and 63 % (one time constant) of the maximal temperature increase.

physema and observed narrowing or obliteration of the intrapulmonary bronchial arteries with diminished branches of the pleural branches. In chronic bronchitis microscopic examination revealed medial hyperplasia and intimal proliferation of varying severity. It was also established that the reduction of blood supply to the lung is the result and not the cause of emphysema (24). When the emphysematous component is less relevant compared to the inflammatory bronchitic component the airway mucosa may show an enlarged vascular bed (25). The blood flow is inversely proportional to the radius of the vessel (law of Bernulli) therefore when the vessels are enlarged they become engorged with blood and the blood flow is reduced when there isn't a proportional increase in the driving pressure along the vessels. Therefore in COPD the bronchial blood flow may be reduced both because of reduced calibre of the bronchial arteries or because of engorgement of the vessels with blood. In both cases the heat transfer across the airway wall may be reduced as reflected in the reduced exhaled breath temperature in these patients.

These findings are in contrast to those seen in patients with asthma who have faster increases of exhaled breath temperature compared to normal subjects. In asthmatic patients, elevated Δe^oT

may be due to the increased vascularity of the bronchial vessels (3) resulting in higher blood supply (26) and therefore heat transfer across the bronchial wall.

Exhaled breath temperature, plateau method

This method requires a slow exhalation from total lung capacity to residual volume while the exhalation flow rate is controlled by diverting the exhaled breath through a fixed resistor. This is in contrast with the $\Delta e^o T$ method where the exhalation flow rate is standardised by visual feedback. The advantage of the latter is an improved control on the effort to exhale and the resulting airway pressure. More specifically, the use of a resistor allows achieving the same exhalation flow rates with efforts of different intensity, this, in turn, may generate different airway pressures. These may not only affect NO production (27) and vasodilatation altering heat exchange, but may also affect the area of respiratory tract to which the exhaled air is exposed to affecting the temperature gradients and $\Delta e^o T$.

The plateau temperature is defined as a period of at least 2 s in the last 20% of the exhalation curve, at least 6 s after the beginning of the expiratory manoeuvre, during which the temperature variations are <0.5°C. This definition raises a number of concerns. Firstly, it is difficult to identify the last 20% of the exhalation reproducibly, indeed patients with different lung volumes will reach residual volume at different times and the exhaled air will therefore reflect different parts of the lung. Secondly, the plateau end exhalation temperatures will more likely reflect air coming from the periphery of the lung which are closer to the body core temperature and less affected by the pathological changes in the airways.

Despite these methodological limitations, it was possible to show a correlation of plateau temperatures with exhaled NO and sputum eosinophil count in a population of asthmatic children (18). The same authors also found a correlation of plateau breath temperature with metalloproteinase, a marker of airway remodelling (28).

Both the $\Delta e^o T$ and the plateau method for the measurement of exhaled breath temperature have shown correlations with other markers of inflammation such as exhaled NO. Hyperemia and tissue temperature may be the final common pathways of inflammation, the measurement of these parameters maybe another non-invasive way to assess the level of inflammation in the airways. However, the use of this techniques is limited by its poor reproducibility, and the large overlap of exhaled breath temperatures in COPD patients compared to normal subjects. The use of more sophisticated thermometers with a faster response time, such as infrared temperature readers, is expected to improve the reproducibility and sensitivity of exhaled breath temperature measurement in the future.

Bronchial Blood Flow

A consistent feature of tissue inflammation is hyperemia and hyperperfusion. Several animal models of airway inflammation including allergen challenge have been shown to have an increased blood flow. In inflammatory lung diseases, like asthma and COPD, airway inflammation involves mainly the subepithelial airway tissue where most of the blood perfusion is localised, therefore, the measurement of bronchial blood flow (Q_{aw}) is of particular importance and maybe a marker of inflammation by itself.

Measurement of bronchial blood flow

Several techniques have been developed to measure bronchial blood flow invasively in animals. Even though there are some relevant anatomical differences compared to humans, these techniques have provided useful information in the understanding of the pathophysiology of airway disease. Bronchial blood flow has recently been measured non-invasively in humans and this has received increasing interest in view of its possible use as a marker of airway inflammation in asthma and COPD (17, 29).

Non-invasive measurement of blood flow

Dimethylether method. The rate at which soluble inert gasses are taken up by the lung has long been used to measure non-invasively pulmonary capillary blood flow as an index of cardiac output (30). The same principle was applied, in a pioneering study, to measure the blood flow of an isolated segment of the airways (31) making use of dimethylether, a gas with high affinity with haemoglobin. This method is based on the theory that the uptake of an inert soluble gas in tissue with capillaries and active flow of blood is determined by the volume of the tissue with which the gas equilibrates and by the blood flow through those capillaries (32). The same method was later modified and validated indirectly with microospheres in the sheep (33), however, the method was never validated in humans.

The dimethylether method requires that the subjects use nose clips and inhale through a mouthpiece a gas mixture of 10% dimethylether (DME), 5% helium, and balance oxygen, hold their breath for 5, 10, 15, and 20s in random order and then exhale into the spirometer. During exhalation, the concentrations of DME, nitrogen, and helium are measured at the airway opening with a mass spectrometer along with the expired gas volume. Anatomic dead s-pace (DS) is determined from the expired nitrogen concentration curve as described by Fowler and co-workers (34). The helium-corrected decrease in the DME concentration over time is obtained by least squares fit using the two measurements per gas for each of the four breath-hold times. From the helium-corrected DME slope multiplied by the DS (V_{DME}), the mean DME concentration in the DS ($F\bar{D}\bar{M}\bar{E}$), and the solubility coefficient for DME in blood and tissue ($\propto$), $\dot{Q}_{aw}$ is calculated using the Fick principle ($\dot{Q}_{aw} = V_{DME}/\propto \cdot F\bar{D}\bar{M}\bar{E}$) (35).

This method, despite being described a number of years ago, has never been used in laboratories other than the one where it was first developed. This may be in part due to complexity of the data it produces, eight breath hold manoeuvres for a single measurement. In addition, the high explosive potential of a gas mixture containing both dimethylether and oxygen has no doubt deterred other researchers. Besides the difficulty of the measurements and the potential risks, it is noteworthy that this technique has never been validated in humans.

In order to address these limitations, the same group that developed the method originally has recently simplified the technique (36) by reducing the breath hold times to two, a short breath hold of 5 seconds and a longer one of 15 seconds. With this approach there is no need for helium and oxygen in the gas mixture, the gas signals do not need to be integrated and dimethylether is not dangerously mixed with oxygen. Because this new simplified method is in agreement with the more complicated old technique, the authors hope to see this new approach used by other research groups.

Acetylene method. This method uses acetylene, a gas with high affinity for oxygen but potentially less explosive than dimethylether

(5, 37). The subjects inhale through a mouthpiece (with nose clips on) initially room air and then a gas mixture from a Teflon bag containing 35% O_2, 0,3% acetylene, 5% sulphur hexafluoride (SF_6), CO 3% and a balance of nitrogen (Figure 3).

During exhalation the concentration of acetylene and SF_6 is measured directly online by a mass spectrometer, the exhaled gas volume is also measured. The area under the curve (AUC) is inversely proportional to bronchial blood flow, therefore multiple breath holds are not required. The exhaled breath acetylene concentration is exhalation flow dependent, therefore, the exhalation flow rate is standardised at 5-6 L/min. To avoid errors due to the recirculation of acetylene from previous measurements, the tests are repeated at least 10 minutes apart. The coefficient of variability is 8%.

This method presents some advantages compared to the previously described dimethylether method. Firstly, multiple breath holds are not required and this method is less time consuming. Secondly, the mixture of acetylene and oxygen is not explosive at the concentrations used. Even though this method has not been validated directly, the effect of vasoactive compounds such as the

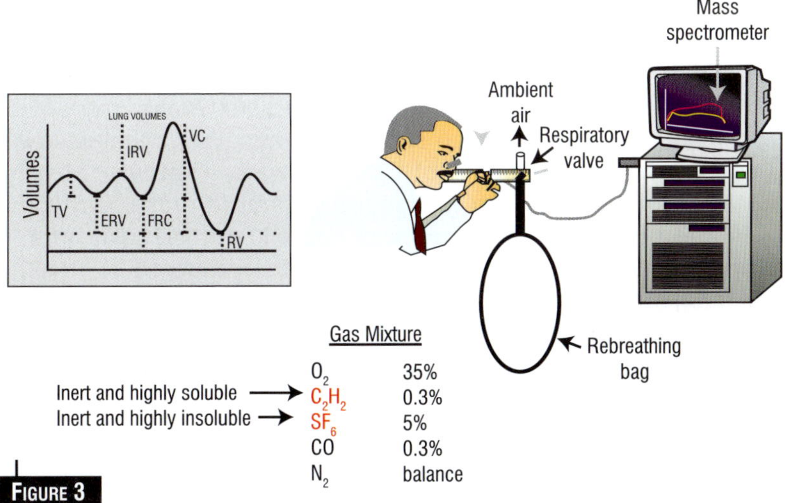

FIGURE 3

Schematic representation of the method for bronchial blood flow measurement, see text for explanation.

vasoconstriction induced by corticosteroids (17), adrenaline (38) and L-NAME (38) and the vasodilatation following the inhalation of β2-agonists (17, 29, 38), and NO (38) support the hypothesis that the method effectively measures bronchial blood flow. It is reassuring that the same method based on the dilution of acetylene has been developed independently by two groups with similar results.

Clinical studies

Contrary to what has been shown in asthma where Q_{AW} is increased (17, 39), patients with COPD have normal bronchial blood flow. This may reflect the normal vascularity of the bronchial vessels (40) and low blood supply caused by intimal proliferation and hyperplasia (23). Initial studies by *Cudkiwicz* et al (23) observed narrowing or obliteration of the intrapulmonary bronchial arteries with diminished pleural branches. In chronic bronchitis microscopic examination revealed medial hyperplasia and intimal proliferation of varying severity. These results are in keeping with our previous investigations showing reduced temperature gradients ($\Delta e^{\circ}T$) of the exhaled breath of COPD patients (16). This may be due to the normal or reduced vascularity of the airways and blunted vascular reactivity (41). More specifically, despite the presence of airway inflammation in COPD patients, the bronchial vessels which are reduced or normal in number, do not respond to the inflammatory vasodilating stimuli, therefore the total bronchial blood flow is unaffected.

A bronchovideoscopic study (42) and the measurement of bronchial blood flow (29) also support the hypothesis that vascular remodelling is not a feature of COPD airways. However, at least two studies have shown increased bronchial vascularity, as measured both as in the number of vessels and vascular area in symptomatic smokers and COPD patients compared to healthy non-smokers (43, 44). This discrepancy has not been explained but it may be due the recruitment of more severe and elderly patients in the last two studies.

Contrary to COPD patients, the bronchial submucosa of asthmatic subjects has a larger number of vessels, occupying a larger percentage of area compared to normal subjects (45, 46). In addition, the vascularity of the airways may be increased not only in the larger, but also the medium and small airways (40) and is also present in patients with mild and moderate disease (3). The use of a high magnification bronchovideoscope allowed the direct visualisation of the of the bronchial wall and quantification of the bronchial vessels (42), confirming the presence of an increased number of vessels in asthmatic subjects as indicated previously by the pathology studies.

The measurement of bronchial blood flow may indirectly reflect airway inflammation and may provide information about angiogenesis. The development of non-invasive methods for the measurement of bronchial blood flow (26) has provided an insight into the pathophysiology of the bronchial circulation.

Volatile Organic Compounds

Ethane and pentane

Oxidative stress is implicated in the pathogenesis and progression of asthma (47, 48) chronic obstructive respiratory disease (COPD) (49) and cystic fibrosis (50). Reactive oxygen species (ROS) are unstable compounds with unpaired electrons, capable of initiating oxidation. Several of the inflammatory cells which participate in the inflammatory response, such as macrophages, neutrophils and eosinophils release increased amounts of ROS (47, 51) exceeding the already reduced tissue antioxidant defences of asthmatic and COPD patients (48).

One mechanism by which oxidants may cause lung injury is through lipid peroxidation. ROS, such as superoxide anion (O_2^-), and hydrogen peroxide (H_2O_2) released by activated immune and inflammatory cells can induce the lipid peroxidation of polyunsaturated membrane fatty acids (52), impair membrane function and inactivate membrane-bound receptors and enzymes, increase tissue permeability (53), and therefore promote airflow limitation.

Volatile hydrocarbons are products of lipid peroxidation and their measurement in the exhaled breath has been proposed as a means to assess lipid peroxidation *in vivo* (52, 54, 55) (Figure 4).

Ethane derived from n-3 polyunsaturated fatty acids (i.e. linolenic acid), and 1-pentane, derived from n-6 fatty acids (i.e. linoleic and arachidonic acids), are non-invasive markers of lipid peroxidation. These alkanes are produced by -scission of the lipoalkoxyl radical to produce the alkyl radical followed by hydrogen abstraction to produce ethane or 1-pentane. Although only a small fraction of the lipid peroxides actually produces ethane or 1-pentane, the production of

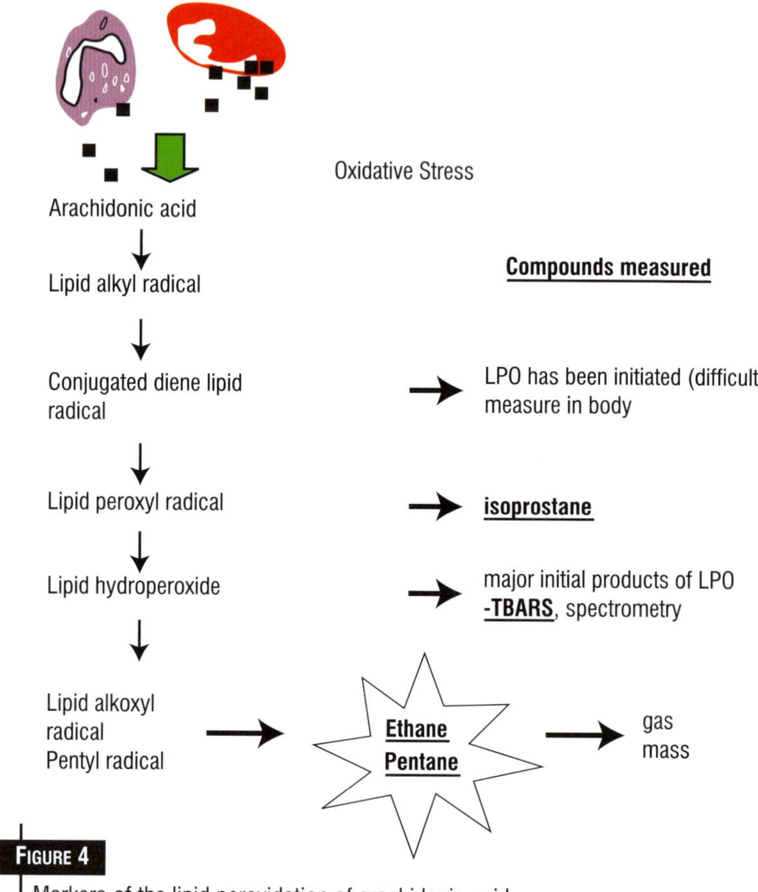

FIGURE 4

Markers of the lipid peroxidation of arachidonic acid.

these alkanes reflects the extent of lipid peroxidation and, thereby, the *in vivo* oxidative stress. In this group of exhaled gases ethane has received more attention because of its easier and faster chromatographic measurement compared to other hydrocarbons (56-58). The exhaled air of human subjects was first analysed for the presence of hydrocarbons in the 1960s (59). Since then, the research in this area has progressed slowly because of technical and practical problems, such as the contamination of ambient hydrocarbons and the need to concentrate exhaled air because of the low concentrations of these volatile compounds.

Two approaches have been used to deal with the problem of ambient air. Some researchers employ washout periods to clear the lungs for four or five minutes (60, 61), alternatively, the problem of ambient contamination is neglected (62) or dealt with correcting for the actual background concentrations (57, 63).

The concentration of the sample of exhaled breath has also been addressed in two different ways. In some studies, exhaled breath was concentrated in cartridges containing adsorbing resins (adsorption/desorption method), in other studies breath was concentrated at low temperatures in a gas sampling loop (the cryofocusing technique).

Our group modified a technique for single breath analysis of exhaled hydrocarbons developed by Zarling et al (56) where the sample does not require concentration and the collection is not preceded by washout with hydrocarbon-free air. Exhaled breath is collected at constant exhalation flow and pressure into a reservoir and later analysed by gas chromatography for the content of hydrocarbons. The levels of ambient ethane are subtracted from exhaled breath concentrations to reduce ambient contamination.

Like other authors (58), we favour ethane over pentane as a measure of lipid peroxidation because of the more rapid metabolism of pentane by animals and man (64). In addition, mass spectroscopic analysis of human exhalate has demonstrated the presence of significant amounts of isoprene, which may be mistaken for pentane during gas chromatographic analysis rendering pentane quantification complex (57).

The measurement of exhaled ethane is non-invasive, it can be repeated and may be applied to children and to patients with severe disease. Measurement of exhaled ethane may provide a means of detecting and monitoring cytokine-mediated inflammation and oxidant stress in the airways and of assessing the efficacy of treatment.

Method

Exhaled ethane is collected into a collapsible reservoir during a single exhalation from total lung capacity to residual volume at a constant flow (10-11 L/min) over 20-30 s against a mild resistance (21) (Figure 5). The inhalation to total lung capacity has to be contin-

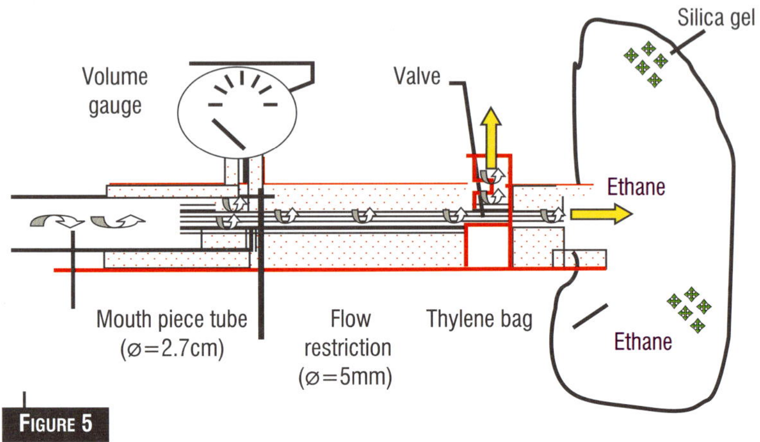

FIGURE 5

Schematic representation of the portable device for exhaled breath collection.

uous without pauses. A breathold can increase the concentration of exhaled ethane.

During exhalation the air coming from the dead space, contaminated with nasal and ambient ethane is discarded in the atmosphere by a three-way valve. The time needed to wash out the dead space (t) is estimated to be 1-2 s (t = dead space volume/exhalation flow where dead space is calculated as weight (lb) + age in years, and exhalation flow is 10-11 L/min) (65). Once the exhalation manoeuvre is finished and the patient has reached residual volume the three-way valve is promptly closed to avoid ambient contamination of the collected air or reflux out of the reservoir.

A sample (2 ml) of the collected expired air is analyzed for ethane content using gas chromatography (Chromatograph model PU 4500; Philips, Eindhoven, The Netherlands); column Poropak Q 1-3-mx4mm; column temperature, 60°C; injector temperature, 140°C; detector temperature, 160°C; signal output to a CR6A integrator (Shimadzu, Kyoto, Japan). The sensitivity of exhaled ethane measurement is 0.4ppb.

With these settings, the retention time for ethane is 1.5 min. The levels of ambient ethane are subtracted from exhaled breath concentrations to reduce ambient contamination.

The reproducibility of this method was proved by the Bland and Altman test (66). The coefficient of variation (standard deviation/mean

value x 100) of exhaled ethane levels measured during two successive collections at five minute intervals (single session variability) was
5.4%, while between sessions variability, (one day interval) was 6.2%.

Clinical studies

Patients with COPD have elevated levels of exhaled ethane which
correlates with disease severity as assessed by FEV_1 (67). In addition, exhaled ethane concentrations are reduced in steroid-treated
patients compared to untreated patients.

Other volatile organic compounds have been studied in COPD
and pentane and isoprene were found to be increased in normal
smokers. Although vitamin E given for 3 wk failed to reduce
exhaled ethane in cigarette smokers, those whose ethane values
fell the most tended to have better-preserved lung function (58).

Taken together these data show that increased levels of volatile
organic compounds in exhaled breath could be used as biochemical markers of exposure to cigarette smoke and oxidative damage
caused by smoking.

As in COPD patients, exhaled ethane is elevated in patients with
asthma compared to normal subjects (68). These results indicate
that there is increased lipid peroxidation in this group of patients
confirming previous studies showing elevated levels of other markers of lipid peroxidation such as thiobarbituric acid-reactive products (69) in exhaled breath condensate. In addition, Olopade et al (70)
showed elevated levels of exhaled pentane, which is also a marker
of lipid peroxidation, during acute asthma attacks.

Other Volatile Organic Compounds and their Measurement

More than 500 different endogenous and exogenous volatile organic compounds (VOCs) can be detected in the human breath and
ethane and pentane may not be the only disease markers in this
group of gases. Only compounds with a relatively low molecular
weight, usually less than 300 Daltons, are sufficiently volatile to be
detected in the exhaled breath (71). Their concentrations range
from below parts per billion by volume (ppbv) to parts per million
by volume (ppmv). Detecting gases in humid breath and quantifying them is a technical challenge and lots of different methods

have been used in order to overcome difficulties such as the high humidity of the sample.

As discussed above, the first pioneering studies used gas chromatography mass spectrometry (GC-MS). More recent techniques such as Ion Mobility Spectrometry (IMS), Proton Transfer Reaction Mass Spectrometry (PTR-MS) and Selected-Ion Flow-Tube Mass spectrometry (SIFT-MS), include the combination of mass spectrometry and fast flow tubes. This arrangement allows the real time analysis of exhaled breath.

The IMS technique is based on ionization of gaseous metabolites, which are separated with short impulses (about 10-100μs) in drift tubes only a few centimeters long and maintained at ambient pressure. The very small electric current (nA to pA) generated at a Faraday plate forms the spectrum of the running time of the ions. The combination of IMS with gas chromatographic columns guarantees a pre-separation of gaseous metabolites before entering the drift tube. The main advantages of IMS are its ability to detect very low gas concentrations without any pre-concentration, and the short time for analysis. Unfortunately IMS does not allow the identification of unknown gases in a gas mixture. Thus, this technique may only be used to identify disease-specific VOCs peaks (72).

The PTR-MS method uses a soft ionization method based on proton transfer from H_3O^+ ions to all compounds with a higher proton affinity than water. The common constituents of air such as N_2, O_2, Ar, and CO_2 have a lower proton affinity than water and are therefore not detected. The reaction products are analyzed using a quadrupole mass spectrometer and detected by a secondary electron multiplier (SEM) (73).

The PTR-MS technique has a response time of 100ms, this allows online real-time measurements which are not possible using GC-MS.

The SIFT-MS method performs real time measurements of complex gas mixtures regardless of the water vapor content and without sample preparation. Instrument reactant ions (precursors) are formed by electron impact (EI) or microwave discharge in a carrier gas (usually helium) in a separate ionization region. The trace gases in the sample react with quadrupole mass-selected H_3O^+, NO^+ or O_2^+ primary positive ions in the sample injection region. The resulting product ions are mass selected by a second downstream quadrupole and detected using a particle multiplier producing the resulting mass spectrum allowing the quantification of gases in the exhaled breath (74).

Clinical studies

VOCs can potentially be used as non-invasive biomarkers of various biochemical pathways in health and disease. Interestingly there are indications of a link between VOCs and lung disorders. Some studies have suggested that the measurement of exhaled VOCs may distinguish between patients with and without lung cancer (75), others, using a technique employing a nanocomposite array of 32 organic polymer sensors, found a distinctive "smellprint" in asthmatic patients (76) compared to normal subjects and different VOCs patterns in COPD compared to lung cancer patients (77). However, the method of sample analysis used in these last two studies does not allow a quantitative assessment of the gases measured but is only a pattern recognition tool.

Studies using more sophisticated breath analysis techniques such as the IMS, PTR-MS and SIFT-MS methods described above are now appearing in the literature (72). Besides providing quantitative VOCs analysis, these new techniques may also allow the on-line direct measurement of exhaled VOCs. These innovative methods are a major advancement in breath analysis and will provide an insight into the pathophysiology of lung disease.

Carbon Monoxide

CO is produced endogenously from the stress protein heme oxygenase-1 (HO-1), which is induced by oxidants, inflammatory cytokines and other forms of cellular stress in a variety of cell types. HO-1 plays an important role in the response to oxidative stress (78). HO-1 converts heme and hemin to biliverdin with the formation of CO. Biliverdin is rapidly converted to bilirubin, which is a potent antioxidant. CO may also be produced by the activity of HO-2, a constitutive enzyme highly expressed in the brain and testes.

The precise mechanisms for anti oxidant protection are not fully understood, but both the degradation of heme with removal of iron and induction of ferritin) and the generation of bilirubin (an antioxidant) may be involved. There is evidence that the deleterious effects of ROS, such as superoxide and H_2O_2, are dependent on the presence of iron. The intracellular pool of free iron can react with both H_2O_2 and superoxide, giving rise to the OH radical via the Fenton reaction. The free iron that is not metabolized intracellularly sequestered in cells as ferritin. Thus, ferritin serves as a reservoir to restrict iron from participating in the Fenton reaction. It has been shown that free iron released from heme by HO may induce ferritin synthesis, and heme-induced HO-1 protein also activates ferritin via mRNA expression. Furthermore, the metabolite of heme degradation, bilirubin, is itself an effective antioxidant of peroxynitrite-mediated protein oxidation and may be even more effective than vitamin E in preventing lipid peroxidation. Moderate overexpression of HO-1 improves the resistance of cells to oxygen toxicity.

Measurement

In most studies CO is measured electrochemically. The sensors used are selective and provide reproducible results. CO can also be measured by laser spectrophotometer and near-infrared CO analysers. Gas chromatography is a reference method for CO measurements, but its use is limited to specialized laboratories.

The exhalation manoeuvre is a single exhalation at a constant flow rate (5-6 L/min) after inspiration to total lung capacity from functional residual capacity. The measurement is completely non-invasive and reproducible. It is well tolerated by patients with poor lung volumes and by children.

Clinical studies

Smoking causes an acute increase in exhaled breath CO making this measurement less useful in COPD patients. However, there are high levels of exhaled CO in ex-smokers COPD patients (67). These levels are further increased during acute exacerbations and decline after recovery.

Heme oxygenase is present in the pulmonary vascular endothelium and alveolar macrophages and can be upregulated by oxidative stress and proinflammatory cytokines, thus increasing the production of CO. The high levels of exhaled CO found in COPD patients may be due to inflammatory cytokines or ROS induced HO-1 expression, therefore, the measurement of exhaled CO may reflect inflammation, oxidative stress, or both.

There is an increase in exhaled CO in patients with asthma (79) which is associated with HO-1 expression in macrophages in induced sputum (80). There is a further increase of CO during allergen challenge, whereas its levels are not modified by methacoline induced bronchocostriction (81) confirming that exhaled CO is a marker of oxidative stress in the airways and is not influenced by bronchocostriction per se.

The CO levels of patients with asthma or COPD largely overlap with those of normal control subjects, and the effect of inhaled corticosteroids on exhaled CO in patients with mild asthma, as it has been reported recently, is negligible (78). Therefore, at least when measured electrochemically, exhaled CO may not be of clinical value. However, the use of more sensitive techniques such as gas chromatography or laser may make the measurement of this gas more appealing in the future.

Conclusions

We have presented a number of new techniques to assess and monitor airway inflammation and oxidative stress in COPD. These methods may provide additional information to induced sputum and exhaled nitric oxide by offering an insight into some pathogenetic pathways of lung disease such as lipid peroxidation and airway remodelling.

The measurement of bronchial blood flow and exhaled ethane are promising methods which have been shown to be reproducible and correlate with other markers of airway inflammation such as exhaled NO. Unfortunately, the measurement of exhaled CO and breath temperature do not show the same degree reproducibility and patients with lung disease have values that largely overlap with normal subjects. The use of more technologically advanced techniques including infrared thermometers and laser carbon monoxide detectors is expected to improve these methods.

Longitudinal studies are required to investigate the usefulness of these measurements in a clinical setting, furthermore, cheaper and more user friendly devices are required to allow the day to day use of these techniques in the clinical management of inflammatory lung diseases.

References

1. Nightingale JA, Rogers DF, Barnes PJ. Effect of repeated sputum induction on cell counts in normal volunteers. Thorax. 1998 Feb;53(2):87-90.

2. Carroll NG, Cooke C, James AL. Bronchial blood vessel dimensions in asthma. Am J Respir Crit Care Med. 1997 Feb;155(2):689-95.

3. Li X, Wilson JW. Increased vascularity of the bronchial mucosa in mild asthma. Am J Respir Crit Care Med. 1997 Jul;156(1):229-33.

4. Gooding CA, Lallemand DP, Brasch RC, Wesbey GE, Davis B. Magnetic resonance imaging in cystic fibrosis. J Pediatr. 1984 Sep;105(3):384-8.

5. Chediak AD, Elsasser S, Csete ME, Gazeroglu H, Wanner A. Effect of histamine on tracheal mucosal perfusion, water content and airway smooth muscle in sheep. Respir Physiol. 1991 May;84(2):231-43.

6. Laitinen LA, Laitinen MA, Widdicombe JG. Dose-related effects of pharmacological mediators on tracheal vascular resistance in dogs. Br J Pharmacol. 1987 Dec;92(4):703-9.

7. McDonald DM. Neurogenic inflammation in the respiratory tract: actions of sensory nerve mediators on blood vessels and epithelium of the airway mucosa. Am Rev Respir Dis. 1987 Dec;136(6 Pt 2):S65-72.

8. Bjork J, Smedegard G. Acute microvascular effects of PAF-acether, as studied by intravital microscopy. Eur J Pharmacol. 1983 Dec 9;96(1-2):87-94.

9. Moreno RH, Hogg JC, Pare PD. Mechanics of airway narrowing. Am Rev Respir Dis. 1986 Jun;133(6):1171-80.

10. Hogg JC, Pare PD, Moreno R. The effect of submucosal edema on airways resistance. Am Rev Respir Dis. 1987 Jun;135(6 Pt 2):S54-6.

11. McFadden ER, Jr. Hypothesis: exercise-induced asthma as a vascular phenomenon. Lancet. 1990 Apr 14;335(8694):880-3.

12. Cabanes LR, Weber SN, Matran R, Regnard J, Richard MO, Degeorges ME, et al. Bronchial hyperresponsiveness to methacholine in patients with impaired left ventricular function. N Engl J Med. 1989 May 18;320(20):1317-22.

13. Rolla G, Scappaticci E, Baldi S, Bucca C. Methacholine inhalation challenge after rapid saline infusion in healthy subjects. Respiration. 1986;50(1):18-22.

14. Fagan KA, Tyler RC, Sato K, Fouty BW, Morris KG, Jr., Huang PL, et al. Relative contributions of endothelial, inducible, and neuronal NOS to tone in the murine pulmonary circulation. Am J Physiol. 1999 Sep;277(3 Pt 1):L472-8.

15. Paredi P, Kharitonov SA, Barnes PJ. Faster rise of exhaled breath temperature in asthma: a novel marker of airway inflammation? Am J Respir Crit Care Med. 2002 Jan 15;165(2):181-4.

16. Paredi P, Caramori G, Cramer D, Ward S, Ciaccia A, Papi A, et al. Slower rise of exhaled breath temperature in chronic obstructive pulmonary disease. Eur Respir J. 2003 Mar;21(3):439-43.

17. Paredi P, Kharitonov SA, Barnes PJ. Correlation of exhaled breath temperature with bronchial blood flow in asthma. Respir Res. 2005;6:15.

18. Piacentini GL, Bodini A, Zerman L, Costella S, Zanolla L, Peroni DG, et al. Relationship between exhaled air temperature and exhaled nitric oxide in childhood asthma. Eur Respir J. 2002 Jul;20(1):108-11.

19. Pifferi M, Ragazzo V, Previti A, Pioggia G, Ferro M, Macchia P, et al. Exhaled air temperature in asthmatic children: a mathematical evaluation. Pediatr Allergy Immunol. 2009 Mar;20(2):164-71.

20. Piacentini GL, Peroni D, Crestani E, Zardini F, Bodini A, Costella S, et al. Exhaled air temperature in asthma: methods and relationship with markers of disease. Clin Exp Allergy. 2007 Mar;37(3):415-9.

21. Paredi P, Loukides S, Ward S, Cramer D, Spicer M, Kharitonov SA, et al. Exhalation flow and pressure-controlled reservoir collection of exhaled nitric oxide for remote and delayed analysis. Thorax. 1998 Sep;53(9):775-9.

22. Reid A, Heard BE. Preliminary studies of human pulmonary capillaries by India ink injection. Med Thorac. 1962;19:215-9.

23. Cudkowicz L, Armstrong JB. The bronchial arteries in pulmonary emphysema. Thorax. 1953 Mar;8(1):46-58.

24. Ricketts HJ, Carrington CB. Experimental bronchial artery occlusion in sheep. Aspen Emphysema Conf. 1968;11:187-9.

25. Boushy SF, North LB, Trice JA. The bronchial arteries in chronic obstructive pulmonary disease. Am J Med. 1969 Apr;46(4):506-15.

26. Kumar SD, Emery MJ, Atkins ND, Danta I, Wanner A. Airway mucosal blood flow in bronchial asthma. Am J Respir Crit Care Med. 1998 Jul; 158(1):153-6.

27. Noda A, Nakata S, Koike Y, Miyata S, Kitaichi K, Nishizawa T, et al. Continuous positive airway pressure improves daytime baroreflex sensitivity and nitric oxide production in patients with moderate to severe obstructive sleep apnea syndrome. Hypertens Res. 2007 Aug;30(8):669-76.

28. Piacentini GL, Peroni DG, Bodini A, Corradi M, Boner AL. Exhaled breath temperature as a marker of airway remodelling in asthma: a preliminary study. Allergy. 2008 Apr;63(4):484-5.

29. Paredi P, Ward S, Cramer D, Barnes PJ, Kharitonov SA. Normal bronchial blood flow in COPD is unaffected by inhaled corticosteroids and correlates with exhaled nitric oxide. Chest. 2007 Apr;131(4):1075-81.

30. Grollman A. The determination of the cardiac output of man by the use of acetylene. Am J Physiol. 1929;88:432-45.

31. Wanner A, Barker JA, Long WM, Mariassy AT, Chediak AD. Measurement of airway mucosal perfusion and water volume with an inert soluble gas. J Appl Physiol. 1988 Jul;65(1):264-71.

32. Cander I, Forster R. Determination of pulmonary parenchymal tissue volume and pulmonary capillary blood flow in man. J Appl Physiol. 1959;14:541-51.

33. Scuri M, McCaskill V, Chediak AD, Abraham WM, Wanner A. Measurement of airway mucosal blood flow with dimethylether: validation with microspheres. J Appl Physiol. 1995 Oct; 79(4):1386-90.

34. Fowler WS, Cornish ER, Jr., Kety SS. Lung function studies. VIII. Analysis of

alveolar ventilation by pulmonary N2 clearance curves. J Clin Invest. 1952 Jan;31(1):40-50.

35. Brieva J, Wanner A. Adrenergic airway vascular smooth muscle responsiveness in healthy and asthmatic subjects. J Appl Physiol. 2001 Feb;90(2):665-9.

36. Wanner A, Mendes ES, Atkins ND. A simplified noninvasive method to measure airway blood flow in humans. J Appl Physiol. 2006 May;100(5):1674-8.

37. Brieva JL, Danta I, Wanner A. Effect of an inhaled glucocorticosteroid on airway mucosal blood flow in mild asthma. Am J Respir Crit Care Med. 2000 Jan;161(1):293-6.

38. Clarke G, Ledbetter C, Greenway S, Simcock D, Greenough A, O'Connor B. The effect of vasoactive substances on airway mucosal blood flow in asthma. Am J Respir Crit Care Med. 2006:A457.

39. Hecht SS. Approaches to cancer prevention based on an understanding of N-nitrosamine carcinogenesis. Proc Soc Exp Biol Med. 1997 Nov;216(2):181-91.

40. Hashimoto M, Tanaka H, Abe S. Quantitative analysis of bronchial wall vascularity in the medium and small airways of patients with asthma and COPD. Chest. 2005 Mar;127(3):965-72.

41. Wanner A, Campos MA, Mendes E. Airway blood flow reactivity in smokers. Pulm Pharmacol Ther. 2007;20(2):126-9.

42. Tanaka H, Yamada G, Saikai T, Hashimoto M, Tanaka S, Suzuki K, et al. Increased airway vascularity in newly diagnosed asthma using a high-magnification bronchovideoscope. Am J Respir Crit Care Med. 2003 Dec 15;168(12):1495-9.

43. Calabrese C, Bocchino V, Vatrella A, Marzo C, Guarino C, Mascitti S, et al. Evidence of angiogenesis in bronchial biopsies of smokers with and without airway obstruction. Respir Med. 2006 Aug;100(8):1415-22.

44. Hiroshima K, Iyoda A, Shibuya K, Hoshino H, Haga Y, Toyozaki T, et al. Evidence of neoangiogenesis and an increase in the number of proliferating cells within the bronchial epithelium of smokers. Cancer. 2002 Oct 1;95(7):1539-45.

45. Hoshino M, Takahashi M, Aoike N. Expression of vascular endothelial growth factor, basic fibroblast growth factor, and angiogenin immunoreactivity in asthmatic airways and its relationship to angiogenesis. J Allergy Clin Immunol. 2001 Feb;107(2):295-301.

46. Salvato G. Quantitative and morphological analysis of the vascular bed in bronchial biopsy specimens from asthmatic and non-asthmatic subjects. Thorax. 2001 Dec;56(12):902-6.

47. Barnes PJ. Reactive oxygen species and airway inflammation. Free Radic Biol Med. 1990;9(3):235-43.

48. Rahman I, Morrison D, Donaldson K, MacNee W. Systemic oxidative stress in asthma, COPD, and smokers. Am J Respir Crit Care Med. 1996 Oct;154(4 Pt 1):1055-60.

49. Repine JE, Bast A, Lankhorst I. Oxidative stress in chronic obstructive pulmonary disease. Oxidative Stress Study Group. Am J Respir Crit Care Med. 1997 Aug;156(2 Pt 1):341-57.

50. Brown RK, Wyatt H, Price JF, Kelly FJ.

Pulmonary dysfunction in cystic fibrosis is associated with oxidative stress. Eur Respir J. 1996 Feb;9(2):334-9.

51. Jarjour NN, Calhoun WJ. Enhanced production of oxygen radicals in asthma. J Lab Clin Med. 1994 Jan;123(1): 131-6.

52. Kneepkens CM, Lepage G, Roy CC. The potential of the hydrocarbon breath test as a measure of lipid peroxidation. Free Radic Biol Med. 1994 Aug;17(2):127-60.

53. Morrison D, Rahman I, Lannan S, MacNee W. Epithelial permeability, inflammation, and oxidant stress in the air spaces of smokers. Am J Respir Crit Care Med. 1999 Feb;159(2):473-9.

54. Habib MP, Clements NC, Garewal HS. Cigarette smoking and ethane exhalation in humans. Am J Respir Crit Care Med. 1995 May;151(5):1368-72.

55. Kazui M, Andreoni KA, Norris EJ, Klein AS, Burdick JF, Beattie C, et al. Breath ethane: a specific indicator of free-radical-mediated lipid peroxidation following reperfusion of the ischemic liver. Free Radic Biol Med. 1992 Nov;13(5): 509-15.

56. Zarling EJ, Clapper M. Technique for gas-chromatographic measurement of volatile alkanes from single-breath samples. Clin Chem. 1987 Jan;33(1): 140-1.

57. Kohlmuller D, Kochen W. Is n-pentane really an index of lipid peroxidation in humans and animals? A methodological reevaluation. Anal Biochem. 1993 May 1;210(2):268-76.

58. Habib MP, Tank LJ, Lane LC, Garewal HS. Effect of vitamin E on exhaled ethane in cigarette smokers. Chest. 1999 Mar;115(3):684-90.

59. Aulik IV. [Gas chromatographic analysis of exhaled air and acetylene mixture]. Biull Eksp Biol Med. 1966 Sep;62(9): 115-7.

60. Lemoyne M, Van Gossum A, Kurian R, Ostro M, Axler J, Jeejeebhoy KN. Breath pentane analysis as an index of lipid peroxidation: a functional test of vitamin E status. Am J Clin Nutr. 1987 Aug;46(2):267-72.

61. Refat M, Moore TJ, Kazui M, Risby TH, Perman JA, Schwarz KB. Utility of breath ethane as a noninvasive biomarker of vitamin E status in children. Pediatr Res. 1991 Nov;30(5): 396-403.

62. Toshniwal PK, Zarling EJ. Evidence for increased lipid peroxidation in multiple sclerosis. Neurochem Res. 1992 Feb;17(2):205-7.

63. Moscarella S, Laffi G, Buzzelli G, Mazzanti R, Caramelli L, Gentilini P. Expired hydrocarbons in patients with chronic liver disease. Hepatogastroenterology. 1984 Apr;31(2):60-3.

64. Jeejeebhoy KN. In vivo breath alkane as an index of lipid peroxidation. Free Radic Biol Med. 1991;10(3-4):191-3.

65. Cotes JE. Lung function. Assessment and application in medicine. 5th ed; 1994.

66. Bland JM, Altman DG. Statistical methods for assessing agreement between two methods of clinical measurement. Lancet. 1986 Feb 8;1(8476):307-10.

67. Paredi P, Kharitonov SA, Leak D, Ward S, Cramer D, Barnes PJ. Exhaled ethane, a marker of lipid peroxidation, is elevated in chronic obstructive pulmonary disease. Am J Respir Crit Care Med. 2000 Aug;162(2 Pt 1):369-73.

68. Paredi P, Kharitonov SA, Barnes PJ. Elevation of exhaled ethane concentration in asthma. Am J Respir Crit Care Med. 2000 Oct;162(4 Pt 1): 1450-4.

69. Antczak A, Nowak D, Shariati B, Krol M, Piasecka G, Kurmanowska Z. Increased hydrogen peroxide and thiobarbituric acid-reactive products in expired breath condensate of asthmatic patients. Eur Respir J. 1997 Jun; 10(6):1235-41.

70. Olopade CO, Zakkar M, Swedler WI, Rubinstein I. Exhaled pentane levels in acute asthma. Chest. 1997 Apr;111(4):862-5.

71. Smith D, Spanel P. The challenge of breath analysis for clinical diagnosis and therapeutic monitoring. Analyst. 2007 May;132(5):390-6.

72. Westhoff M, Litterst P, Freitag L, Urfer W, Bader S, Baumbach JI. Ion mobility spectrometry for the detection of volatile organic compounds in exhaled breath of lung cancer patients. Thorax. 2009 Jan 21.

73. Steeghs MM, Cristescu SM, Munnik P, Zanen P, Harren FJ. An off-line breath sampling and analysis method suitable for large screening studies. Physiol Meas. 2007 May;28(5):503-14.

74. Buszewski B, Kesy M, Ligor T, Amann A. Human exhaled air analytics: biomarkers of diseases. Biomed Chromatogr. 2007 Jun;21(6):553-66.

75. Phillips M, Gleeson K, Hughes JM, Greenberg J, Cataneo RN, Baker L, et al. Volatile organic compounds in breath as markers of lung cancer: a cross-sectional study. Lancet. 1999 Jun 5;353(9168):1930-3.

76. Dragonieri S, Schot R, Mertens BJ, Le Cessie S, Gauw SA, Spanevello A, et al. An electronic nose in the discrimination of patients with asthma and controls. J Allergy Clin Immunol. 2007 Oct;120(4):856-62.

77. Dragonieri S, Annema JT, Schot R, van der Schee MP, Spanevello A, Carratu P, et al. An electronic nose in the discrimination of patients with non-small cell lung cancer and COPD. Lung Cancer. 2009 May;64(2):166-70.

78. Choi AM, Alam J. Heme oxygenase-1: function, regulation, and implication of a novel stress-inducible protein in oxidant-induced lung injury. Am J Respir Cell Mol Biol. 1996 Jul;15(1):9-19.

79. Zayasu K, Sekizawa K, Okinaga S, Yamaya M, Ohrui T, Sasaki H. Increased carbon monoxide in exhaled air of asthmatic patients. Am J Respir Crit Care Med. 1997 Oct;156(4 Pt 1):1140-3.

80. Horvath I, Donnelly LE, Kiss A, Paredi P, Kharitonov SA, Barnes PJ. Raised levels of exhaled carbon monoxide are associated with an increased expression of heme oxygenase-1 in airway macrophages in asthma: a new marker of oxidative stress. Thorax. 1998 Aug;53(8):668-72.

81. Paredi P, Leckie MJ, Horvath I, Allegra L, Kharitonov SA, Barnes PJ. Changes in exhaled carbon monoxide and nitric oxide levels following allergen challenge in patients with asthma. Eur Respir J. 1999 Jan;13(1):48-52.

Perspective: Can Non-Invasive Biomarkers Replace the Invasive Assessment of Airways Inflammation?

Mina Gaga • Eleftherios Zervas

osinophilic inflammation in asthma was observed for the first time more than a hundred years ago (1, 2) however invasive assessment of inflammation in the bronchi through bronchoscopy and bronchial biopsies started in the 1980's (3-6). Those landmark studies helped us recognize the role of eosinophils and T cells as well as structural changes, later termed remodeling (7-14). These studies were followed by studies involving various challenges and serial biopsies which helped us understand the pathophysiology of asthma and the time course of the inflammatory reaction (7, 15-19). As immunohistochemical and molecular methodologies evolved, more and more elaborate studies could be performed and they could be coupled with functional assays, genetic studies and a multitude of tests to help us form and confirm a theory of asthma pathophysiology and phenotypes. The effect of treatment has al-

Correspondence

Dr. Mina Gaga

7th Respiratory Medicine Dept. and Asthma Centre, Athens Chest Hospital, Mesogeion 152, Athens 11527, Greece

e-mail: minagaga@yahoo.com

so been examined and confirmed through bronchial biopsies and those studies established the role of anti-inflammatory treatment and especially ICS in asthma (20-22). Asthma lends itself particularly to time-course studies as it can be provoked by stimuli such as allergens and the reaction is quick (within hours to a few days) so it is easy to observe in a study setting. This is different to the situation in most other chronic diseases such as COPD where the disease develops much more slowly and changes appear after years of stimulation or exposure.

On the other hand, the approach to COPD has been rather nihilistic and studies examining inflammatory changes and the possible effect of treatment, started later than those in asthma (23, 24). In COPD, invasive assessment of the pathology of the bronchi led to the recognition of inflammation that is mostly CD8 cell driven (25). However, COPD is not only a disease of the bronchi but also involves the lung parenchyma. Although information about changes has been received through biopsies taken at bronchoscopy with bronchial or transbronchial sampling (26-28), a lot of information has been provided by studies that have used tissue taken at surgery for other reasons, such as lung cancer (29, 30) This has the additional benefit of obtaining large samples and a clearer idea of the changes in both the airways and the parenchyma. Although as previously stated it is difficult to experimentally provoke time changes and examine the time course of inflammatory changes the effect of treatment can be tested. Bronchial biopsies have been used to assess the state of the bronchi and the effect of treatment and changed the approach to COPD management (20, 31, 32). Currently, the definition of COPD is that the disease is a chronic inflammatory disease that is preventable and treatable.

What Have we Learned from Biopsies and BAL?

Asthma

The chronic inflammatory response in the airway in asthma is characterized by the presence of increased numbers of Th2 lymphocytes, eosinophils, and activated mast cells (7, 33, 34). In addition to the presence of inflammatory cells in the airway, the airways of patients with asthma exhibit varying levels of structural changes termed airway remodeling (9, 10, 13, 14, 35-37). Characteristic structural changes of airway remodeling include increased goblet cell cells and mucus gland hypertrophy (mucus metaplasia), smooth muscle hypertrophy/hyperplasia, thickening of the basement membrane and subepithelial collagen deposition/fibrosis, and increased angiogenesis (10, 14, 35-37). Although it is well recognized that airway inflammation is a prominent feature of asthma, the relationship between airway inflammation and the progression to remodeling of the airways in asthma is not well understood (38) The use of fiberoptic bronchoscopy and bronchial biopsies have helped us not only characterize the presence of inflammatory cells and mediators but also correlate levels of individual cell types, cytokines and mediators with levels of airway remodeling (12, 39-42) Asthma is a disease that lends itself particularly to experimental studies as both the early and late phase reactions are expressed within hours. Bronchial biopsies have been used to examine the pathology of asthma compared to healthy control biopsies. Furthermore, the time course of the asthmatic reaction after allergen challenge has been established through serial biopsies pre- and post- challenge (19, 43-45). Moreover, simultaneous biopsies in the bronchial and nasal mucosa in asthma and/or rhinitis have shown inflammatory as well as histological similarities and have helped formulate the one airway- one disease hypothesis (46-49). It has thus been determined that allergen challenge leads to increased cellular infiltration, initially with neutrophils and then with eosinophils and T cells and that markers of remodeling such as tenascin or heat shock proteins can appear fairly early (49). *In situ* hybridization studies have proved the presence of Th2 type cytokines, even in non-atopic asthma (50, 51).

Furthermore, bronchial biopsies have been taken pre and post-treatment to examine the effect of specific medications. Early bronchial biopsy studies showed that steroid treatment reduces cellular infiltration and leads to regression of remodeling changes (22), while more recent ones show the anti-inflammatory effect is maintained or indeed enhanced even with lower ICS dose when ICS/LABA are used in combination (52, 53). Other medications such as anti IgE and anti IL-5 may lead to reduced eosinophilic infiltration (44, 54). Moreover, bronchial biopsies in severe asthma have shown that infiltration may be eosinophilic, neutrophilic, mixed or paucigranulocytic and the assessment is important in guiding treatment decisions(55). Currently, bronchial biopsies are recommended in severe and difficult to treat asthma to exclude other diagnoses such as Churg-Strauss disease and to help guide treatment (56, 57).

Bronchoscopy with bronchial biopsy and BAL sampling has provided us with invaluable information, has helped us define the inflammatory nature of the disease and lead to a more cognitive approach to treatment. A limitation of these studies of human bronchial biopsies is that a cause and effect relationship between expression of a particular cell, cytokine, or mediator and the pathogenesis of airway inflammation and remodeling cannot be established unless functional studies are performed or specific cells have been depleted and specific cytokine/mediators neutralized. So findings from biopsy studies have been coupled with findings from animal models of asthma, human skin models of asthma and studies of non-invasive markers and have helped us form a clearer picture.

COPD

Clinicaly, COPD has two distinct phenotypes, emphysema and chronic bronchitis but, most often, there is overlap. The airways of patients with chronic obstructive pulmonary disease (COPD) show squamous cell metaplasia, loss of epithelial cilia, goblet cell hyperplasia, mucus gland enlargement and smooth muscle hypertrophy while in the lung parenchyma destruction of alveolar walls and attachments is observed (58-61). Increase in smooth muscle mass is more predominant in smaller airways where airway wall fibrosis and stenotic lesions are also observed (30). Recent studies in COPD using immunohistochemistry, in situ hybridization and other newly available techniques showed that inflammation is characterised by increased macrophages, CD8+ T-cells and neutrophils and have helped us understand the inflammatory and immunological aspect of the disease (60, 62, 63). In smokers, the number of CD8+ T-lymphocytes in the peripheral airways is significantly correlated with the degree of airflow limitation, suggesting an important role for these cells in the pathophysiology of COPD (58, 60). In contrast to asthma, T cells in the bronchial mucosa of COPD patients predominantly express IFN-γ and CXCR3 but do not express IL-4 and CCR4 (64, 65). The lack of IL-4 expression by infiltrating T cells confirms the non-atopic nature of COPD, while the expression of CXCR3 suggest that this specific chemocine axis may be involved in the T cell recruitment that occurs in peripheral airways of COPD patients and that these T cells may have a type-1 profile (65). This is in agreement with a number of published in vitro and in vivo studies in which CXCR3 was consistently found associated with Th1-type responses (66, 67). These specific histopatho-logical differences can help us to differentiate patients with COPD or severe asthma with fixed airway obstruction and treated them accordingly (68).

Smooth muscle alterations have been demonstrated in COPD patients. Airway smooth muscle increases significantly in the small airways in COPD (69, 70) and this is likely to be the most important abnormality responsible for the increased airflow resistance ob-served in response to bronchoconstricting stimuli in both obstructive lung diseases (asthma and COPD) (71). Peripheral muscle abnor-malities have also been observed in COPD in relation to the systemic inflammatory component of the disease. Studies have shown in-creased expression of different cytokines, especially TNFa, in respi-ratory and periphery muscles, associated with muscle weakness and dysfunction (72, 73). Furthermore, vascular abnormalities have been associated with the development of COPD (74, 75). An increase in wall area of small pulmonary vessels in patients with mild to moder-ate COPD and medial thickening in severe cases as well been corre-lated with a decline in FEV1 (76). Furthermore, recent observations have indicated that muscular pulmonary and bronchiolar arteries have increased adventitial infiltration of CD8+ T lymphocytes and have intimal thickening that is correlated with the amount of total col-lagen deposition (75, 77). In addition, emphysema may lead to loss of the pulmonary vascular bed and induce angiogenesis (78). One of the potent proteins involved in vascular remodeling is vascular en-dothelial growth factor (VEGF) and many researchers have found that VEGF expression is increased in COPD (79, 80).

Moreover, currently COPD is considered a systemic disease and markers of systemic inflammation can be used to assess and mon-itor this component of the disease (81).

Correlations with Non-Invasive Markers

Studies of invasive assessment of the bronchi give us invaluable in-formation on the disease phenotype, confirm or exclude our diagno-sis and have helped us define the effects of treatment. However, it is not possible, practical or even safe to monitor patients using serial bronchoscopic biopsies. As several non-invasive markers have be-come available for the assessment of inflammation, it is important to examine how these correlate to biopsy findings and how they can be used longitudinally. Markers that can be assessed non invasively are mainly markers related to inflammation while markers of remodeling and structural changes are still assessed only directly in bronchial tissue.

Induced Sputum

Induced sputum is a relatively noninvasive method and fairly easy as a technique to perform. It is used to assess airway inflammation of the central airways (82) and guidelines about the procedure have been published (83). Cell differential count in the cell pellet and mediator measurements in sputum supernatant are well validated and normal ranges derived from large adult populations have been published (84).

The presence of sputum eosinophils has been considered a feature of asthma. Recent studies have shown that monitoring of sputum eosinophils (in addition to guideline-recommended monitoring of symptoms and lung function) helps better assessment and management and leads to fewer exacerbations (85, 86). On the other hand, sputum neutrophilia may indicate infection but may also imply the specific neutrophilic phenotype of severe asthma (87, 88) and the presence of sputum neutrophils is currently used in studies that examine novel treatments for this specific phenotype. Analysis of inflammatory cells in induced sputum provides similar data to secretions obtained through bronchial wash and bronchoalveolar lavage, but only to some extent with bronchial biopsies (89, 90). This may be due to the fact that sputum and BAL sample the airway lumen, whereas the cellular inflammation in the airway submucosa may be distinct. Induced sputum therefore could be used to monitor luminal eosinophilic inflammation but probably not mucosal inflammation in asthma (91). In accordance with this, in a recent study in severe asthmatics the vast majority of subjects with high sputum eosinophil counts did not have high mucosal eosinophil counts (92).

In COPD, an increase in number of total inflammatory cells, in the percentage of neutrophils and in some patients eosinophils, have been observed in induced sputum differential cell count (93, 94). CD8+ T cells are increased in induced sputum of patients with COPD, while CD8+-IL4 and CD8+-IFNgamma cells were reduced suggesting an imbalance both in T-lymphocyte subpopulation

(CD4/CD8) and in CD8+ cell subsets (Tc1/Tc2) that characterize the inflammatory responses of smokers with established COPD (95). An increased number of eosinophils may be a sign of exacerbation or concomitant asthma or "asthmatic" phenotype of the disease. Studies suggest that this eosinophilic airway inflammation may contribute to airflow obstruction and symptoms in some patients with COPD and that the favourable short-term effects of corticosteroids are due to modification of this feature of the inflammatory response (96, 97). Several studies have reported the effects of drugs on sputum neutrophils or eosinophils with conflicting results (98-101). However, the use of induced sputum differential cell counts in the monitoring and tailoring of treatment in COPD has not been tested in large clinical trials and is not used in clinical practice. Comparisons of induced sputum to bronchial wash (BW), bronchoalveolar lavage (BAL) and bronchial biopsies in COPD have shown that differential cell counts in sputum did not correlate with the counts in BW or BAL fluid or biopsies suggesting that induced sputum is derived from a d-ifferent compartment than bronchoscopicaly obtained samples (102).

Many cytokines, chemokines, pro-inflammatory proteins, soluble remodelling-associated proteins, such as MMPs, TIMPs and cytokines can be detected in the sputum supernatants of asthma and COPD patients (29, 94). However, sputum processing requires the addition of a reducing mucolytic agent to help the release of the cellular components from the mucus. This significantly reduces the concentration of inflammatory cytokines in the sputum and directly interferes with the immunoassay (29, 103). This is one of the major limitations in studying mediators in induced sputum. Other limitations include the inconsistency of the dilution factor and the difficulty of obtaining adequate specimen. As already mentioned for cell counts, again, a rather poor correlation exists between induced sputum data and those obtained with invasive techniques (103).

Therefore, although induced sputum can provide information regarding the ongoing overall inflammation, it might not be the ideal method for studying the exact pathophysiological events that occur within the airway wall (104). On the other hand, induced sputum it is a relatively noninvasive technique, well tolerated and easy to perform, although it is time-consuming. Sputum induction can moreover be performed repeatedly, before and after challenge/treatment, and even in children and exacerbated patients. For these reasons, the assessment of airway diseases through induced sputum analyses is gaining popularity in research.

Exhaled Nitric Oxide (eNO)

Measuring biomarkers in exhaled air is a very attractive approach to monitoring inflammation, as it is noninvasive and can be done repeatable (105). The fraction of nitric oxide (NO) in exhaled air (FeNO) is the most extensively studied exhaled marker and abnormalities in exhaled NO have been documented in several lung diseases. The cellular source of NO in the lower respiratory tract is not yet certain but NO seems to originate at the alveolar surface. In inflammatory diseases such as asthma and COPD, the increase in exhaled NO reflects further induction of the enzyme NO synthase (NOS) in response to inflammatory signals (105). Normal ranges from large adult populations have been reported (106, 107) and guidelines about the procedure have been published both by European Respiratory Society and American Thoracic Society (108).

FeNO has been extensively investigated in asthma and increased levels have been demonstrated (105, 109). NO measurements have been used as a diagnostic but also as a screening tool in asthma - especially in children - showing superiority to conventional approaches (110-112). Studies have shown that NO levels can not differentiate asthma severity (113) but can identify a subgroup of subjects with persistent eosinophilia despite steroid therapy (114). Furthermore, exhaled NO has been widely used to monitor the effect of anti-inflammatory treatment (115, 116) and also to guide treatment in chronic asthma. The first studies implicated NO monitoring in asthma management plans have shown promising results (117, 118), but more recent and larger trials failed to confirm these findings (119, 120). On the other hand, the relationship between exhaled NO and asthmatic inflammation is still uncertain and in some studies, no significant relationship is seen between exhaled NO and eosinophils or other inflammatory cells in bronchial biopsies or bronchoalveolar lavage (121, 122). This may indicate that increased exhaled NO reflects some, but not all, aspects of airway inflammation in asthma, and further work is needed to determine how it relates to some other markers of airway inflammation

In COPD, FeNO measurement is less useful, as a wide range of FeNO levels and a high variability of FeNO over time have been observed; levels reported usually normal or only slightly elevated, except during exacerbations (123-125). This is likely due to the increase in oxidative stress, observed in the airways of COPD patients. This also explains why FeNO is reduced in normal smokers (126). In patients with stable COPD an increase in FeNO, correlated with increased numbers of eosinophils, an increased bronchodilator response and steroid responsiveness, suggesting that these patients may have a different response to treatment (97). There are only few studies examining the relationship between NO and other non-invasive markers of inflammation in COPD (105), but no studies have checked the possible association of this marker with inflammatory indices in bronchial biopsies or BAL. For the time being, NO does not seem to be a very useful biomarker of COPD inflammation, but further studies on reproducibility, relationship to disease severity and the effects of treatments are certainly needed.

Exhaled Breath Condensate

Exhaled breath condensate (EBC) is another widely used method to study inflammatory markers in exhaled air. EBC is collected by cooling or freezing exhaled air and is totally noninvasive. The collection procedure has no influence on airway function or inflammation, and there is evidence that abnormalities in condensate composition may reflect biochemical changes of airway lining fluid (105). EBC contains large number of mediators including adenosine, ammonia, hydrogen peroxide, isoprostanes, leukotrienes, nitrogen oxides, peptides and cytokines. Concentrations of these mediators are influenced by lung diseases and modulated by therapeutic interventions (127). Methodological issues regarding EBC collection and recommendations for the measurements off all these mediators have recently been published (127) and efforts to identify references values have started (128).

EBC from asthmatic patients is characterized by increased concentrations of markers expressing oxidative stress, leukotrienes, products of NO metabolism, and cytokines (105, 129). Elevated exhaled condensate levels of cysteinyl-leukotrienes (cys-LTs) LTC4, LTD4 and LTE4 have been observed in patients with asthma (130, 131) and increase with disease severity (131). Moreover, levels increase during both the early and late phase reactions as shown in studies examining early asthmatic responses (EARs) after allergen (132), as well as asthmatic exacerbations (133). Some pharmaceutical interventions have been shown to decrease these elevated CysLTs levels (130, 133). In a recent pilot study there was a significant relationship between EBC cysLTs and RBM thickness in the subgroup of children who were not treated with montelukast, suggesting an association of EBC cysLTs with remodeling changes in asthma (134). A marker of oxidative stress, 8-isoprostane has also been reported to be elevated in asthmatic patients and increased with disease severity (131, 135). But as the measurement of all these markers still remains a time-consuming procedure, recently published data suggest that EBC pH is the only rapid marker, which reflects a significant part of asthma pathophysiology and is measurable on-site with standardized methodology (129).

EBC has also been used in COPD and markers of oxidative stress such as H_2O_2, 8-isoprostane, pH as well as inflammatory mediators have been measured (136). Studies have shown higher levels of E-BC 8-isoprostane in stable COPD patients compared with healthy controls (137, 138) with evidence of further increase during exacerbation (139). However, no correlations have been observed between 8-isoprostane and FEV_1 or sputum cells in COPD studies (137, 140). Also 8-isoprostane levels have varied considerably within the same subject group of COPD patients despite the use of identical methods (136). EBC pH is another extensively used marker of airways oxidation in COPD patient. COPD patients exhibit a very low pH of EBC which may be indicative of a specific COPD phenotype (141, 142). Studies focusing on relationships of pH EBC with other markers of inflammation, like induced sputum differential cell count, has given conflicting results (141, 142).

Unfortunately, studies examining possible correlations between markers assessed with EBC and those assessed via invasive methods have shown negative results (143), raising questions about correlations of EBC markers and on site inflammation. Moreover, many issues regarding both sample collection and analysis have to been solved (127).

Bronchial Hyperresponsiveness

Bronchial hyperresponsiveness (BHR) is defined as excessive narrowing of the airways to various inhaled direct or indirect stimuli. Guidelines for both "direct" and "indirect" methods of BHR measurement has been published (144, 145).

BHR to a variety of bronchoconstrictor stimuli is a crucial feature of asthma and its measure can be of great importance in diagnosis and evaluation of asthma severity (146). Methacholine is currently the gold standard for the assessment of BHR (145), as it is more sensitive than exercise or cold air challenge and produces less side effects than histamine. In addition, it has been shown that BHR measurement using methacholine challenge was the most sensitive predictor of an asthma exacerbation (147) and a sensitive marker to adjust anti-inflammatory treatment (148, 149). On the other hand AMP, an indirect stimulus of airway narrowing (150), has been also used to measure bronchial hyperresponsiveness in asthmatic patients. There are studies showing that asthmatics and atopic individuals are very sensitive to AMP challenge whereas non-atopic subjects are not (151). Additionally ICS treatment reported to have a significantly greater effect on AMP induced airway responsiveness than on methacholine induced BHR (152). BHR is used as an indirect method to assess airway inflammation and remodeling in asthma (153, 154) and it has been shown that increased BHR correlates to airway eosinophilia, basement membrane thickness and airway remodeling (153-156). BHR is both an innate characteristic of asthma and a result of inflammatory and remodeling changes and therefore, although time-consuming, it can be used in the monitoring of a specific patient. However, BHR cannot identify the underlying pathogenetic mechanisms leading to changes in the bronchi and in the patient's clinical outcome. Lastly, BHR is not a disease specific measurement: BHR is quite commonly found in general population samples with a reported prevalence ranging between 6% and 35%, according to various studies (157, 158). In the Lung Health Study, BHR to methacholine was identified in 25% of men and 48% of women with COPD (159). BHR is a risk factor for the development of respiratory symptoms and COPD (160, 161) while current smokers with BHR show increased annual loss in FEV1 (162). ICS have been shown to reduce bronchial hyper-responsiveness in COPD patients but the measurement of BHR cannot predict which patient will benefit by this treatment (163, 164). In COPD patients, hyperresponsiveness to AMP is associated with airway inflammation that is characterized by increased numbers of mucosal CD8 + cells and higher percentages of sputum eosinophils (165) but its significance in the clinical course of the disease remains to be determined.

Conclusions

Non-invasive assessment of inflammation cannot replace the invasive assessment nor does it provide the same information. However, some markers such as BHR, sputum eosinophils and NO have been shown to predict the upcoming loss of control in asthma and help us guide treatment. This is not the case in COPD where good markers for monitoring in clinical practice are still awaited. Lastly, although non-invasive markers may become available for the monitoring of inflammation, structural changes need to be directly assessed in histological samples.

References

1. Ellis GA. The pathological anatomy of bronchial asthma. Am J Med Sci 1908;136:407-29.
2. Charcot JM, Robin C. Mem Soc Biol. 1853;5:44-50.
3. Foresi A, Bertorelli G, Pesci A, Chetta A, Olivieri D. Inflammatory markers in bronchoalveolar lavage and in bronchial biopsy in asthma during remission. Chest. 1990 Sep;98(3):528-35.
4. Laitinen LA, Heino M, Laitinen A, Kava T, Haahtela T. Damage of the airway epithelium and bronchial reactivity in patients with asthma. Am Rev Respir Dis. 1985 Apr;131(4):599-606.
5. Laursen LC, Taudorf E, Borgeskov S, Kobayasi T, Jensen H, Weeke B. Fiberoptic bronchoscopy and bronchial mucosal biopsies in asthmatics undergoing long-term high-dose budesonide aerosol treatment. Allergy. 1988 May;43(4):284-8.
6. Lundgren R, Soderberg M, Horstedt P, Stenling R. Morphological studies of bronchial mucosal biopsies from asthmatics before and after ten years of treatment with inhaled steroids. Eur Respir J. 1988 Dec;1(10):883-9.
7. Azzawi M, Bradley B, Jeffery PK, Frew AJ, Wardlaw AJ, Knowles G, et al. Identification of activated T lymphocytes and eosinophils in bronchial biopsies in stable atopic asthma. Am Rev Respir Dis. 1990 Dec;142(6 Pt 1):1407-13.
8. Bousquet J, Chanez P, Lacoste JY, Barneon G, Ghavanian N, Enander I, et al. Eosinophilic inflammation in asthma. N Engl J Med. 1990 Oct 11; 323(15):1033-9.
9. Brewster CE, Howarth PH, Djukanovic R, Wilson J, Holgate ST, Roche WR. Myofibroblasts and subepithelial fibrosis in bronchial asthma. Am J Respir Cell Mol Biol. 1990 Nov;3(5): 507-11.
10. Chetta A, Foresi A, Del Donno M, Bertorelli G, Pesci A, Olivieri D. Airways remodeling is a distinctive feature of asthma and is related to severity of disease. Chest. 1997 Apr;111(4):852-7.
11. Djukanovic R, Wilson JW, Britten KM, Wilson SJ, Walls AF, Roche WR, et al. Quantitation of mast cells and eosinophils in the bronchial mucosa of symptomatic atopic asthmatics and healthy control subjects using immunohistochemistry. Am Rev Respir Dis. 1990 Oct;142(4):863-71.
12. Djukanovic R, Roche WR, Wilson JW, Beasley CR, Twentyman OP, Howarth

RH, et al. Mucosal inflammation in asthma. Am Rev Respir Dis. 1990 Aug;142(2):434-57.

13. Jeffery PK, Wardlaw AJ, Nelson FC, Collins JV, Kay AB. Bronchial biopsies in asthma. An ultrastructural, quantitative study and correlation with hyperreactivity. Am Rev Respir Dis. 1989 Dec;140(6):1745-53.

14. Roche WR, Beasley R, Williams JH, Holgate ST. Subepithelial fibrosis in the bronchi of asthmatics. Lancet. 1989 Mar 11;1(8637):520-4.

15. Aalbers R, Kauffman HF, Vrugt B, Koeter GH, de Monchy JG. Allergen-induced recruitment of inflammatory cells in lavage 3 and 24 h after challenge in allergic asthmatic lungs. Chest. 1993 Apr;103(4):1178-84.

16. Bentley AM, Meng Q, Robinson DS, Hamid Q, Kay AB, Durham SR. Increases in activated T lymphocytes, eosinophils, and cytokine mRNA expression for interleukin-5 and granulocyte/macrophage colony-stimulating factor in bronchial biopsies after allergen inhalation challenge in atopic asthmatics. Am J Respir Cell Mol Biol. 1993 Jan;8(1):35-42.

17. Montefort S, Gratziou C, Goulding D, Polosa R, Haskard DO, Howarth PH, et al. Bronchial biopsy evidence for leukocyte infiltration and upregulation of leukocyte-endothelial cell adhesion molecules 6 hours after local allergen challenge of sensitized asthmatic airways. J Clin Invest. 1994 Apr;93(4):1411-21.

18. Paggiaro P, Bacci E, Paoletti P, Bernard P, Dente FL, Marchetti G, et al. Bronchoalveolar lavage and morphology of the airways after cessation of exposure in asthmatic subjects sensitized to toluene diisocyanate. Chest. 1990 Sep;98(3):536-42.

19. Frew AJ, St-Pierre J, Teran LM, Trefilieff A, Madden J, Peroni D, et al. Cellular and mediator responses twenty-four hours after local endobronchial allergen challenge of asthmatic airways. J Allergy Clin Immunol. 1996 Jul;98(1):133-43.

20. Chanez P, Bourdin A, Vachier I, Godard P, Bousquet J, Vignola AM. Effects of inhaled corticosteroids on pathology in asthma and chronic obstructive pulmonary disease. Proc Am Thorac Soc. 2004;1(3):184-90.

21. Howarth PH, Beckett P, Dahl R. The effect of long-acting beta2-agonists on airway inflammation in asthmatic patients. Respir Med. 2000 Oct;94 Suppl F:S22-5.

22. Laitinen LA, Laitinen A, Haahtela T. A comparative study of the effects of an inhaled corticosteroid, budesonide, and a beta 2-agonist, terbutaline, on airway inflammation in newly diagnosed asthma: a randomized, double-blind, parallel-group controlled trial. J Allergy Clin Immunol. 1992 Jul;90(1):32-42.

23. Di Stefano A, Turato G, Maestrelli P, Mapp CE, Ruggieri MP, Roggeri A, et al. Airflow limitation in chronic bronchitis is associated with T-lymphocyte and macrophage infiltration of the bronchial mucosa. Am J Respir Crit Care Med. 1996 Feb;153(2):629-32.

24. Saetta M, Di Stefano A, Maestrelli P, Ferraresso A, Drigo R, Potena A, et al. Activated T-lymphocytes and macrophages in bronchial mucosa of subjects with chronic bronchitis. Am Rev Respir Dis. 1993 Feb;147(2):301-6.

25. O'Shaughnessy TC, Ansari TW, Barnes NC, Jeffery PK. Inflammation in bronchial biopsies of subjects with chronic bronchitis: inverse relationship of CD8+ T lymphocytes with FEV1. Am J Respir Crit Care Med. 1997 Mar;155(3):852-7.

26. Di Stefano A, Caramori G, Ricciardolo FL, Capelli A, Adcock IM, Donner CF. Cellular and molecular mechanisms in chronic obstructive pulmonary disease: an overview. Clin Exp Allergy. 2004 Aug;34(8):1156-67.

27. Di Stefano A, Caramori G, Oates T, Capelli A, Lusuardi M, Gnemmi I, et al. Increased expression of nuclear factor-kappaB in bronchial biopsies from smokers and patients with COPD. Eur Respir J. 2002 Sep;20(3):556-63.

28. Lams BE, Sousa AR, Rees PJ, Lee TH. Subepithelial immunopathology of the large airways in smokers with and without chronic obstructive pulmonary disease. Eur Respir J. 2000 Mar;15(3):512-6.

29. Bergeron C, Tulic MK, Hamid Q. Tools used to measure airway remodelling in research. Eur Respir J. 2007 Mar;29(3):596-604.

30. Saetta M, Ghezzo H, Kim WD, King M, Angus GE, Wang NS, et al. Loss of alveolar attachments in smokers. A morphometric correlate of lung function impairment. Am Rev Respir Dis. 1985 Oct;132(4):894-900.

31. Barnes NC, Qiu YS, Pavord ID, Parker D, Davis PA, Zhu J, et al. Antiinflammatory effects of salmeterol/fluticasone propionate in chronic obstructive lung disease. Am J Respir Crit Care Med. 2006 Apr 1;173(7):736-43.

32. Gamble E, Grootendorst DC, Brightling CE, Troy S, Qiu Y, Zhu J, et al. Antiinflammatory effects of the phosphodiesterase-4 inhibitor cilomilast (Ariflo) in chronic obstructive pulmonary disease. Am J Respir Crit Care Med. 2003 Oct 15;168(8):976-82.

33. Cohn L, Elias JA, Chupp GL. Asthma: mechanisms of disease persistence and progression. Annu Rev Immunol. 2004;22:789-815.

34. Robinson DS, Hamid Q, Ying S, Tsicopoulos A, Barkans J, Bentley AM, et al. Predominant TH2-like bronchoalveolar T-lymphocyte population in atopic asthma. N Engl J Med. 1992 Jan 30;326(5):298-304.

35. Boulet LP, Sterk PJ. Airway remodelling: the future. Eur Respir J. 2007 Nov;30(5):831-4.

36. Mauad T, Bel EH, Sterk PJ. Asthma therapy and airway remodeling. J Allergy Clin Immunol. 2007 Nov;120(5):997-1009; quiz 10-1.

37. Pascual RM, Peters SP. Airway remodeling contributes to the progressive loss of lung function in asthma: an overview. J Allergy Clin Immunol. 2005 Sep;116(3):477-86; quiz 87.

38. Gaga M. Fixed obstruction in severe asthma: not just a matter of time. Eur Respir J. 2004 Jul;24(1):8-10.

39. Pepe C, Foley S, Shannon J, Lemiere C, Olivenstein R, Ernst P, et al. Differences in airway remodeling between subjects with severe and moderate asthma. J Allergy Clin Immunol. 2005 Sep;116(3):544-9.

40. Davies DE, Wicks J, Powell RM, Puddicombe SM, Holgate ST. Airway remodeling in asthma: new insights. J Allergy Clin Immunol. 2003 Feb;111(2):215-25; quiz 26.

41. Vignola AM, Kips J, Bousquet J. Tissue remodeling as a feature of persis-

tent asthma. J Allergy Clin Immunol. 2000 Jun;105(6 Pt 1):1041-53.

42. Chu HW, Halliday JL, Martin RJ, Leung DY, Szefler SJ, Wenzel SE. Collagen deposition in large airways may not differentiate severe asthma from milder forms of the disease. Am J Respir Crit Care Med. 1998 Dec;158(6):1936-44.

43. Beasley R, Roche WR, Roberts JA, Holgate ST. Cellular events in the bronchi in mild asthma and after bronchial provocation. Am Rev Respir Dis. 1989 Mar;139(3):806-17.

44. van Rensen EL, Evertse CE, van Schadewijk WA, van Wijngaarden S, Ayre G, Mauad T, et al. Eosinophils in bronchial mucosa of asthmatics after allergen challenge: effect of anti-IgE treatment. Allergy. 2009 Jan;64(1): 72-80.

45. Macfarlane AJ, Kon OM, Smith SJ, Zeibecoglou K, Khan LN, Barata LT, et al. Basophils, eosinophils, and mast cells in atopic and nonatopic asthma and in late-phase allergic reactions in the lung and skin. J Allergy Clin Immunol. 2000 Jan;105(1 Pt 1):99-107.

46. Cruz AA, Popov T, Pawankar R, Annesi-Maesano I, Fokkens W, Kemp J, et al. Common characteristics of upper and lower airways in rhinitis and asthma: ARIA update, in collaboration with GA(2)LEN. Allergy. 2007;62 Suppl 84:1-41.

47. Djukanovic R, Wilson SJ, Howarth PH. Pathology of rhinitis and bronchial asthma. Clin Exp Allergy. 1996 May;26 Suppl 3:44-51.

48. Gaga M, Lambrou P, Papageorgiou N, Koulouris NG, Kosmas E, Fragakis S, et al. Eosinophils are a feature of upper and lower airway pathology in non-atopic asthma, irrespective of the presence of rhinitis. Clin Exp Allergy. 2000 May;30(5):663-9.

49. Kariyawasam HH, Aizen M, Barkans J, Robinson DS, Kay AB. Remodeling and airway hyperresponsiveness but not cellular inflammation persist after allergen challenge in asthma. Am J Respir Crit Care Med. 2007 May 1;175(9):896-904.

50. Humbert M, Durham SR, Ying S, Kimmitt P, Barkans J, Assoufi B, et al. IL-4 and IL-5 mRNA and protein in bronchial biopsies from patients with atopic and nonatopic asthma: evidence against "intrinsic" asthma being a distinct immunopathologic entity. Am J Respir Crit Care Med. 1996 Nov;154(5):1497-504.

51. Ying S, Humbert M, Meng Q, Pfister R, Menz G, Gould HJ, et al. Local expression of epsilon germline gene transcripts and RNA for the epsilon heavy chain of IgE in the bronchial mucosa in atopic and nonatopic asthma. J Allergy Clin Immunol. 2001 Apr;107(4):686-92.

52. Pavord ID, Jeffery PK, Qiu Y, Zhu J, Parker D, Carlsheimer A, et al. Airway inflammation in patients with asthma with high-fixed or low-fixed plus as-needed budesonide/formoterol. J Allergy Clin Immunol. 2009 May;123(5): 1083-9, 9 e1-7.

53. Jarjour NN, Wilson SJ, Koenig SM, Laviolette M, Moore WC, Davis WB, et al. Control of airway inflammation maintained at a lower steroid dose with 100/50 microg of fluticasone propionate/salmeterol. J Allergy Clin Immunol. 2006 Jul;118(1):44-52.

54. Flood-Page P, Menzies-Gow A, Phipps S, Ying S, Wangoo A, Ludwig

MS, et al. Anti-IL-5 treatment reduces deposition of ECM proteins in the bronchial subepithelial basement membrane of mild atopic asthmatics. J Clin Invest. 2003 Oct;112(7):1029-36.

55. Wenzel SE, Schwartz LB, Langmack EL, Halliday JL, Trudeau JB, Gibbs RL, et al. Evidence that severe asthma can be divided pathologically into two inflammatory subtypes with distinct physiologic and clinical characteristics. Am J Respir Crit Care Med. 1999 Sep;160(3):1001-8.

56. Chanez P, Wenzel SE, Anderson GP, Anto JM, Bel EH, Boulet LP, et al. Severe asthma in adults: what are the important questions? J Allergy Clin Immunol. 2007 Jun;119(6):1337-48.

57. Chung KF, Godard P, Adelroth E, Ayres J, Barnes N, Barnes P, et al. Difficult/therapy-resistant asthma: the need for an integrated approach to define clinical phenotypes, evaluate risk factors, understand pathophysiology and find novel therapies. ERS Task Force on Difficult/Therapy-Resistant Asthma. European Respiratory Society. Eur Respir J. 1999 May;13(5): 1198-208.

58. Baraldo S, Turato G, Badin C, Bazzan E, Beghe B, Zuin R, et al. Neutrophilic infiltration within the airway smooth muscle in patients with COPD. Thorax. 2004 Apr;59(4):308-12.

59. Maestrelli P, Saetta M, Mapp CE, Fabbri LM. Remodeling in response to infection and injury. Airway inflammation and hypersecretion of mucus in smoking subjects with chronic obstructive pulmonary disease. Am J Respir Crit Care Med. 2001 Nov 15; 164(10 Pt 2):S76-80.

60. Saetta M, Di Stefano A, Turato G, Facchini FM, Corbino L, Mapp CE, et al. CD8+ T-lymphocytes in peripheral airways of smokers with chronic obstructive pulmonary disease. Am J Respir Crit Care Med. 1998 Mar;157 (3 Pt 1):822-6.

61. Saetta M, Turato G, Maestrelli P, Mapp CE, Fabbri LM. Cellular and structural bases of chronic obstructive pulmonary disease. Am J Respir Crit Care Med. 2001 May;163(6):1304-9.

62. Snoeck-Stroband JB, Lapperre TS, Gosman MM, Boezen HM, Timens W, ten Hacken NH, et al. Chronic bronchitis sub-phenotype within COPD: inflammation in sputum and biopsies. Eur Respir J. 2008 Jan;31(1):70-7.

63. Gamble E, Grootendorst DC, Hattotuwa K, O'Shaughnessy T, Ram FS, Qiu Y, et al. Airway mucosal inflammation in COPD is similar in smokers and ex-smokers: a pooled analysis. Eur Respir J. 2007 Sep;30(3):467-71.

64. Panina-Bordignon P, Papi A, Mariani M, Di Lucia P, Casoni G, Bellettato C, et al. The C-C chemokine receptors C-CR4 and CCR8 identify airway T cells of allergen-challenged atopic asthmatics. J Clin Invest. 2001 Jun;107(11): 1357-64.

65. Saetta M, Mariani M, Panina-Bordignon P, Turato G, Buonsanti C, Baraldo S, et al. Increased expression of the chemokine receptor CXCR3 and its ligand CXCL10 in peripheral airways of smokers with chronic obstructive pulmonary disease. Am J Respir Crit Care Med. 2002 May 15; 165(10):1404-9.

66. Loetscher P, Uguccioni M, Bordoli L, Baggiolini M, Moser B, Chizzolini C, et al. CCR5 is characteristic of Th1 lym-

phocytes. Nature. 1998 Jan 22;391 (6665):344-5.

67. Qin S, Rottman JB, Myers P, Kassam N, Weinblatt M, Loetscher M, et al. The chemokine receptors CXCR3 and CCR5 mark subsets of T cells associated with certain inflammatory reactions. J Clin Invest. 1998 Feb 15; 101(4): 746-54.

68. Fabbri LM, Romagnoli M, Corbetta L, Casoni G, Busljetic K, Turato G, et al. Differences in airway inflammation in patients with fixed airflow obstruction due to asthma or chronic obstructive pulmonary disease. Am J Respir Crit Care Med. 2003 Feb 1;167(3):418-24.

69. Saetta M, Turato G, Baraldo S, Zanin A, Braccioni F, Mapp CE, et al. Goblet cell hyperplasia and epithelial inflammation in peripheral airways of smokers with both symptoms of chronic bronchitis and chronic airflow limitation. Am J Respir Crit Care Med. 2000 Mar;161(3 Pt 1):1016-21.

70. Bosken CH, Wiggs BR, Pare PD, Hogg JC. Small airway dimensions in smokers with obstruction to airflow. Am Rev Respir Dis. 1990 Sep;142(3): 563-70.

71. Lambert RK, Wiggs BR, Kuwano K, Hogg JC, Pare PD. Functional significance of increased airway smooth muscle in asthma and COPD. J Appl Physiol. 1993 Jun;74(6):2771-81.

72. Casadevall C, Coronell C, Ramirez-Sarmiento AL, Martinez-Llorens J, Barreiro E, Orozco-Levi M, et al. Up-regulation of pro-inflammatory cytokines in the intercostal muscles of COPD patients. Eur Respir J. 2007 Oct;30(4):701-7.

73. Barreiro E, Schols AM, Polkey MI, Galdiz JB, Gosker HR, Swallow EB, et al. Cytokine profile in quadriceps muscles of patients with severe COPD. Thorax. 2008 Feb;63(2):100-7.

74. Dinh-Xuan AT, Higenbottam TW, Clelland CA, Pepke-Zaba J, Cremona G, Butt AY, et al. Impairment of endothelium-dependent pulmonary-artery relaxation in chronic obstructive lung disease. N Engl J Med. 1991 May 30;324(22):1539-47.

75. Peinado VI, Barbera JA, Abate P, Ramirez J, Roca J, Santos S, et al. Inflammatory reaction in pulmonary muscular arteries of patients with mild chronic obstructive pulmonary disease. Am J Respir Crit Care Med. 1999 May;159(5 Pt 1):1605-11.

76. Magee F, Wright JL, Wiggs BR, Pare PD, Hogg JC. Pulmonary vascular structure and function in chronic obstructive pulmonary disease. Thorax. 1988 Mar;43(3):183-9.

77. Santos S, Peinado VI, Ramirez J, Melgosa T, Roca J, Rodriguez-Roisin R, et al. Characterization of pulmonary vascular remodelling in smokers and patients with mild COPD. Eur Respir J. 2002 Apr;19(4):632-8.

78. Jeffery PK. Remodeling in asthma and chronic obstructive lung disease. Am J Respir Crit Care Med. 2001 Nov 15;164(10 Pt 2):S28-38.

79. Kranenburg AR, de Boer WI, Alagappan VK, Sterk PJ, Sharma HS. Enhanced bronchial expression of vascular endothelial growth factor and receptors (Flk-1 and Flt-1) in patients with chronic obstructive pulmonary disease. Thorax. 2005 Feb;60(2):106-13.

80. Santos S, Peinado VI, Ramirez J, Morales-Blanhir J, Bastos R, Roca J, et al. Enhanced expression of vascular

endothelial growth factor in pulmonary arteries of smokers and patients with moderate chronic obstructive pulmonary disease. Am J Respir Crit Care Med. 2003 May 1;167(9):1250-6.

81. Agusti A. Systemic effects of chronic obstructive pulmonary disease: what we know and what we don't know (but should). Proc Am Thorac Soc. 2007 Oct 1;4(7):522-5.

82. Pavord ID, Pizzichini MM, Pizzichini E, Hargreave FE. The use of induced sputum to investigate airway inflammation. Thorax. 1997 Jun;52(6):498-501.

83. Efthimiadis A, Spanevello A, Hamid Q, Kelly MM, Linden M, Louis R, et al. Methods of sputum processing for cell counts, immunocytochemistry and in situ hybridisation. Eur Respir J Suppl. 2002 Sep;37:19s-23s.

84. Belda J, Leigh R, Parameswaran K, O'Byrne PM, Sears MR, Hargreave FE. Induced sputum cell counts in healthy adults. Am J Respir Crit Care Med. 2000 Feb;161(2 Pt 1):475-8.

85. Green RH, Brightling CE, McKenna S, Hargadon B, Parker D, Bradding P, et al. Asthma exacerbations and sputum eosinophil counts: a randomised controlled trial. Lancet. 2002 Nov 30;360(9347):1715-21.

86. Petsky HL, Kynaston JA, Turner C, Li AM, Cates CJ, Lasserson TJ, et al. Tailored interventions based on sputum eosinophils versus clinical symptoms for asthma in children and adults. Cochrane Database Syst Rev. 2007(2):CD005603.

87. Louis R, Lau LC, Bron AO, Roldaan AC, Radermecker M, Djukanovic R. The relationship between airways inflammation and asthma severity. Am J Respir Crit Care Med. 2000 Jan; 161(1):9-16.

88. ten Brinke A, Zwinderman AH, Sterk PJ, Rabe KF, Bel EH. Factors associated with persistent airflow limitation in severe asthma. Am J Respir Crit Care Med. 2001 Sep 1;164(5):744-8.

89. Grootendorst DC, Sont JK, Willems LN, Kluin-Nelemans JC, Van Krieken JH, Veselic-Charvat M, et al. Comparison of inflammatory cell counts in asthma: induced sputum vs bronchoalveolar lavage and bronchial biopsies. Clin Exp Allergy. 1997 Jul;27(7): 769-79.

90. Kim CK, Hagan JB. Sputum tests in the diagnosis and monitoring of asthma. Ann Allergy Asthma Immunol. 2004 Aug;93(2):112-22; quiz 22-4, 84.

91. Silkoff PE, Trudeau JB, Gibbs R, Wenzel S. The relationship of induced-sputum inflammatory cells to BAL and biopsy. Chest. 2003 Mar;123(3 Suppl):371S-2S.

92. Lemiere C, Ernst P, Olivenstein R, Yamauchi Y, Govindaraju K, Ludwig MS, et al. Airway inflammation assessed by invasive and noninvasive means in severe asthma: eosinophilic and noneosinophilic phenotypes. J Allergy Clin Immunol. 2006Nov;118(5):1033-9.

93. Peleman RA, Rytila PH, Kips JC, Joos GF, Pauwels RA. The cellular composition of induced sputum in chronic obstructive pulmonary disease. Eur Respir J. 1999 Apr;13(4):839-43.

94. Barnes PJ, Chowdhury B, Kharitonov SA, Magnussen H, Page CP, Postma D, et al. Pulmonary biomarkers in chronic obstructive pulmonary disease. Am J Respir Crit Care Med. 2006 Jul 1;174(1):6-14.

95. Tzanakis N, Chrysofakis G, Tsoumakidou M, Kyriakou D, Tsiligianni J, Bouros D, et al. Induced sputum CD8+ T-lymphocyte subpopulations in chronic obstructive pulmonary disease. Respir Med. 2004 Jan;98(1): 57-65.

96. Brightling CE, Monteiro W, Ward R, Parker D, Morgan MD, Wardlaw AJ, et al. Sputum eosinophilia and short-term response to prednisolone in chronic obstructive pulmonary disease: a randomised controlled trial. Lancet. 2000 Oct 28;356(9240): 1480-5.

97. Papi A, Romagnoli M, Baraldo S, Braccioni F, Guzzinati I, Saetta M, et al. Partial reversibility of airflow limitation and increased exhaled NO and sputum eosinophilia in chronic obstructive pulmonary disease. Am J Respir Crit Care Med. 2000 Nov; 162(5): 1773-7.

98. Brightling CE, McKenna S, Hargadon B, Birring S, Green R, Siva R, et al. Sputum eosinophilia and the short term response to inhaled mometasone in chronic obstructive pulmonary disease. Thorax. 2005 Mar; 60(3):193-8.

99. Culpitt SV, Maziak W, Loukidis S, Nightingale JA, Matthews JL, Barnes PJ. Effect of high dose inhaled steroid on cells, cytokines, and proteases in induced sputum in chronic obstructive pulmonary disease. Am J Respir Crit Care Med. 1999 Nov;160(5 Pt 1):1635-9.

100. Culpitt SV, de Matos C, Russell RE, Donnelly LE, Rogers DF, Barnes PJ. Effect of theophylline on induced sputum inflammatory indices and neutrophil chemotaxis in chronic obstructive pulmonary disease. Am J Respir Crit Care Med. 2002 May 15;165(10):1371-6.

101. Perng DW, Tao CW, Su KC, Tsai CC, Liu LY, Lee YC. Anti-inflammatory effects of salmeterol/fluticasone, tiotropium/fluticasone or tiotropium in COPD. Eur Respir J. 2009 Apr;33(4):778-84.

102. Rutgers SR, Timens W, Kaufmann HF, van der Mark TW, Koeter GH, Postma DS. Comparison of induced sputum with bronchial wash, bronchoalveolar lavage and bronchial biopsies in COPD. Eur Respir J. 2000 Jan;15(1):109-15.

103. Kelly MM, Keatings V, Leigh R, Peterson C, Shute J, Venge P, et al. Analysis of fluid-phase mediators. Eur Respir J Suppl. 2002 Sep;37:24s-39s.

104. Kips JC, Inman MD, Jayaram L, Bel EH, Parameswaran K, Pizzichini MM, et al. The use of induced sputum in clinical trials. Eur Respir J Suppl. 2002 Sep;37:47s-50s.

105. Kharitonov SA, Barnes PJ. Exhaled markers of pulmonary disease. Am J Respir Crit Care Med. 2001 Jun;163(7):1693-722.

106. Olin AC, Bake B, Toren K. Fraction of exhaled nitric oxide at 50 mL/s: reference values for adult lifelong never-smokers. Chest. 2007 Jun;131(6): 1852-6.

107. Travers J, Marsh S, Aldington S, Williams M, Shirtcliffe P, Pritchard A, et al. Reference ranges for exhaled nitric oxide derived from a random community survey of adults. Am J Respir Crit Care Med. 2007 Aug 1;176(3):238-42.

108. ATS/ERS recommendations for stan-

dardized procedures for the online and offline measurement of exhaled lower respiratory nitric oxide and nasal nitric oxide, 2005. Am J Respir Crit Care Med. 2005 Apr 15;171(8): 912-30.

109. Kharitonov SA, Yates D, Robbins RA, Logan-Sinclair R, Shinebourne EA, Barnes PJ. Increased nitric oxide in exhaled air of asthmatic patients. Lancet. 1994 Jan 15;343(8890): 133-5.

110. Smith AD, Cowan JO, Filsell S, McLachlan C, Monti-Sheehan G, Jackson P, et al. Diagnosing asthma: comparisons between exhaled nitric oxide measurements and conventional tests. Am J Respir Crit Care Med. 2004 Feb 15;169(4):473-8.

111. Kostikas K, Papaioannou AI, Tanou K, Koutsokera A, Papala M, Gourgoulianis KI. Portable exhaled nitric oxide as a screening tool for asthma in young adults during pollen season. Chest. 2008 Apr;133(4): 906-13.

112. Moeller A, Diefenbacher C, Lehmann A, Rochat M, Brooks-Wildhaber J, Hall GL, et al. Exhaled nitric oxide distinguishes between subgroups of preschool children with respiratory symptoms. J Allergy Clin Immunol. 2008 Mar;121(3):705-9.

113. Moore WC, Bleecker ER, Curran-Everett D, Erzurum SC, Ameredes BT, Bacharier L, et al. Characterization of the severe asthma phenotype by the National Heart, Lung, and Blood Institute's Severe Asthma Research Program. J Allergy Clin Immunol. 2007 Feb;119(2):405-13.

114. Silkoff PE, Lent AM, Busacker AA, Katial RK, Balzar S, Strand M, et al.

Exhaled nitric oxide identifies the persistent eosinophilic phenotype in severe refractory asthma. J Allergy Clin Immunol. 2005 Dec;116(6): 1249-55.

115. Kharitonov SA, Yates DH, Barnes PJ. Inhaled glucocorticoids decrease nitric oxide in exhaled air of asthmatic patients. Am J Respir Crit Care Med. 1996 Jan;153(1):454-7.

116. Montuschi P, Mondino C, Koch P, Ciabattoni G, Barnes PJ, Baviera G. Effects of montelukast treatment and withdrawal on fractional exhaled nitric oxide and lung function in children with asthma. Chest. 2007 Dec;132(6):1876-81.

117. Pijnenburg MW, Bakker EM, Hop WC, De Jongste JC. Titrating steroids on exhaled nitric oxide in children with asthma: a randomized controlled trial. Am J Respir Crit Care Med. 2005 Oct 1;172(7):831-6.

118. Smith AD, Cowan JO, Brassett KP, Herbison GP, Taylor DR. Use of exhaled nitric oxide measurements to guide treatment in chronic asthma. N Engl J Med. 2005 May 26;352(21): 2163-73.

119. Szefler SJ, Mitchell H, Sorkness CA, Gergen PJ, O'Connor GT, Morgan WJ, et al. Management of asthma based on exhaled nitric oxide in addition to guideline-based treatment for inner-city adolescents and young adults: a randomised controlled trial. Lancet. 2008 Sep 20;372(9643): 1065-72.

120. Shaw DE, Berry MA, Thomas M, Green RH, Brightling CE, Wardlaw AJ, et al. The use of exhaled nitric oxide to guide asthma management: a randomized controlled trial. Am J

Respir Crit Care Med. 2007 Aug 1;176(3):231-7.

121. Turktas H, Oguzulgen K, Kokturk N, Memis L, Erbas D. Correlation of exhaled nitric oxide levels and airway inflammation markers in stable asthmatic patients. J Asthma. 2003 Jun;40(4):425-30.

122. Lim S, Jatakanon A, Meah S, Oates T, Chung KF, Barnes PJ. Relationship between exhaled nitric oxide and mucosal eosinophilic inflammation in mild to moderately severe asthma. Thorax. 2000 Mar;55(3):184-8.

123. Agusti AG, Villaverde JM, Togores B, Bosch M. Serial measurements of exhaled nitric oxide during exacerbations of chronic obstructive pulmonary disease. Eur Respir J. 1999 Sep;14(3):523-8.

124. Rutgers SR, Meijer RJ, Kerstjens HA, van der Mark TW, Koeter GH, Postma DS. Nitric oxide measured with single-breath and tidal-breathing methods in asthma and COPD. Eur Respir J. 1998 Oct;12(4):816-9.

125. Maziak W, Loukides S, Culpitt S, Sullivan P, Kharitonov SA, Barnes PJ. Exhaled nitric oxide in chronic obstructive pulmonary disease. Am J Respir Crit Care Med. 1998 Mar;157(3 Pt 1):998-1002.

126. Kharitonov SA, Robbins RA, Yates D, Keatings V, Barnes PJ. Acute and chronic effects of cigarette smoking on exhaled nitric oxide. Am J Respir Crit Care Med. 1995 Aug;152(2):609-12.

127. Horvath I, Hunt J, Barnes PJ, Alving K, Antczak A, Baraldi E, et al. Exhaled breath condensate: methodological recommendations and unresolved questions. Eur Respir J. 2005 Sep;26(3):523-48.

128. Koutsokera A, Loukides S, Gourgoulianis KI, Kostikas K. Biomarkers in the exhaled breath condensate of healthy adults: mapping the path towards reference values. Curr Med Chem. 2008;15(6):620-30.

129. Kostikas K, Koutsokera A, Papiris S, Gourgoulianis KI, Loukides S. Exhaled breath condensate in patients with asthma: implications for application in clinical practice. Clin Exp Allergy. 2008 Apr;38(4):557-65.

130. Antczak A, Montuschi P, Kharitonov S, Gorski P, Barnes PJ. Increased exhaled cysteinyl-leukotrienes and 8-isoprostane in aspirin-induced asthma. Am J Respir Crit Care Med. 2002 Aug 1;166(3):301-6.

131. Samitas K, Chorianopoulos D, Vittorakis S, Zervas E, Economidou E, Papatheodorou G, et al. Exhaled cysteinyl-leukotrienes and 8-isoprostane in patients with asthma and their relation to clinical severity. Respir Med. 2009 May;103(5):750-6.

132. Ono E, Mita H, Taniguchi M, Higashi N, Tsuburai T, Hasegawa M, et al. Increase in inflammatory mediator concentrations in exhaled breath condensate after allergen inhalation. J Allergy Clin Immunol. 2008 Oct;122(4):768-73 e1.

133. Baraldi E, Carraro S, Alinovi R, Pesci A, Ghiro L, Bodini A, et al. Cysteinyl leukotrienes and 8-isoprostane in exhaled breath condensate of children with asthma exacerbations. Thorax. 2003 Jun;58(6):505-9.

134. Lex C, Zacharasiewicz A, Payne DN, Wilson NM, Nicholson AG,

Kharitonov SA, et al. Exhaled breath condensate cysteinyl leukotrienes and airway remodeling in childhood asthma: a pilot study. Respir Res. 2006;7:63.

135. Montuschi P, Corradi M, Ciabattoni G, Nightingale J, Kharitonov SA, Barnes PJ. Increased 8-isoprostane, a marker of oxidative stress, in exhaled condensate of asthma patients. Am J Respir Crit Care Med. 1999 Jul;160(1):216-20.

136. Borrill ZL, Roy K, Singh D. Exhaled breath condensate biomarkers in COPD. Eur Respir J. 2008 Aug;32(2):472-86.

137. Montuschi P, Collins JV, Ciabattoni G, Lazzeri N, Corradi M, Kharitonov SA, et al. Exhaled 8-isoprostane as an in vivo biomarker of lung oxidative stress in patients with COPD and healthy smokers. Am J Respir Crit Care Med. 2000 Sep;162(3 Pt 1):1175-7.

138. Loukides S, Bouros D, Papatheodorou G, Panagou P, Siafakas NM. The relationships among hydrogen peroxide in expired breath condensate, airway inflammation, and asthma severity. Chest. 2002 Feb;121(2):338-46.

139. Biernacki WA, Kharitonov SA, Barnes PJ. Increased leukotriene B4 and 8-isoprostane in exhaled breath condensate of patients with exacerbations of COPD. Thorax. 2003 Apr;58(4):294-8.

140. Kostikas K, Papatheodorou G, Psathakis K, Panagou P, Loukides S. Oxidative stress in expired breath condensate of patients with COPD. Chest. 2003 Oct;124(4):1373-80.

141. Borrill Z, Starkey C, Vestbo J, Singh D. Reproducibility of exhaled breath condensate pH in chronic obstructive pulmonary disease. Eur Respir J. 2005 Feb;25(2):269-74.

142. Kostikas K, Papatheodorou G, Ganas K, Psathakis K, Panagou P, Loukides S. pH in expired breath condensate of patients with inflammatory airway diseases. Am J Respir Crit Care Med. 2002 May 15;165(10):1364-70.

143. Jackson AS, Sandrini A, Campbell C, Chow S, Thomas PS, Yates DH. Comparison of biomarkers in exhaled breath condensate and bronchoalveolar lavage. Am J Respir Crit Care Med. 2007 Feb 1;175(3):222-7.

144. Joos GF, O'Connor B, Anderson SD, Chung F, Cockcroft DW, Dahlen B, et al. Indirect airway challenges. Eur Respir J. 2003 Jun;21(6):1050-68.

145. Crapo RO, Casaburi R, Coates AL, Enright PL, Hankinson JL, Irvin CG, et al. Guidelines for methacholine and exercise challenge testing-1999. This official statement of the American Thoracic Society was adopted by the ATS Board of Directors, July 1999. Am J Respir Crit Care Med. 2000 Jan;161(1):309-29.

146. Hargreave FE, O'Byrne PM, Ramsdale EH. Mediators, airway responsiveness, and asthma. J Allergy Clin Immunol. 1985 Aug;76(2 Pt 2):272-6.

147. Leuppi JD, Salome CM, Jenkins CR, Anderson SD, Xuan W, Marks GB, et al. Predictive markers of asthma exacerbation during stepwise dose reduction of inhaled corticosteroids. Am J Respir Crit Care Med. 2001 Feb;163(2):406-12.

148. Nuijsink M, Hop WC, Sterk PJ, Duiverman EJ, de Jongste JC. Long-

term asthma treatment guided by airway hyperresponsiveness in children: a randomised controlled trial. Eur Respir J. 2007 Sep;30(3):457-66.

149. Sont JK, Willems LN, Bel EH, van Krieken JH, Vandenbroucke JP, Sterk PJ. Clinical control and histopathologic outcome of asthma when using airway hyperresponsiveness as an additional guide to long-term treatment. The AMPUL Study Group. Am J Respir Crit Care Med. 1999 Apr;159(4 Pt 1):1043-51.

150. Van Schoor J, Joos GF, Pauwels RA. Indirect bronchial hyperresponsiveness in asthma: mechanisms, pharmacology and implications for clinical research. Eur Respir J. 2000 Sep;16(3):514-33.

151. Ludviksdottir D, Janson C, Bjornsson E, Stalenheim G, Boman G, Hedenstrom H, et al. Different airway responsiveness profiles in atopic asthma, nonatopic asthma, and Sjogren's syndrome. BHR Study Group. Bronchial hyperresponsiveness. Allergy. 2000 Mar;55(3):259-65.

152. Prosperini G, Rajakulasingam K, Cacciola RR, Spicuzza L, Rorke S, Holgate ST, et al. Changes in sputum counts and airway hyperresponsiveness after budesonide: monitoring anti-inflammatory response on the basis of surrogate markers of airway inflammation. J Allergy Clin Immunol. 2002 Dec;110(6):855-61.

153. Chetta A, Foresi A, Del Donno M, Consigli GF, Bertorelli G, Pesci A, et al. Bronchial responsiveness to distilled water and methacholine and its relationship to inflammation and remodeling of the airways in asthma.

Am J Respir Crit Care Med. 1996 Mar;153(3):910-7.

154. Ward C, Pais M, Bish R, Reid D, Feltis B, Johns D, et al. Airway inflammation, basement membrane thickening and bronchial hyperresponsiveness in asthma. Thorax. 2002 Apr;57(4):309-16.

155. Ali FR, Kay AB, Larche M. Airway hyperresponsiveness and bronchial mucosal inflammation in T cell peptide-induced asthmatic reactions in atopic subjects. Thorax. 2007 Sep;62(9):750-57.

156. Ward C, Reid DW, Orsida BE, Feltis B, Ryan VA, Johns DP, et al. Inter-relationships between airway inflammation, reticular basement membrane thickening and bronchial hyper-reactivity to methacholine in asthma; a systematic bronchoalveolar lavage and airway biopsy analysis. Clin Exp Allergy. 2005 Dec;35(12):1565-71.

157. Jansen DF, Timens W, Kraan J, Rijcken B, Postma DS. (A)symptomatic bronchial hyper-responsiveness and asthma. Respir Med. 1997 Mar;91(3):121-34.

158. Kolnaar BG, Folgering H, van den Hoogen HJ, van Weel C. Asymptomatic bronchial hyperresponsiveness in adolescents and young adults. Eur Respir J. 1997 Jan;10(1):44-50.

159. Kanner RE, Connett JE, Altose MD, Buist AS, Lee WW, Tashkin DP, et al. Gender difference in airway hyperresponsiveness in smokers with mild COPD. The Lung Health Study. Am J Respir Crit Care Med. 1994 Oct;150(4):956-61.

160. Brutsche MH, Downs SH, Schindler C, Gerbase MW, Schwartz J, Frey M,

et al. Bronchial hyperresponsiveness and the development of asthma and COPD in asymptomatic individuals: SAPALDIA cohort study. Thorax. 2006 Aug;61(8):671-7.

161. Xu X, Rijcken B, Schouten JP, Weiss ST. Airways responsiveness and development and remission of chronic respiratory symptoms in adults. Lancet. 1997 Nov 15;350(9089): 1431-4.

162. Tashkin DP, Altose MD, Connett JE, Kanner RE, Lee WW, Wise RA. Methacholine reactivity predicts changes in lung function over time in smokers with early chronic obstructive pulmonary disease. The Lung Health Study Research Group. Am J Respir Crit Care Med. 1996 Jun;153(6 Pt 1):1802-11.

163. Effect of inhaled triamcinolone on the decline in pulmonary function in chronic obstructive pulmonary disease. N Engl J Med. 2000 Dec 28;343(26):1902-9.

164. Burge PS, Calverley PM, Jones PW, Spencer S, Anderson JA. Prednisolone response in patients with chronic obstructive pulmonary disease: results from the ISOLDE study. Thorax. 2003 Aug;58(8):654-8.

165. Rutgers SR, Timens W, Tzanakis N, Kauffman HF, van der Mark TW, Koeter GH, et al. Airway inflammation and hyperresponsiveness to adenosine 5'-monophosphate in chronic obstructive pulmonary disease. Clin Exp Allergy. 2000 May; 30(5):657-62.

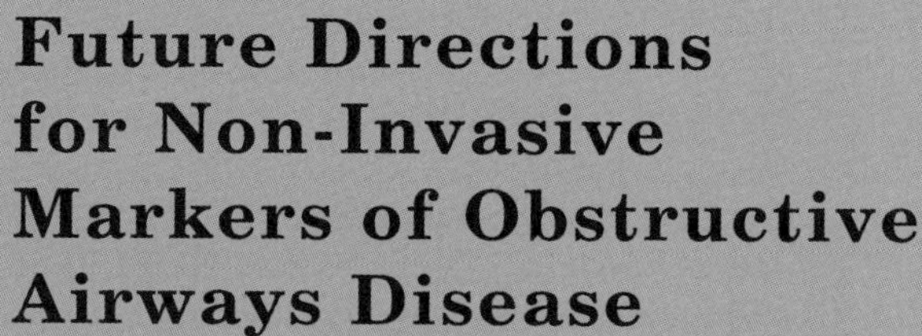

Future Directions for Non-Invasive Markers of Obstructive Airways Disease

Peter J. Barnes

Introduction

Inflammation plays a central role in the pathogenesis of asthma and COPD and underlies symptoms and exacerbations. Monitoring of inflammation ("inflammometry") has therefore become a growing area of research and this book brings together the current approaches to non-invasive monitoring. There is emerging evidence that inflammometry may improve clinical outcomes in carefully selected patients and it is likely that more sophisticated measurements will aid diagnosis and therapy even more in the future(1). Cluster analysis of patients with asthma shows that while most patients show a concordance between increased sputum eosinophils and increased sputum, there are groups of patients that have excessive symptoms compared to their eosinophil counts who

Correspondence

Prof. Peter J. Barnes

Airway Disease Section, National Heart and Lung Institute, Imperial College London, Dovehouse St, London SW3 6LY, UK
e-mail: p.j.barnes@imperial.ac.uk

tend to be overtreated, whereas other patients have increased sputum eosinophils and few symptoms indicating undertreatment (2) (Figure 1). It is likely that non-invasive measurements of inflammation are only going to be of added value in these patients

Induced Sputum

Induced sputum has provided important insights into the inflammatory mechanisms of asthma and COPD and there is now evidence that it may be useful in guiding therapy in both asthma and COPD.

Methodological issues

Sputum induction following nebulization of hypertonic saline is successful in many patients but may be not be used in asthmatic patients with FEV_1 <50% predicted, although it can be used safely in COPD patients with lower FEV_1 values (3). One problem with this approach is that the nebulized hypertonic saline itself induces a neutrophilic inflammation for at least 24h so cannot be repeated frequently (4, 5). Induced sputum gives reasonably reproducible cell differ-

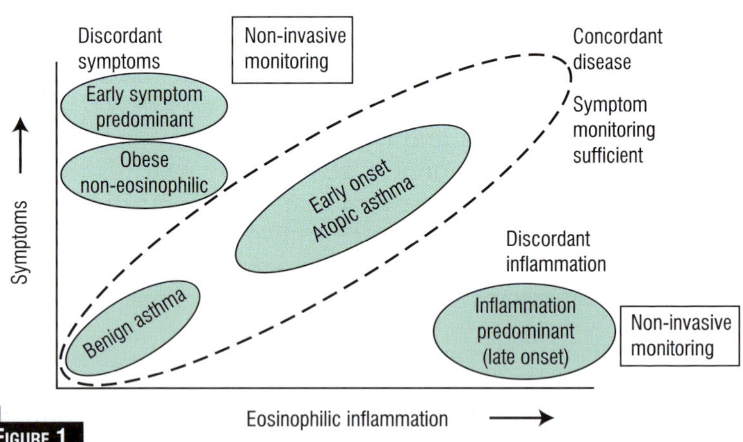

FIGURE 1

Cluster analysis of asthma patients indicating groups of patients who are over- and under-treated who may benefit from non-invasive monitoring of inflammation. Adapted after permission from reference 2.

ential counts, but there is usually a much greater variation in concentrations of mediators and proteases detected in the sol fluid. Many protein mediators may be undetectable as solubilisation of the sputum with dithiothreitol (DTT) cross-links cysteine residues so that many cytokines and chemokines cannot be recognised by conventional antibodies. It is possible to overcome this by ultracentrifugation to separate the sol phase, but this is very time consuming. An alternative approach is to dialyse the sputum sample after solubilisation to remove DTT and to use protease inhibitors and protein renaturing solutions to restore immunogenicity of proteins (6). This makes it possible to detect mediators that were previously unmeasurable. Development of more sensitive assays for proteins may also make it possible to detect more mediators and enzymes with a greater degree of certainly.

Clinical application

Use of induced sputum can be used to assess inflammation relatively non-invasively, but at the present time it is used mainly as a research tool. Sputum induction may be difficult in clinical practice because of the time needed for successful measurement and the high demand on the time of a skilled technician. However, a recent cost analysis study has shown that sputum induction may prove to be cost-effective in preventing exacerbations (7). However, research has now focussed on less invasive techniques, particularly those that could be used in patients with more severe disease and in children. Prospective assessment of sputum eosinophils has been convincingly shown to improve control of asthma and reduce exacerbations in patients with elevated sputum eosinophils and to achieve control at lower doses of inhaled corticosteroids, particularly in patients with more severe asthma (8, 9). Similar, but less convincing data, have been demonstrated in patients with COPD, where eosinophil counts have been used to assess the need for inhaled corticosteroids and to reduce severe exacerbations (10).

The recognition that some asthmatic patients have a predominantly neutrophilic rather than eosinophilic pattern of asthma may be important in highlighting the need for alternative anti-inflammatory treatments, since thee patients appear to be less responsive to corticosteroids than the eosinophil-predominant asthmatics (11, 12). New treatments that target neutrophilic inflammation are needed for these patients, although current therapies, such as long-acting $\beta2$-

agonists, appear to have anti-neutrophilic effects through inhibition of interleukin-8 (CXCL8) secretion from airway epithelial cells (13, 14). It does not appear to be possible to clinically distinguish asthmatic patients with neutrophilic inflammation from those with predominantly eosinophilic pattern of inflammation and the same patients may switch from one type of inflammation to the other. For example, exacerbations of asthma may be neutrophilic or eosinophilic on different occasions, presumably reflecting different causal mechanisms (15).

In the future it is likely that induced sputum will be used to select patients for specific therapies. For example, anti-interleukin(IL)-5 antibody (mepolizumab) reduces eosinophils in induced sputum, yet has no effect on any clinical parameters in unselected symptomatic asthmatic patients (16, 17). However, if patients are selected who have high sputum eosinophil counts despite high doses of inhaled corticosteroids and a history of exacerbations, mepolizumab is able to significantly reduce exacerbations (while having no effect on symptoms or lung function) (18, 19) . This suggests that careful selection of patients may be needed when assessing more specific therapies.

Research application

Induced sputum is increasingly used in the assessment of novel anti-inflammatory drugs in asthma and COPD, with measurements of inflammatory cells and mediators (20, 21). Induced sputum may also be used to select which patients are suitable for studying particular drugs. For example, in studying the effect of an anti-IL-13 antibody patients who have elevated IL-13 concentrations in sputum should be selected as they would be most likely to benefit from this therapy.

Exhaled Nitric Oxide

There has been an explosion of research into the measurement of exhaled nitric oxide (eNO) in airway disease, particularly asthma (22, 23). The measurement is easy to perform, reproducible and may be repeated, even in patients with severe obstruction and in young children. The recent availability of a hand-held device for the electrochemical detection of NO (NIOX MINO) has made it possible to make eNO measurements in clinical trials, in a general practice setting, in children and in the home (24-28). This device appears to be cost-effective in informing the diagnosis of asthma in general practice (29).

Clinical use

Although an initial study showing that monitoring of eNO was able to reduce the need of inhaled corticosteroids and reduce (although not significantly) the number of exacerbations compared to recommended clinical practice (30), three other studies have suggested that it does not improve asthma management in adults or children compared to routine management (28, 31, 32), although the patients were poorly controlled originally so improved with routine management. This stresses the importance of careful selection of patients, and as discussed above, eNO should be useful in patients who are under- or over-treated.

Exhaled NO is also useful in clinical practice as a diagnostic test in patients who present with cough, since an elevated NO is relatively specific for asthma (including so-called cough variant asthma), and excludes non-asthmatic eosinophilic bronchitis and oesophageal reflux (33, 34). Exhaled NO is also useful in measuring compliance with inhaled corticosteroids therapy in asthmatic patients, as elevated eNO values usually indicate that patients are not taking inhaled corticosteroids (35). Elevated eNO despite treatment with high doses of inhaled or oral corticosteroids may also indicate corticosteroid resistance (36) and may be a useful means of quantifying corticosteroids resistance in the future. Exhaled NO is not usually elevated in patients with COPD because of increased oxidative stress, which may result in the formation of peroxynitrite, thus removing NO from the gaseous phase (37). However, in patients with COPD who have bronchodilator reversibility ($>15\%$ increase in FEV_1 after inhaled salbutamol 400 µg), there is evidence of increased eNO and sputum eosinophils (38). This is likely to indicate concomitant asthma and the likelihood of a good response to inhaled corticosteroids, but eNO is easier to measure in clinical practice than induced sputum analysis (39).

Partitioned exhaled NO

Measurement of eNO as several exhaled flows makes it possible to partition eNO into a peripheral (alveolar) and central (bronchial) components and this may provide additional useful information about peripheral lung inflammation(40). Partitioned NO is reproducible and may also be measured in children(41). Peripheral NO is increased in COPD, whereas central NO is low or normal (Figure 2) (42). This is likely to reflect the peripheral lung inflammation and the increased expression of induced and neuronal NO synthases in small airways and lung parenchyma seen in COPD patients (43). In patients with asthma elevated peripheral NO is seen in patients with severe disease and is correlated with nocturnal symptoms (40, 44). Inhaled corticosteroids are less effective in reducing peripheral compared to central NO, which may indicate that the drug does not reach peripheral airways in high enough concentrations (45) and this is confirmed by the fact that oral prednisolone reduces peripheral NO in patients with refractory asthma not controlled on inhaled corticosteroids (46).

Future directions

The ease of measuring eNO makes it an attractive non-invasive biomarker and it is already proving to be useful in diagnosis and

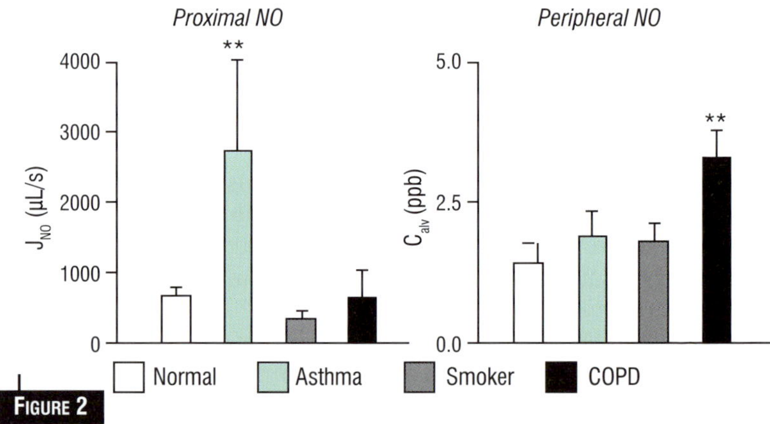

FIGURE 2

Partitioning of exhaled nitric oxide makes it possible to calculate proximal ("bronchial", JNO) and peripheral ("alveolar", Calv) fractions. In asthma patients proximal NO is elevated, whereas peripheral NO is usually normal (although elevated in severe asthma. By contrast in COPD patients central NO is normal or low, whereas peripheral NO is increased. Smokers have a reduction in proximal NO but normal peripheral NO. ** = p<0.01. Adapted after permission from reference 42.

monitoring compliance. As an aid to improve asthma control more studies are needed in selected populations that are likely to benefit. The introduction of hand-held monitoring devices has extended the measurements to general practice and to home monitoring, although the expense of these devices may preclude their widespread use. In the future it may be possible to develop devices that are cheaper and smaller, using different detector systems such as porphyrins or bacterial NO detector proteins, making the devices more readily available for home monitoring (47-49). In a study which examined increasing inflammation with loss of control of asthma induced by reducing the maintenance dose of inhaled corticosteroids we found that eNO increased before symptoms or rescue inhaler use increased or peak expiratory flow fell. This suggests that monitoring of eNO may be useful in the early detection of exacerbations of asthma so that appropriate intervention may be instituted earlier (50).

Partitioning eNO provides further information, particularly about inflammation in the lung periphery and therefore may be used in the future to study the effects of new therapies in treating peripheral inflammation in COPD and severe asthma. Several new therapies are now in development so this technique provides a non-invasive way to monitor their anti-inflammatory profile. Corticosteroids reduce eNO rapidly but do not appear to have a direct inhibitory effect on human inducible NO synthase in marked contrast to rodents, but rather work by reducing the inflammatory signals that active inducible NO synthase (51). This suggests that eNO should also be useful in detecting other anti-inflammatory therapies that are now in development for the treatment of severe asthma and COPD (21).

Exhaled Breath Condensate

The technique of exhaled breath condensate (EBC) has the virtue of simplicity and ease of collection as it is dependent on tidal breathing. Many different inflammatory mediators and biomarkers of oxidative and nitrative stress have now been detected in EBC (52, 53).

Problems

However, a major limitation of this technique is the variability of many of the markers with detection levels close to the limits of the available assays. This is likely to reflect enormous dilution of epithelial lining fluid by the condensation of water vapour in exhaled air. So far there has not been any acceptable way to correct for this dilution using ion conductance or lyophilisation, so it remains a problem for the measurement of most soluble mediators. However, several lipid mediators, such as leukotriene B_4 (LTB_4) and 8-isoprostane appear to be reliably and reproducibly measured and this might reflect the fact that these mediators have some volatility as body temperature.

Use in clinical practice

EBC is a simple entirely non-invasive procedure that can be used in patients with severe disease and in children over the age of 4 years. The apparatus is relatively simple to use and operate and inexpensive, making it possible to conduct studies in a general practice setting that may be particularly appropriate for common lung diseases, such as asthma and COPD. For example, COPD patients were studied in a general practice study during and following an acute exacerbation and an increase in exhaled 8-isoprostane and LTB_4, presumably reflecting the increased oxidative stress and neutrophilic inflammation, was found (54). Interestingly, a very slow recovery to baseline values was observed in this study, indicating that the increase in inflammation associated with an acute exacerbation is very prolonged in COPD consistent with the very prolonged reduction in quality of life measurements after an exacerbation. EBC measurements may be repeated frequently so that the kinetics of drugs can be investigated. The measurement of specific mediators and biomarkers means that it may be used to explore the effects of specific inhibitors, as well as anti-inflammatory effects. For example, measurement of LTB_4 or cysteinyl-leukotrienes can be used to study the efficacy of 5-lipoxygenase inhibitors, or exhaled 8-isoprostane to study the effect of antioxidants.

Increased sensitivity of assays

One of the current limitations of EBC measurements is the low concentration of many biomarkers so that their measurement is limited by the sensitivity of assays. It is likely that ever more sensitive assays will be developed as more potent antibodies are developed and new molecular detection techniques are introduced. Several commercially available multiplex detection systems are now available with increased sensitivity for detecting proteins, compared to ELISA and radioimmunoassays. Different patterns of cytokines have been reported in COPD patients using a multiplex array system, with differences between smokers and COPD patients (55).

Metabolomics

Metabolomics (sometimes called metabonomics) involves the detection of hundred of thousands of metabolites in a biological fluid usually using high resolution nuclear magnetic resonance (NMR) spectrometry or liquid chromatography/mass spectrometry (56). Powerful pattern recognition computer programs recognise patters of metabolites that are sensitive to disease, effects of treatment and disease severity. Metabolomics of EBC (a "breathogram") may therefore prove to be useful in screening lung diseases, following disease progression, predicting responses to treatment and in monitoring of response to therapy. Several studies have recently applied metabolomics to EBC in order to detect specific patterns that differentiate patients with disease from normal subjects. In children with asthma it was possible to discriminate a particular pattern of NMR spectra, particularly in oxidised and acetylated metabolites (Figure 3)(57). NMR spectra of EBC are clearly different from saliva and are reasonably reproducible so have potential to discriminate and monitor airway diseases in the future (58).

Proteomics

Proteomics is able to measure a spectrum of proteins by 2-dimenional electrophoresis combined with mass spectrometry and is increasingly used to identify abnormal patterns of protein expression in disease and in identifying novel targets for diagnosis and therapy (59). Proteomics has been applied to EBC samples and has shown a pattern in normal subjects that is dominated by cytokeratins (60). In COPD there are increased concentrations of several proteins, including cytokines and cytokeratins (61). Variable dilution and contamination with salivary proteins is a major problem in applying proteomic analysis to EBC samples so that it will be necessary to be very careful in collection techniques. Even so that pattern of proteins in E-BC is very similar to that found in saliva (62).

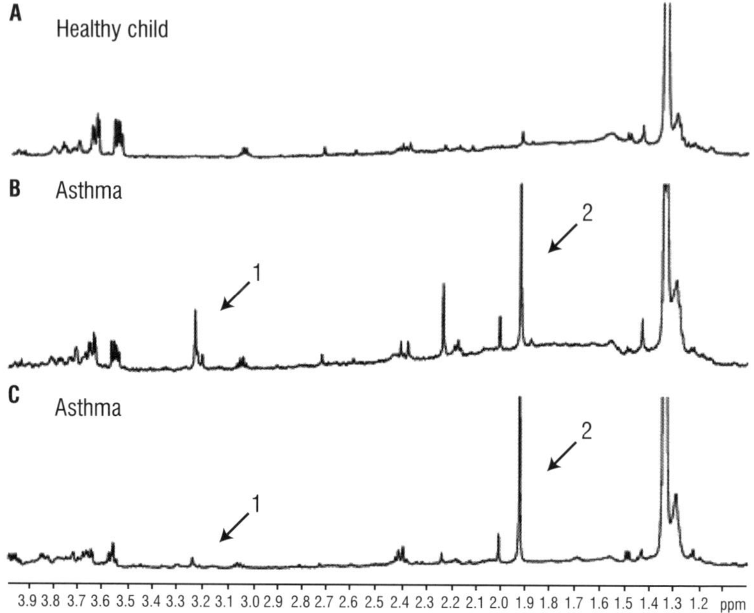

FIGURE 3

Metabolomics of exhaled breath condensate. Examples of nuclear magnetic resonance spectra obtained in healthy children (A) and children with asthma (B and C). Children with asthma are characterized by the presence of signals in the 3.2- to 3.4-ppm regions indicative of the presence of oxidized compounds (1). Significant signals are also found in the 1.7- to 2.2-ppm region in children with asthma compared with healthy subjects, suggesting the presence of acetylated compounds (2). Reproduced after permission from reference 57.

Genomics

It is possible to detect DNA in EBC samples making it possible to look at different patterns of gene expression or to detect microbial D-NA for diagnosis using PCR amplification. This approach has so far been applied to lung cancer, with detection of point mutations in p53 in patients with lung cancer (63) and an increase in microsatellite instability compared to controls, which correspond to the abnormal patterns seen in the resected tumours (64). This technique may therefore be useful for lung cancer screening is susceptible patients, such as those with COPD. Little progress has been made in detecting lung infections and applying DNA analysis of EBC to detect *Mycobacterium tuberculosis* infection using the IS6110 repetitive DNA element has been disappointing so far (65). In the future it might be possible to identify DNA or RNA from viruses infecting the respiratory tract in order to diagnose or predict acute exacerbations of asthma and COPD.

On-line measurements

A relative disadvantage of EBC measurements is that they require a subsequent analysis and it is likely that there will be important advances in on-line detection of particular biomarkers using sensitive biosensors. For example it is possible to detect hydrogen peroxide on-line (real-time) using a silver electrode or by coating a platinum electrode or polymer with horseradish peroxidase (66, 67). Similar enzyme detector systems may also be developed for real time monitoring of various lipid mediators, including 8-isoprostane, prostaglandins and leukotrienes. It is relatively easy to monitor pH of EBC and this is readily amenable to real-time detection. Several molecular biosensors are now in development and have the potential to detect very low concentrations of various relevant biomarkers (68). Ultimately it may be desirable to collect EBC to monitor patients in clinical practice using disposable detector sticks similar to currently used urinalysis sticks.

Exhaled Volatile Compounds

In view of the methodological problems with EBC compared with the relative success of measuring exhaled NO it is logical to explore the measurement of other volatile chemicals in the breath. It is already known that many volatile organic compounds are detectable in the breath using gas chromatography-mass spectrometry (GC/MS) (69). These include the lipid peroxidation product ethane, which is increased in asthma, COPD and cystic fibrosis and is related to disease severity (70-72). There is evidence that exhaled ethane concentrations are flow-dependent in patients with asthma compared to normal subjects, but most of the exhaled ethane is flow-independent suggesting that it is of systemic origin (73). Another hydrocarbon n-pentane is also increased in exhaled breath of patients during acute exacerbations of asthma and in cystic fibrosis (74, 75), but this is not flow-dependent so likely to be derived systemically (73). High concentrations of isoprene are also detectable in the breath in normal subjects, but this is also likely to be derived from the circulation (76).

Electronic nose

Electronic noses with multiple nano-sensors are able to detect patterns of VOCs, although it may be difficult to identify specific compounds. The wide availability of electronic noses using various detector systems has allowed the investigation of discriminant profiles in different airway diseases and lung cancer using pattern recognition algorithms, such as principle component, canonic discriminant and fuzzy logic analyses to differentiate patterns associated with different diseases (77-80). The detection of lung cancer is promising as a screening method in patients at high risk such as smokers with COPD. The VOCs that account for these differences have been analysed by GC/MS and in lung cancer patients increased concentrations of the hydrocarbons acetone, butane, benzene, decane, isoprene and pentane have been detected (81). Using solid-phase microextraction and gas chromatography it has been possible to identify VOCs in the headspace above lung caner cells *in vitro* that are also found in the breath of lung cancer patients, including isoprene and undecane (82). A similar procedure could be applied to tissue from asthma and COPD patients. Using thermal desorption and GC/MS it has been possible to discriminate VOCs in smokers and non-smokers, namely 2,5-dimethyl hexane, dodecane, 2,5-dimethylfuran and 2-methylfuran(83). Selected ion flow tube mass spectrometry (SIFT-MS) has been used to identify several VOCs in exhaled breath in real time (84). Field asymmetric ion mobility spectrometry (FAIMS) has been used to detect very low concentrations of multiple chemicals, including proteins, on a small (1 cm^2) silicon chips, raising the possibility that this type of detector could be used as a portable means of measuring breath VOCs (85).

VOCs may also be useful in detecting infections, but so far this has been little explored. Patients with confirmed *M. tuberculosis* infection can be discriminated from non-infected subjects with a high level of specificity and the prominent discriminant molecules were naphthalene, 1-methyl- and cyclohexane, 1,4-dimethyl-, which are also produced in the headspace above *M. tuberculosis* cultures (86). Pseudomonas infection generates hydrogen cyanide (HCN) gas *in vitro* and therefore may be a biomarker of pulmonary Pseudomonas infection in cystic fibrosis and other diseases (87). Higher concentrations of HCN have been detected in the breath of children with CF who are infected with Pseudomonas (~13 ppb) compared to normal control children (~2 ppb) (88). It is likely that bacteria emit different volatile substances that may be detectable in the breath, so that exhaled breath may be a means of non-invasively diagnosing pulmonary infections and following their response to antibiotic therapy. This approach might also be used to distinguish between infective exacerbations with bacteria or viruses in COPD patients in order to decide which patients should be treated with antibiotics, which are currently used indiscriminately.

Breathomics

There is a rapid development in detectors that are able to measure multiple volatile chemicals, including electronic nose devices, GC/MS and FAIMS. As discriminant patterns between different airway disease are further refined it may be possible to develop detectors that are specifically designed to diagnose airway diseases, detect lung infections and to monitor therapy. This "breathomic" approach may be able to discriminate different phenotypes of asthma and COPD and to predict responses to therapy. Animals such as dogs have a highly developed sense of smell which may be harnessed to the development of even more sensitive detector devices in the future. Olfactory receptors are G-protein coupled receptors that are able to discriminate thousands of different volatile molecules. Volatile odorant molecules bind to olfactory receptor proteins resulting in an increase in calcium ion flux and depolarisation, which may be detectable with electrodes. Human kidney cell lines transfected with specific olfactory receptors and exposed to their specific odorant generate a detectable electrical current so that it may be possible to construct an array of odorant detectors as a cell-based olfactory biosensor to measure complex mixtures of volatile substances as in the breath (89). Recently it has been found that single-stranded DNA sequences dried on to surfaces are able to bind different odorants and if labelled fluorescently can be used to detect odours and may provide sensors to detect multiple volatile molecules (90).

Conclusions

There have been major developments in non-invasive monitoring approaches. Sputum induction has provided valuable information about the inflammatory process in asthma and COPD and has considerable research potential. However, it is technically demanding and difficult to use in clinical practice so it may be restricted to a few specialist centres.

Breath analysis is more feasible in the clinic and eNO is already widely used in the clinic for diagnosis and monitoring of asthma. However, it has so far proved difficult to demonstrate a clinical advantage and further studies in more selected patients are now needed. Partitioning of eNO may be more useful for monitoring COPD and severe asthma in the future. The development of cheap and sensitive NO detectors to allow home monitoring is now proceeding.

EBC has potential to measure semi-volatile lipid mediators as well as pH and there are novel electrochemical assays that may allow on-line detection. However, a major problem that limits the usefulness of this technique is variable dilution with water vapour. Many VOCs have now been detected in the breath and the pattern of molecules can now be characterised with various electronic nose devices. Use of smaller and more sensitive mass spectrometry approaches allows the identification of the discriminatory chemicals so that more selective detectors may be developed in the future. Harnessing olfactory receptors and solid state DNA sequences hold hope for the future development of even more sensitive sensors so that breathomics may become a reality in the clinic.

References

1. Pavord ID, Shaw DE, Gibson PG, Taylor DR. Inflammometry to assess airway diseases. Lancet 2008 Sep 20; 372 (9643):1017-9.

2. Haldar P, Pavord ID, Shaw DE, Berry MA, Thomas M, Brightling CE, et al. Cluster analysis and clinical asthma phenotypes. Am J Respir Crit Care Med 2008 Aug 1;178(3):218-24.

3. Makris D, Tzanakis N, Moschandreas J, Siafakas NM. Dyspnea assessment and adverse events during sputum induction in COPD. BMC Pulm Med2006; 6:17.

4. Nightingale JA, Rogers DF, Barnes PJ. Effect of repeated sputum induction on cell counts in normal volunteers. Thorax1998 Feb;53(2):87-90.

5. Holz O, Richter K, Jorres RA, Speckin P, Mucke M, Magnussen H. Changes in sputum composition between two inductions performed on consecutive days. Thorax1998 Feb;53(2):83-6.

6. Erin EM, Jenkins GR, Kon OM, Zacharasiewicz AS, Nicholson GC, Neighbour H, et al. Optimized dialysis and protease inhibition of sputum dithiothreitol supernatants. Am J Respir Crit Care Med 2008 Jan 15; 177(2):132-41.

7. D'Silva L, Gafni A, Thabane L, Jayaram L, Hassack P, Hargreave FE, et al. Cost analysis of monitoring asthma treatment using sputum cell counts. Can Respir J2008 Oct;15(7):370-4.

8. Green RH, Brightling CE, McKenna S, Hargadon B, Parker D, Bradding P, et al. Asthma exacerbations and sputum eosinophil counts: a randomised controlled trial. Lancet 2002 Nov 30;360 (9347):1715-21.

9. Jayaram L, Pizzichini MM, Cook RJ, Boulet LP, Lemiere C, Pizzichini E, et al. Determining asthma treatment by monitoring sputum cell counts: effect on exacerbations. Eur Respir J2006 Mar; 27(3):483-94.

10. Siva R, Green RH, Brightling CE, Shelley M, Hargadon B, McKenna S, et al. Eosinophilic airway inflammation and exacerbations of COPD: a randomised controlled trial. Eur Respir J 2007 May; 29(5):906-13.

11. Simpson JL, Scott R, Boyle MJ, Gibson PG. Inflammatory subtypes in asthma: assessment and identification using induced sputum. Respirology2006 Jan;11(1):54-61.

12. Jatakanon A, Uasuf C, Maziak W, Lim S, Chung KF, Barnes PJ. Neutrophilic inflammation in severe persistent asthma. Am J Respir Crit Care Med 1999 Nov;160(5 Pt 1):1532-9.

13. Maneechotesuwan K, Essilfie-Quaye S, Meah S, Kelly C, Kharitonov SA, Adcock IM, et al. Formoterol attenuates neutrophilic airway inflammation in asthma. Chest 2005 Oct;128(4): 1936-42.

14. Barnes PJ. New molecular targets for the treatment of neutrophilic diseases. J Allergy Clin Immunol 2007 May; 119(5):1055-62; quiz 63-4.

15. D'Silva L, Cook RJ, Allen CJ, Hargreave FE, Parameswaran K. Changing pattern of sputum cell counts during successive exacerbations of airway disease. Respir Med 2007 Oct;101 (10): 2217-20.

16. Leckie MJ, ten Brinke A, Khan J, Diamant Z, O'Connor BJ, Walls CM, et al. Effects of an interleukin-5 blocking monoclonal antibody on eosinophils, airway hyper-responsiveness, and the late asthmatic response. Lancet 2000 Dec 23-30;356(9248):2144-8.

17. Flood-Page P, Swenson C, Faiferman I, Matthews J, Williams M, Brannick L, et al. A study to evaluate safety and efficacy of mepolizumab in patients with moderate persistent asthma. Am J Respir Crit Care Med2007 Dec 1; 176(11):1062-71.

18. Nair P, Pizzichini MM, Kjarsgaard M, Inman MD, Efthimiadis A, Pizzichini E, et al. Mepolizumab for prednisone-dependent asthma with sputum eosinophilia. N Engl J Med 2009 Mar 5;360 (10):985-93.

19. Haldar P, Brightling CE, Hargadon B, Gupta S, Monteiro W, Sousa A, et al. Mepolizumab and exacerbations of refractory eosinophilic asthma. N Engl J Med 2009 Mar 5;360(10):973-84.

20. Adcock IM, Caramori G, Chung KF. New targets for drug development in asthma. Lancet 2008 Sep 20;372 (9643):1073-87.

21. Barnes PJ. Emerging pharmacothera-

pies for COPD. Chest 2008 Dec; 134 (6):1278-86.

22. Ricciardolo FL, Sterk PJ, Gaston B, Folkerts G. Nitric oxide in health and disease of the respiratory system. Physiol Rev 2004 Jul;84(3):731-65.

23. Kharitonov SA, Barnes PJ. Exhaled biomarkers. Chest 2006 Nov; 130(5): 1541-6.

24. Maniscalco M, de Laurentiis G, Weitzberg E, Lundberg JO, Sofia M. Validation study of nasal nitric oxide measurements using a hand-held electrochemical analyser. Eur J Clin Invest 2008 Mar;38(3):197-200.

25. de Laurentiis G, Maniscalco M, Cianciulli F, Stanziola A, Marsico S, Lundberg JO, et al. Exhaled nitric oxide monitoring in COPD using a portable analyzer. Pulm Pharmacol Ther 2008 Aug;21(4):689-93.

26. Pijnenburg MW, Floor SE, Hop WC, De Jongste JC. Daily ambulatory exhaled nitric oxide measurements in asthma. Pediatr Allergy Immunol 2006 May;17(3):189-93.

27. Torre O, Olivieri D, Barnes PJ, Kharitonov SA. Feasibility and interpretation of FE(NO) measurements in asthma patients in general practice. Respir Med 2008 Oct;102(10):1417-24.

28. de Jongste JC, Carraro S, Hop WC, Baraldi E. Daily telemonitoring of exhaled nitric oxide and symptoms in the treatment of childhood asthma. Am J Respir Crit Care Med 2009 Jan 15;179(2):93-7.

29. Price D, Berg J, Lindgren P. An economic evaluation of NIOX MINO airway inflammation monitor in the United Kingdom. Allergy 2009 Mar;64 (3):431-8.

30. Smith AD, Cowan JO, Brassett KP, Herbison GP, Taylor DR. Use of exhaled nitric oxide measurements to guide treatment in chronic asthma. N Engl J Med 2005 May 26;352(21): 2163-73.

31. Shaw DE, Berry MA, Thomas M, Green RH, Brightling CE, Wardlaw AJ, et al. The use of exhaled nitric oxide to guide asthma management: a randomized controlled trial. Am J Respir Crit Care Med 2007 Aug 1;176(3): 231-7.

32. Szefler SJ, Mitchell H, Sorkness CA, Gergen PJ, O'Connor GT, Morgan WJ, et al. Management of asthma based on exhaled nitric oxide in addition to guideline-based treatment for inner-city adolescents and young adults: a randomised controlled trial. Lancet 2008 Sep 20;372(9643):1065-72.

33. Sato S, Saito J, Sato Y, Ishii T, Xintao W, Tanino Y, et al. Clinical usefulness of fractional exhaled nitric oxide for diagnosing prolonged cough. Respir Med2008 Oct;102(10):1452-9.

34. Oh MJ, Lee JY, Lee BJ, Choi DC. Exhaled nitric oxide measurement is useful for the exclusion of nonasthmatic eosinophilic bronchitis in patients with chronic cough. Chest 2008 Nov;134(5):990-5.

35. Katsara M, Donnelly D, Iqbal S, Elliott T, Everard ML. Relationship between exhaled nitric oxide levels and compliance with inhaled corticosteroids in asthmatic children. Respir Med 2006 Sep;100(9):1512-7.

36. Stirling RG, Kharitonov SA, Campbell D, Robinson DS, Durham SR, Chung KF, et al. Increase in exhaled nitric oxide levels in patients with difficult asthma and correlation with symptoms and disease severity despite treatment

with oral and inhaled corticosteroids. Asthma and Allergy Group. Thorax 1998 Dec;53(12):1030-4.

37. Maziak W, Loukides S, Culpitt S, Sullivan P, Kharitonov SA, Barnes PJ. Exhaled nitric oxide in chronic obstructive pulmonary disease. Am J Respir Crit Care Med1998 Mar;157(3 Pt 1):998-1002.

38. Papi A, Romagnoli M, Baraldo S, Braccioni F, Guzzinati I, Saetta M, et al. Partial reversibility of airflow limitation and increased exhaled NO and sputum eosinophilia in chronic obstructive pulmonary disease. Am J Respir Crit Care Med 2000 Nov;162 (5):1773-7.

39. Brightling CE, Monteiro W, Ward R, Parker D, Morgan MD, Wardlaw AJ, et al. Sputum eosinophilia and short-term response to prednisolone in chronic obstructive pulmonary disease: a randomised controlled trial. Lancet 2000 Oct 28;356(9240):1480-5.

40. Lehtimaki L, Kankaanranta H, Saarelainen S, Hahtola P, Jarvenpaa R, Koivula T, et al. Extended exhaled NO measurement differentiates between alveolar and bronchial inflammation. Am J Respir Crit Care Med 2001 Jun; 163(7):1557-61.

41. Paraskakis E, Brindicci C, Fleming L, Krol R, Kharitonov SA, Wilson NM, et al. Measurement of bronchial and alveolar nitric oxide production in normal children and children with asthma. Am J Respir Crit Care Med2006 Aug 1;174(3):260-7.

42. Brindicci C, Ito K, Resta O, Pride NB, Barnes PJ, Kharitonov SA. Exhaled nitric oxide from lung periphery is increased in COPD. Eur Respir J2005 Jul;26(1):52-9.

43. Ricciardolo FL, Caramori G, Ito K, Capelli A, Brun P, Abatangelo G, et al. Nitrosative stress in the bronchial mucosa of severe chronic obstructive pulmonary disease. J Allergy Clin Immunol 2005 Nov;116(5):1028-35.

44. Brindicci C, Ito K, Barnes PJ, Kharitonov SA. Differential flow analysis of exhaled nitric oxide in patients with asthma of differing severity. Chest 2007 May;131(5):1353-62.

45. Lehtimaki L, Kankaanranta H, Saarelainen S, Turjanmaa V, Moilanen E. Inhaled fluticasone decreases bronchial but not alveolar nitric oxide output in asthma. Eur Respir J 2001 Oct;18(4): 635-9.

46. Berry M, Hargadon B, Morgan A, Shelley M, Richter J, Shaw D, et al. Alveolar nitric oxide in adults with asthma: evidence of distal lung inflammation in refractory asthma. Eur Respir J 2005 Jun;25(6):986-91.

47. Hrbac J, Gregor C, Machova M, Kralova J, Bystron T, Ciz M, et al. Nitric oxide sensor based on carbon fiber covered with nickel porphyrin layer deposited using optimized electropolymerization procedure. Bioelectrochemistry 2007 Sep;71(1):46-53.

48. Lim MH, Lippard SJ. Fluorescence-based nitric oxide detection by ruthenium porphyrin fluorophore complexes. Inorg Chem 2004 Oct 4;43 (20):6366-70.

49. Boon EM, Marletta MA. Sensitive and selective detection of nitric oxide using an H-NOX domain. J Am Chem Soc 2006 Aug 9;128(31):10022-3.

50. Jatakanon A, Lim S, Barnes PJ. Changes in sputum eosinophils predict loss of asthma control. Am J Respir Crit Care Med 2000 Jan;161(1): 64-72.

51. Donnelly LE, Barnes PJ. Expression and regulation of inducible nitric oxide synthase from human primary airway epithelial cells. Am J Respir Cell Mol Biol 2002 Jan;26(1):144-51.

52. Montuschi P, Barnes PJ. Analysis of exhaled breath condensate for monitoring airway inflammation. Trends Pharmacol Sci 2002 May;23(5):232-7.

53. Hunt J. Exhaled breath condensate: an overview. Immunol Allergy Clin North Am 2007 Nov;27(4):587-96; v.

54. Biernacki WA, Kharitonov SA, Barnes PJ. Increased leukotriene B4 and 8-isoprostane in exhaled breath condensate of patients with exacerbations of COPD. Thorax 2003 Apr;58(4):294-8.

55. Gessner C, Scheibe R, Wotzel M, Hammerschmidt S, Kuhn H, Engelmann L, et al. Exhaled breath condensate cytokine patterns in chronic obstructive pulmonary disease. Respir Med 2005 Oct;99(10):1229-40.

56. Giovane A, Balestrieri A, Napoli C. New insights into cardiovascular and lipid metabolomics. J Cell Biochem 2008 Oct 15;105(3):648-54.

57. Carraro S, Rezzi S, Reniero F, Heberger K, Giordano G, Zanconato S, et al. Metabolomics applied to exhaled breath condensate in childhood asthma. Am J Respir Crit Care Med 2007 May 15;175(10):986-90.

58. de Laurentiis G, Paris D, Melck D, Maniscalco M, Marsico S, Corso G, et al. Metabonomic analysis of exhaled breath condensate in adults by nuclear magnetic resonance spectroscopy. Eur Respir J 2008 Nov;32(5):1175-83.

59. Bowler RP, Ellison MC, Reisdorph N. Proteomics in pulmonary medicine. Chest 2006 Aug;130(2):567-74.

60. Kurova VS, Anaev EC, Kononikhin AS, Fedorchenko KY, Popov IA, Kalupov TL, et al. Proteomics of exhaled breath: methodological nuances and pitfalls. Clin Chem Lab Med 2009;47(6): 706-12.

61. Fumagalli M, Dolcini L, Sala A, Stolk J, Fregonese L, Ferrari F, et al. Proteomic analysis of exhaled breath condensate from single patients with pulmonary emphysema associated to alpha1-antitrypsin deficiency. J Proteomics 2008 Jul 21;71(2):211-21.

62. Griese M, Noss J, von Bredow C. Protein pattern of exhaled breath condensate and saliva. Proteomics 2002 Jun;2(6):690-6.

63. Gessner C, Kuhn H, Toepfer K, Hammerschmidt S, Schauer J, Wirtz H. Detection of p53 gene mutations in exhaled breath condensate of non-small cell lung cancer patients. Lung Cancer 2004 Feb;43(2):215-22.

64. Carpagnano GE, Foschino-Barbaro MP, Spanevello A, Resta O, Carpagnano F, Mule G, et al. 3p microsatellite signature in exhaled breath condensate and tumor tissue of patients with lung cancer. Am J Respir Crit Care Med 2008 Feb 1;177(3):337-41.

65. Jain R, Schriever CA, Danziger LH, Cho SH, Rubinstein I. The IS6110 repetitive DNA element of Mycobacterium tuberculosis is not detected in exhaled breath condensate of patients with active pulmonary tuberculosis. Respiration 2007;74(3):329-33.

66. Razola SS, Ruiz BL, Diez NM, Mark HB, Jr., Kauffmann JM. Hydrogen peroxide sensitive amperometric biosensor based on horseradish peroxidase entrapped in a polypyrrole electrode.

Biosens Bioelectron 2002 Dec;17(11-12):921-8.

67. Thanachasai S, Rokutanzono S, Yoshida S, Watanabe T. Novel hydrogen peroxide sensors based on peroxidase-carrying poly[pyrrole-co-[4-(3-pyrrolyl)butanesulfonate]] copolymer films. Anal Sci 2002 Jul;18(7):773-7.

68. Nakamura H, Karube I. Current research activity in biosensors. Anal Bioanal Chem 2003 Oct;377(3):446-68.

69. Moser B, Bodrogi F, Eibl G, Lechner M, Rieder J, Lirk P. Mass spectrometric profile of exhaled breath--field study by PTR-MS. Respir Physiol Neurobiol 2005 Feb 15;145(2-3):295-300.

70. Paredi P, Kharitonov SA, Barnes PJ. Elevation of exhaled ethane concentration in asthma. Am J Respir Crit Care Med 2000 Oct;162(4 Pt 1): 1450-4.

71. Paredi P, Kharitonov SA, Leak D, Ward S, Cramer D, Barnes PJ. Exhaled ethane, a marker of lipid peroxidation, is elevated in chronic obstructive pulmonary disease. Am J Respir Crit Care Med 2000 Aug;162(2 Pt 1):369-73.

72. Paredi P, Kharitonov SA, Leak D, Shah PL, Cramer D, Hodson ME, et al. Exhaled ethane is elevated in cystic fibrosis and correlates with carbon monoxide levels and airway obstruction. Am J Respir Crit Care Med 2000 Apr;161(4 Pt 1):1247-51.

73. Larstad MA, Toren K, Bake B, Olin AC. Determination of ethane, pentane and isoprene in exhaled air--effects of breath-holding, flow rate and purified air. Acta Physiol (Oxf)2007 Jan; 189 (1):87-98.

74. Olopade CO, Zakkar M, Swedler WI, Rubinstein I. Exhaled pentane levels in acute asthma. Chest 1997 Apr; 111 (4):862-5.

75. Barker M, Hengst M, Schmid J, Buers HJ, Mittermaier B, Klemp D, et al. Volatile organic compounds in the exhaled breath of young patients with cystic fibrosis. Eur Respir J 2006 May;27(5):929-36.

76. Kushch I, Arendacka B, Stolc S, Mochalski P, Filipiak W, Schwarz K, et al. Breath isoprene--aspects of normal physiology related to age, gender and cholesterol profile as determined in a proton transfer reaction mass spectrometry study. Clin Chem Lab Med 2008;46(7):1011-8.

77. Machado RF, Laskowski D, Deffenderfer O, Burch T, Zheng S, Mazzone PJ, et al. Detection of lung cancer by sensor array analyses of exhaled breath. Am J Respir Crit Care Med 2005 Jun 1;171(11):1286-91.

78. Mazzone PJ, Hammel J, Dweik R, Na J, Czich C, Laskowski D, et al. Diagnosis of lung cancer by the analysis of exhaled breath with a colorimetric sensor array. Thorax 2007 Jul;62(7): 565-8.

79. Dragonieri S, Schot R, Mertens BJ, Le Cessie S, Gauw SA, Spanevello A, et al. An electronic nose in the discrimination of patients with asthma and controls. J Allergy Clin Immunol 2007 Oct;120(4):856-62.

80. Dragonieri S, Annema JT, Schot R, van der Schee MP, Spanevello A, Carratu P, et al. An electronic nose in the discrimination of patients with non-small cell lung cancer and COPD. Lung Cancer 2009 May;64(2):166-70.

81. Phillips M, Gleeson K, Hughes JM,

Greenberg J, Cataneo RN, Baker L, et al. Volatile organic compounds in breath as markers of lung cancer: a cross-sectional study. Lancet 1999 Jun 5;353(9168):1930-3.

82. Chen Y, Shu W, Chen W, Wu Q, Liu H, Cui G. Curcumin, both histone deacetylase and p300/CBP-specific inhibitor, represses the activity of nuclear factor kappa B and Notch 1 in Raji cells. Basic Clin Pharmacol Toxicol 2007 Dec;101(6):427-33.

83. Van Berkel JJ, Dallinga JW, Moller GM, Godschalk RW, Moonen E, Wouters EF, et al. Development of accurate classification method based on the analysis of volatile organic compounds from human exhaled air. J Chromatogr B Analyt Technol Biomed Life Sci 2008 Jan 1;861(1):101-7.

84. Turner C, Parekh B, Walton C, Spanel P, Smith D, Evans M. An exploratory comparative study of volatile compounds in exhaled breath and emitted by skin using selected ion flow tube mass spectrometry. Rapid Commun Mass Spectrom 2008;22(4):526-32.

85. Shvartsburg AA, Smith RD. Optimum waveforms for differential ion mobility spectrometry (FAIMS). J Am Soc Mass Spectrom 2008 Sep;19(9): 1286-95.

86. Phillips M, Cataneo RN, Condos R, Ring Erickson GA, Greenberg J, La Bombardi V, et al. Volatile biomarkers of pulmonary tuberculosis in the breath. Tuberculosis (Edinb)2007 Jan; 87(1):44-52.

87. Carroll W, Lenney W, Wang T, Spanel P, Alcock A, Smith D. Detection of volatile compounds emitted by Pseudomonas aeruginosa using selected ion flow tube mass spectrometry. Pediatr Pulmonol 2005 May;39(5):452-6.

88. Enderby B, Smith D, Carroll W, Lenney W. Hydrogen cyanide as a biomarker for Pseudomonas aeruginosa in the breath of children with cystic fibrosis. Pediatr Pulmonol 2009 Feb;44(2):142-7.

89. Lee SH, Jun SB, Ko HJ, Kim SJ, Park TH. Cell-based olfactory biosensor using microfabricated planar electrode. Biosens Bioelectron 2009 Apr 15;24 (8):2659-64.

90. White J, Truesdell K, Williams LB, Atkisson MS, Kauer JS. Solid-state, dye-labeled DNA detects volatile compounds in the vapor phase. PLoS Biol 2008 Jan;6(1):e9.

Index

mass spectrometry, 178, 276, 319
Gastrooesophageal reflux, 68, 313
Genomics, 248, 318
GINA, 41
Glutathione, 143, 183, 187
  peroxidase, 143

H

H_2O_2, 155, 157, 160, 187, 294
Healthy smokers, 214
Heptanal, 218, 221, 244
Hexanal, 218, 221, 244
Histamine, 126, 143
Horseradish peroxidase, 319
Hydrogen peroxide (H_2O_2), 166, 214, 216, 221, 246, 293, 319
Hydroxyl radical, 208
Hypertonic saline, 310
  normal, 238

I

ICS, 64, 69, 70, 72
IFN, 247
IFN-γ, 288
IL-4, 247, 288
IL-5, 247
IL-6, 219, 247
IL-8, 146, 219, 238
Immunochemistry, 108
Immunocytochemistry, 104, 108
In situ hybridization, 108
Induced sputum, 97, 125, 126, 144, 290
  asthma
    diagnosis, 132
    monitoring, 133
  cell counts, 107
    normal ranges, 127
    repeatability, 127
  comparison with BAL and bronchial biopsies, 117

in asthma, 125
in COPD, 141
patterns, 129
processing phase, 105
reference values, 115
supernatant, 146
technical considerations, 99
towards normal values, 113
Induces sputum, 141, 238
Inducible NO synthase (iNOS), 83
Inflammatory
  cells in induced sputum, 290
  mediators, 142
Inflammometer, 205, 233
Inflammometry, 132, 309
Inhaled
  corticosteroids, 64, 90
iNOS, 24, 83, 87, 217, 235
Interleukin, 155, 183, 219
  -4, 247
  -8, 126
Ion mobility spectrometry, 276
Isoprostanes, 178, 215, 293

L

L-arginine, 24, 25, 235
L-citrulline, 235
Leptin, 143, 146
Leukotriene, 126, 174, 208, 214, 241, 293, 319
Limit of detection, 166
Lipid peroxidation products, 244
Liquid chromatography
  mass spectrometry, 178, 317
  tandem mass sapectrometry, 218
LTB4, 143, 155, 178, 187, 214, 221, 243, 316
LTC4, 241
LTD4, 187, 241
LTE4, 187, 221, 241, 293
Lymphocytes, 115, 126, 127, 143